# Handbuch der experimentellen Pharmakologie

Begründet von A. Heffter

Ergänzungswerk · Vierter Band

## General Pharmacology
A. J. Clark-Edinburgh

Reprint

Springer-Verlag · Berlin · Heidelberg · New York 1973

1st Reprint 1970
2nd Reprint 1973

ISBN -13:978-3-642-80557-8     e-ISBN -13:978-3-642-80555-4
DOI:  10.1007/978-3-642-80555-4

Library of Congress Catalog Card Number 75-105699.

Softcover reprint of the hardcover 1st  edition 1970

# HANDBUCH
# DER EXPERIMENTELLEN
# PHARMAKOLOGIE

BEGRÜNDET VON A. HEFFTER

## ERGÄNZUNGSWERK

HERAUSGEGEBEN VON

W. HEUBNER     UND     J. SCHÜLLER
PROFESSOR DER PHARMAKOLOGIE          PROFESSOR DER PHARMAKOLOGIE
AN DER UNIVERSITÄT BERLIN            AN DER UNIVERSITÄT KÖLN

## VIERTER BAND

## GENERAL PHARMACOLOGY

BY

A. J. CLARK-EDINBURGH

WITH 79 FIGURES

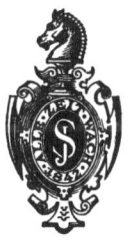

BERLIN
VERLAG VON JULIUS SPRINGER
1937

## Preface.

The author's general aim has been to survey as wide a field of evidence as possible and this had involved excursions into subjects of which he has little first hand knowledge. This width of range also has necessitated a somewhat arbitrary selection of evidence and has prevented full discussion of any individual problem.

The author trusts that he has not misrepresented anyone's results or opinions, and if this has occurred, he can only plead in excuse the peculiar difficulty of giving a brief and yet accurate account of evidence of such a wide variety.

The diagrams reproduced in the article have all been redrawn and in many cases the original figures or diagrams have been modified as, for instance, by recalculating dosage on the logarithmic scale. The original authors therefore have no direct responsibility for the diagrams in their present form.

The author desires to thank Messrs Arnold and Co. for permitting the reproduction of Figs. 9 and 23 from similar figures which appeared in his book „The Mode of Action of Drugs on Cells"; portions of other figures from this book also have been reproduced in modified form.

The author also desires to thank Dr. J. M. ROBSON for help in correction of the proofs.

Edinburgh, July, 1937.

A. J. CLARK.

# Contents.

# Introduction.

Pharmacology may be defined as the study of the manner in which the functions of living organisms can be modified by chemical substances. The subject actually developed in a narrower field because its chief original aim was to provide a scientific basis for therapeutics. This study required as its basis an adequate knowledge of the functions of the normal organism (physiology) and the derangements of these by disease (pathology), hence pharmacology developed later than the other medical sciences.

The first task of the young science was to sift the traditional beliefs of therapeutic practice and to discover how much of this was based on fact and how much was merely a legacy from mediaeval superstition. The energy of pharmacologists during the second half of the nineteenth century was largely expended on this task which was both wearisome and thankless. Neither the clinicians nor the drug manufacturers were grateful to the pharmacologist who hampered their freer flights of fancy by captious criticism. On the other hand the physiologists regarded the pharmacologists as mere collectors of uncorrelated data.

The present situation is very different because it is now recognised that many if not most of the functions of the body are regulated by drug action and hence the manner in which drugs exert their action on cells has become one of the most important fundamental problems in physiology.

The discovery of hormones first suggested that the activities of the body were regulated by chemical agents, and the significance of this advance was recognised by ERNEST STARLING who at the Naturforscherversammlung at Stuttgart concluded a famous address on the then new subject of hormones with the following words (quoted from HEUBNER, 1934[1]):

„Jedes physiologische Problem ist in letzter Linie auf ein chemisches zurückzuführen. Hier reichen sich Physiologie und Pharmakologie die Hände, und die älteste unter den Forschungen, die in Verbindung mit der Heilkunde erscheinen, nämlich jene, welche sich mit der Wirkung der Arzneikörper befaßt, wird uns vielleicht die Handhabe zur Aufklärung der fundamentalen Lebensprobleme liefern."

As HEUBNER (1934) says:

„Man darf wohl sagen, daß STARLINGS prophetische Worte in der seither verflossenen Zeit Erfüllung gefunden haben: mehr und mehr haben sich die Probleme der Physiologie auf chemische reduziert, größer und größer ist die Zahl eigentümlicher und höchst wirksamer Substanzen geworden, die wir als unentbehrliche Werkzeuge im Getriebe des lebendigen Körpers kennengelernt haben; sind wir doch fast schon so weit, als das Wesentliche bei der Übertragung einer Nervenerregung auf das Erfolgsorgan die Produktion eines Pharmakons ansehen zu dürfen."

The development of organic chemistry also has had important consequences, since today the number of organic compounds with possible pharmacological actions is practically unlimited. This has opened new fields in therapeutics but also has opened unpleasant new possibilities in toxicology because all kinds of new compounds are being introduced into industrial and domestic use. Hence accurate knowledge of the possibilities of cumulative poisoning and of drug idiosyncrasy has become of increasing importance.

---

[1] HEUBNER, W.: Klin. Wschr. **13**, 1633 (1934).

Partly as a result of these advances in organic chemistry human society is relying more and more on drugs for the control of parasites and pests. The remarkable development in chemotherapy which has followed the pioneer work of EHRLICH is the chief of such advances, and the discovery of prontosil justifies the hope that, after many decades of fruitless endeavour, corresponding advances are commencing in the control of bacterial infections. The disinfectants, trypanocides, spirochaeticides and anthelmintics form a large and important section of modern therapeutics, and apart from therapeutics agriculture is relying more and more on insecticides and fungicides for the protection of crops. Finally one must recognise the unfortunate fact that poison gases have proved to be weapons of great efficacy in warfare, and apart altogether from the study of poison gases as offensive weapons, it is necessary for medical science to study the means of prevention and cure of poisoning by war gases.

The mode of action of drugs upon organisms is therefore to-day of ever increasing importance, and this subject is of such outstanding importance in physiology that the question is now raised whether pharmacology has any claims to be regarded as a separate branch of science or whether it should not be considered a special branch of physiology or biochemistry.

The objection to this view is that although all the other biological sciences use drugs as useful agents to produce desired effects, yet none of them are prepared to study the action of drugs in a systematic manner. The bacteriologist for instance is satisfied when he discovers that the addition of a small quantity of dye to a medium will inhibit the growth of certain bacteria, but usually he is not interested in studying the manner in which the dye produces this remarkable specific action. The physiologist is content to know that a fraction of a microgram of acetylcholine will produce actions simulating the effect of parasympathetic activity and that this effect is abolished by similar quantity of atropine, but is disinclined to study the possible physico-chemical mechanisms by which these remarkable actions and antagonisms can be produced. For these reasons the writer believes that there is a need for a science which devotes itself primarily to the study of the mode of action of drugs. This science can most conveniently be designated "general pharmacology". It must borrow its methods largely from physical chemistry, biochemistry and physiology, but its task is a distinctive one, namely to discover the mode by which chemical agents alter the functions of living cells.

The study of the mode of action of drugs on cells is of course dependent on our knowledge of the physical chemistry of cells, and this subject owes much to the works of HOEBER (1902)[1] and BECHHOLD (1911)[2] who were some of the first authors to give a systematic account of the physico-chemical properties of cells.

ARRHENIUS (1915)[3] was one of the first to attempt a general interpretation of drug action by means of the laws of physical chemistry. His conclusions are subject to the general criticism that he attempted to explain reactions occurring in complex colloidal systems by laws derived from the simplest homogeneous systems. This fact does not however lessen the importance of his work as a pioneer in a field that had previously been neglected. STORM VAN LEEUWEN (1923)[4] described in a systematic manner the variety of relations between drug concentration and biological response that can be observed with intact animals and

[1] HOEBER, R.: Physikalische Chemie der Zelle und Gewebe. Berlin: Engelmann 1902.
[2] BECHHOLD, H.: Die Kolloide in Biologie und Medizin. Dresden: Steinkopff 1911.
[3] ARRHENIUS, S.: Quantitative Laws in Biological Chemistry. London: Bell and Sons 1915.
[4] STORM VAN LEEUWEN, W.: Grondbegins. d. alg. Pharmacol. Den Haag: Wolters 1923.

with isolated tissues. HEUBNER (1922)[1] defined the outstanding problems of general pharmacology, whilst LOEWE (1927, 1928)[2] formulated certain general laws of drug synergism and drug antagonism. ZUNZ (1930)[3] has more recently provided a review of general pharmacology.

The present article deals with many problems that have been discussed by the author in an earlier work (CLARK, 1933)[4]. In certain cases where problems were discussed fully in this book, and no important new evidence has appeared, the author, in order to avoid repetition has referred to his previous work and in such cases the reference is given in the form (CLARK, 1933)[4]. Similar references are given to such books as those of ARRHENIUS and of STORM VAN LEEUWEN, to which frequent reference is also made.

With regard to the subject matter of this article, it is obvious that this covers a large proportion of pharmacology and hence it is only possible to refer to a small fraction of the work done in the fields that are considered. Considerations of space also have necessitated a somewhat arbitrary curtailment of the problems dealt with.

One of the most serious omissions is the problem of the relation between chemical constitution and pharmacological action. The possibility of establishing general laws in this field was indicated at an early date by the remarkable pioneer work of CRUM BROWN and FRASER (1869)[5] who showed that quaternary ammonium bases possessed the common property of a curareform action. The problems in this field are however so numerous and intricate that the author considered it to be impossible to discuss them profitably within the limits of the present article.

The subject of general pharmacology presents the serious difficulty that there is no basis of generally accepted theory. Almost all relations found between the exposure to drugs and the cell response are capable of more than one explanation, and the various explanations differ fundamentally. For example the rate at which a population of bacteria is killed by a disinfectant may be interpreted either as a monomolecular reaction in which one organism unites with one molecule of drug, or as a simple expression of individual variation, or as the result of a complex chain process acting on a variable population.

The author believes that the living cell is such a complex system that the number of uncontrolled variables and unknown factors influencing its response are too great to permit of definite proof of any theory regarding the mode of action of drugs being obtained directly from its study. Fortunately however it is possible to compare the action of drugs on cells with their action on simpler systems such as enzymes. It will be shown in this monograph that there are striking similarities between the action of drugs on cells and their action on active proteins and hence the former action can be partly interpreted as the expression of processes similar to those which are known to occur in the simpler systems. The relative probability of various hypotheses regarding the nature of drug action has to a certain extent been judged by considering whether the hypothesis relates the action of drugs on cells with their action on simpler systems, and particularly whether the hypothesis involves the assumption of processes unknown in physical chemistry. This attitude is perhaps illogical because the author does not wish to maintain the thesis that all functions of living cells can

---

[1] HEUBNER, W.: Klin. Wschr. **1**, 1289, 1349 (1922).
[2] LOEWE, S.: Klin. Wschr. **6**, 1077 (1927) — Erg. Physiol. **27**, 47 (1928).
[3] ZUNZ, E.: Eléments de Pharmacodynamie Générale. Paris: Masson et Cie. 1930.
[4] CLARK, A. J.: The Mode of Action of Drugs on Cells. London: Arnold and Co. 1933.
[5] CRUM BROWN, A., and T. R. FRASER: Proc. roy. Soc. Edinburgh **1869**, 560.

be interpreted by those laws of physical chemistry which happen to be known at present, but the obvious primary task of a new science is to determine how far its phenomena can be interpreted by the laws that have been established in older sciences which have already acquired a large body of exact knowledge.

Chapter 1

# Methods of General Pharmacology.

**General Considerations.** The aim of general pharmacology is to discover the nature of the chemical reactions that occur when drugs act upon cells, and the obvious line of approach is to apply the methods used in physical chemistry, but any such attempt at once reveals the following fundamental difficulties. In the first place the simplest cell is a far more complex structure than any system studied by physical chemists. This complexity greatly reduces the significance of simple quantitative estimations. Even if it is known that the fixation of a certain number of molecules by a cell produces a certain derangement of function, yet we still do not know what proportion of the drug fixed is responsible for the actions observed. In the second place the entrance of a drug into a cell is in most cases a complex process involving adsorption and diffusion and finally resulting in a response which is measured. It is obvious that the time relations between the introduction of the drug and the appearance of the biological response provide extremely uncertain information, because the delay measured may be due to so many different causes. In the third place, investigations are limited by the fact that normal functions of living cells can only be maintained within a narrow range of physico-chemical conditions, hence it is not possible to test the validity of possible physico-chemical explanations over wide ranges of temperature etc. Fourthly, it must be remembered that all living cells show both static and dynamic variation. A uniform population of cells is an unknown phenomenon, and living cells are usually changing in some manner, a fact which makes it difficult to obtain accurate controls.

If the pharmacologist uses the methods of physical chemistry he must always remember that he is putting these methods to uses for which they were never intended. The dangers of such a procedure ought to be obvious but a study of the literature shows that they are apt to be forgotten.

The usual methods for determining the nature of a chemical reaction are firstly the quantitative determination of the amounts of chemicals taking part in the reaction, and secondly the determination of the kinetics of the reaction. Unfortunately the value of these methods in pharmacology is limited on account of the complications already mentioned. The living cell is so complex that it is very improbable that all the molecules of a drug fixed by a cell exert a similar action. Micro-injection experiments have indeed provided direct evidence in the case of several drugs that these produce different actions according to whether they are applied to the outside of the cell or injected into a cell. Moreover the study of enzyme poisons has shown that even in this relatively simple system the specific action of the poison may be produced by only a small fraction of the drug that is fixed by the enzyme. The chief fact that can be established by quantitative analysis is that a particular action can be produced by not more than a certain quantity of drug, but it is not possible in the vast majority of cases to say what proportion of the drug fixed has actually produced the action observed.

The study of kinetics also presents special difficulties because it is rarely possible to be certain what process in a chain of processes is causing the delay that is being measured.

Quantitative pharmacology is forced therefore to use somewhat indirect methods to investigate the nature of the reactions that occur between drugs and cells. In general the most useful data are those relating the concentration or dose of a drug with the amount of action produced when time is allowed for equilibrium to be established. In this case many of the sources of error that beset kinetic measurements are reduced in importance.

In view of the complexity of the material studied it is unreasonable to expect formal proof for any hypothesis and the best that can be hoped for is the establishment of a reasonable probability.

The writer's aim has been to determine how far the actions produced by drugs on cells can be explained by the known laws of physical chemistry, without making assumptions that are obviously absurd, and without postulating vital processes of unknown nature. Such a method will of course leave many phenomena unexplained, but in view of the uncertainty and difficulty of the subject this is only to be expected.

**Selection of Material.** The chief difficulty in the study of general pharmacology is that the simplest living cell offers a host of unsolved problems as regards its structure and functions, hence it is obviously desirable to choose for study the simplest material available.

Two types of living material are particularly suitable.

(a) Unicellular organisms suspended in water, such as bacteria, yeast, amoebae etc.

(b) Isolated tissues of higher animals, e. g. red blood corpuscles, muscles, etc.

The latter class has certain advantages because owing to specialization of function, the cells are to a certain extent simplified. Furthermore isolated tissues usually are more sensitive to drugs than are unicellular organisms because these latter frequently have complex defence mechanisms.

Another general principle is that it is advantageous to choose living cells whose properties have been studied fairly extensively because in such cases there is the largest amount of information available concerning the structure and the chemical and physical properties of the cells. Examples of such cell populations are B. coli, anthrax spores, sea urchin eggs, yeast cells, red blood corpuscles, and the skeletal and heart muscles of frogs. Similarly it is most profitable to study the common drugs which have been used extensively in quantitative experimental work on a wide variety of cell systems. e. g. phenol, mercuric chloride, narcotics, acetylcholine, adrenaline, etc.

When an eclectic method of this type is used it is however necessary to be very cautious in postulating general rules because every different cell-drug system represents a separate problem and an attractive hypothesis which explains one case may be ridiculously impossible in other cases.

**Employment of Physico-chemical Methods.** The dangers associated with the use of these methods have already been mentioned. The physical chemist when studying heterogeneous systems takes care to obtain the simplest possible system. For example he prefers to study adsorption on a surface of polished metal rather than on pure charcoal, because the latter is inconveniently complex.

Furthermore the physical chemist can test the validity of his conclusions by varying such factors as temperature over a wide range. The pharmacologist is forced to work on an extremely complex system, and is further handicapped by the fact that many conditions such as temperature, osmotic pressure, reaction etc. can only be varied over a narrow range. Consequently when a relation is established between the concentration of a drug and the amount of action and this relation follows some formula that expresses a particular physico-chemical

process, it rarely is possible to vary experimental conditions sufficiently widely
to test adequately the hypothesis that the drug action depend on this process.

**The Mathematical Interpretation of Biological Data.** As a general rule the
accuracy of biological data is very low in comparison with physico-chemical data.
In many cases the significance of the measurements made is uncertain because
they express the relation between a cause and an effect which are divided by a
complex chain of physical and chemical events. Even when the significance of
the measurements is fairly clear yet the data are subject to certain sources of
error such as cell variation, which have already been enumerated. For these
and other reasons it is rare to obtain results which when repeated show a scatter
of less than 10 per cent.

If for instance it is found that concentrations of 1 and of 10 units of drug
respectively produce actions of 20 and 60 per cent. of the maximum possible
effect these figures probably mean that the results lie between the limits of
17—23 and 55—65 per cent. respectively and accuracy greater than this can
very seldom be obtained. Furthermore it usually is particularly difficult to
measure accurately effects less than 10 per cent. and more than 90 per cent. of
the maximum action.

The consequence of these facts is that data very frequently give ambiguous
results because they can be fitted approximately by several different formulae.
The writer's experience is that the chief difficulty is not the finding of a formula
which will fit data but the choice between several alternative formulae all of
which give an approximate fit.

The author has shown for example (CLARK, 1933)[1] that a curve of a type
that is commonly found to relate drug concentrations ($x$) and biological response
($y$) can be fitted over a range of action from 0 up to 70 p.c. of the maximum
action almost equally well by the formula $Kx = \dfrac{y}{100 - y}$, which expresses a
particular form of monomolecular reaction, or by the WEBER's law formula
$Ky = \log(ax + 1)$. Moreover the curve between 20 and 60 p.c. action is also
fitted by FREUNDLICH's empirical adsorption formula $Kx^n = y$. (The value of
$K$ is of course different in each case.) It was indeed found possible to adjust
the constants in these three different formulae so that the curves obtained did
not diverge more than 10 per cent. within the limits mentioned above, and since
in actual practice it is only in exceptionally favourable circumstances that relations
between concentration and action can be established with less than this error,
therefore the calculation referred to above gives a fair indication of the uncertain
results yielded by the mathematical analysis of pharmacological relations.

JACOBS (1935)[2] has given the following clear summary of the limitations of
the use of mathematics in biology:

"In the first place it is utterly hopeless for the biologist with the means at present at
his disposal, to reduce the variables that enter into his problems to the small number usually
encountered in physical investigation. He is compelled therefore, regretfully, but of necessity,
to be content with a lesser degree of precision in his results than that attainable in the so-called
'exact sciences'. It follows that in dealing with most biological problems it is not only useless,
but actually unscientific, to carry mathematical refinements beyond a certain point, just
as it would be both useless and unscientific to employ an analytical balance of the highest
precision for obtaining the growth curve of a rat."

"In the second place, the field of biology is so vast that the biologist is still in the position
of an explorer in a newly discovered continent. His first task is to map out more or less
roughly the main topographical features of the country—after which accurate geodetic

[1] CLARK, A. J.: The Mode of Action of Drugs on Cells. London: Arnold and Co. 1933.
[2] JACOBS, M. H.: Erg. Biol. **12**, 1 (1935).

surveys may profitably be undertaken. The biologist is still for the most part an explorer rather than a surveyor."

In accordance with this general conception of the problem we are unlikely to obtain definite mathematical proof of the occurrence of any particular physico-chemical process in pharmacology. If certain data are fitted by a formula this may suggest the probability of the occurrence of some process. It must however be remembered that a formula is merely a form of shorthand which is convenient but nevertheless dangerous because it may conceal wildly improbable assumptions, which would at once be rejected if stated in words.

Another important point is that care should be used when formulae are employed, which although convenient, yet imply impossibilities. For example the simple kinetic formula: concentration × time = constant, implies that an infinite dilution produces an action in infinite time, and that a sufficiently strong concentration will produce instantaneous action. Both these postulates are untrue in the case of most cell-drug systems, since there is usually a minimum threshold active concentration and also a minimum time needed for the production of a response. A formula of this type may be a convenience in practice because it permits the approximate estimation of the time required for the production of an effect, but obviously it has a limited theoretical value.

These points have been emphasised because it has frequently happened that physicists and chemists have applied mathematical methods of analysis to data obtained by biologists without realising the inaccuracy of the data which they have treated, and have obtained proofs of the occurrence of biological impossibilities, and these proofs have been accepted by biologists who have been impressed if not mesmerised by the imposing formula provided.

It is important always to remember the aphorism of HUXLEY, that no mathematical treatment has yet been devised which will convert inaccurate experimental results into accurate data.

**Favourable Factors in Pharmacological Measurements.** Although the living cell is such a highly complex and variable system that it is difficult to make accurate quantitative studies of its activity, yet it has one striking advantage, namely that its activities can be modified in a remarkable manner by drugs. A wide variety of chemical substances produce specific actions on the living cell, and in a large number of cases the drugs act in very high dilutions. The recent advances in physiology, which have revealed the fact that the animal body is a machine whose activities are normally regulated by drugs, have provided a partial explanation for the striking susceptibility of living cells to drug action.

Another important point is that the pharmacological activity of chemical substances is frequently extremely specific and can be abolished or greatly changed by small alterations in their constitution or even in their molecular configuration.

These facts make quantitative studies in pharmacology intensely interesting and also make them a very promising line of approach to the great problem of the mode of organisation of the living cell. In spite of all modern advances in physical chemistry the living cell is still able to detect in chemical substances differences that elude the physical chemist. Even though the quantitative study of drug action provides information that is often very inexact, yet the information provided is sometimes unique, since it cannot be obtained in any other manner.

**Curves Relating Exposure to Drugs with Biological Effect.** The amount of exposure of cells to a drug can be varied in two ways: firstly, by varying the duration of the exposure, and secondly by varying the concentration of the drug.

The amount of biological response can be estimated in two ways. Firstly by the measurement of the amount of change in some activity such as respiration or movement and secondly by the measurement of the proportion of a cell population which shows some selected response, such for instance as death. These two types of measurement are termed "graded actions" and "all-or-none effects" respectively.

Usually it is fairly certain which type of effect is being measured but sometimes this is doubtful. For example when a drug causes the release of half the haemoglobin contained in a population of red blood corpuscles this effect might be due to each corpuscle losing half its haemoglobin or to half the corpuscles being completely haemolysed. In this case our knowledge of haemolysis informs us that the latter is the true explanation and that the action is of an all-or-none character. Similarly a partial contraction of a skeletal muscle produced by caffeine might be due to a portion of the fibres being fully stimulated or to all the fibres receiving a submaximal stimulation. In this case it is probable that the effect is of a graded character. These cases are relatively simple problems, but cases occur in which it is not possible to decide whether the action is of a graded or all-or-none character.

The following general rules can be applied to these two types of response.

(1) An all-or-none effect, such as death cannot be measured as a graded action. The only partial exception to this rule is that the effect may be roughly subdivided into such classes of response as moribund and dead.

(2) Any graded response can be measured as an all-or-none effect, provided that the fate of each individual cell or organism can be measured. For example the inhibition of the frog's heart by acetylcholine is a simple graded response but if a selected concentration of drug be applied to an adequately large population of hearts then the population can be divided into two groups, those showing and those failing to show some selected response (e.g. 50 per cent. inhibition). The graded action is thus measured as an all-or-none effect.

**Classes of Curves.** Curves expressing drug action can be divided into the following five classes:

(1) Curves relating time and the production of some graded action, e.g. the contraction curve of a smooth muscle in response to a drug such as acetylcholine (time-graded action curves).

(2) Curves relating time and incidence of some all-or-none effect, e.g. destruction of bacteria or haemolysis of red blood corpuscles (time-all-or-none action curves).

(3) Curves relating concentration and time of appearance of some selected action (time-concentration curves). The curves can be derived from time-action curves of either of the two classes already mentioned.

(4) Curves relating concentration and amount of graded action (concentration-action curves). These curves express the relation between concentration and amount of action when time is allowed for equilibrium to be obtained. These can be derived from curves of the first class, when the time-action curves reach equilibrium at a submaximal effect.

(5) Curves relating concentration and incidence of all-or-none effect (characteristic curves). These curves express the incidence of some all-or-none effect (usually death) when varying concentrations or doses of a drug are applied to a population. These curves express the individual variation of the population.

Curves of classes 1, 2 and 3 are kinetic curves which express the rate of action of drugs on cells, whilst curves of classes 4 and 5 express equilibria between drugs and cells.

The kinetic curves which measure the rate of action of drugs present a difficulty which will be discussed in detail in a later chapter but which may be mentioned briefly at this point. These curves are of two types because some measure the time until a drug produces some recognised action, whilst others measure the time required for a tissue to take up a dose of drug which will ultimately produce a certain action.

This difference is obvious in the case of drugs with which there is a long latent period before the action occurs. For example the uptake of curarine by an isolated muscle occurs in less than a minute, whilst the paralysis may not appear for an hour (Военм, 1910[1]). In such a case it is clear that the curve relating concentration and time of uptake will follow a completely different time scale from the curve relating concentration and time of appearance of paralysis. The curves relating concentration with duration of exposure needed to produce death are the most important class of time-concentration curves, and in such cases it is usual to measure the time of exposure which will ultimately produce death and not the time of exposure until death appears. Measurements of the time of exposure until an effect is observed usually provide data of very uncertain significance, and are chiefly of value in cases where it is certain that the time taken by the drug to be absorbed is longer than the time it takes to produce its effects after it has been absorbed.

A large proportion of the evidence available in quantitative pharmacology is in the form of one or other of the five curves described above, but unfortunately the interpretation of most of these five types of curve is the subject of controversy. For example it has been argued that the shape of the time × all-or-none action curves proves that the reaction between drugs and cells is monomolecular. That is to say that one molecule of drug kills one cell as an all-or-none effect. The concentration × graded action curves on the other hand can be interpreted as expressing chemical equilibria or as expressing a peculiar form of individual variation.

A consideration of the nature of these various types of curves shows that the actions they express are very different. In practice however the form of the curves obtained is often very similar in the different classes. These curious resemblances between curves which express completely different processes constitute one of the chief difficulties in quantitative pharmacology. In practice it is very easy to forget that two curves of similar shape are in reality quite different, and if a formula provides a rational explanation of a curve of one class there is a great temptation to apply it to similarly shaped curves of other classes, but in many cases such a procedure is quite unjustifiable.

In general it may be said that it is impossible to sustain any reasoned argument concerning quantitative pharmacology unless great care is exercised in discriminating between the various types of curves, and confusion in this matter is certainly the most frequent source of serious error.

**Discussion.** The chief aim of the present article is to try to establish probable hypotheses for the mode of action of certain classes of drugs on cells. The mode of approach chosen by the writer has been to consider first the outstanding features of cell size and structure, secondly to consider the evidence regarding the action of drugs on simple systems such as proteins and enzymes, and finally to see how far the mode of action of drugs on cells can be interpreted by the facts known regarding the reactions in these simpler systems.

The general outlook of the author is that the living cell is an extremely complex colloidal system, the structure and functions of which are very imperfectly known. Owing to the fortunate chance that the functions of the cell are

[1] Военм, R.: Arch. f. exper. Path. **63**, 219 (1910).

regulated by chemical agents, the study of the mode of action of drugs is one of the most favourable methods for analysing cell functions. Any interpretation of pharmacological data must however take into account the known complexity of the living cell. The writer therefore assumes as a general principle that, if a reaction between a drug and a cell appears to follow simpler laws than those applicable to relatively simple colloidal systems, this apparent simplicity is an accident and is probably due to the mutual cancellation of uncontrolled variables.


## Chapter 2

## The Cell as a Physico-chemical System.

The physical chemistry of cell structures is one of the most important funda-mental problems in biology which is still unsolved. It is impossible even to summarise adequately the evidence relating to a controversial problem of this magnitude, but since this monograph deals with the action of drugs on cells it is necessary to formulate some working hypothesis of cell structure. In compiling the following account of current views the author has been largely guided by the opinions expressed at a recent discussion on the properties and functions of membranes[1].

Some of the problems of cell structure which are of special interest in relation to pharmacology are (1) the structure of protoplasm, (2) the organisation and properties of the cell surface, and (3) the selective permeability of the cell surface to drugs.

**(1) The Structure of Protoplasm.** The nucleus in all cells is a semi-rigid structure but in many cells the mass of the protoplasm is obviously in a fluid condition. For example many plant cells are characterised by streaming movements in the protoplasm. In the case of amoebae, MARSLAND (1934)[2] argued that the protoplasm must be fluid because aqueous media when injected mixed freely with the cell contents, and if the cell surface were destroyed the internal protoplasm mixed with the external aqueous medium. Moreover globules of non-aqueous media did not mix with protoplasm but could move freely in the cell interior.

CHAMBERS (1926)[3] showed in the case of echinoderm eggs that the protoplasmic surface was reformed when torn, but that the presence of calcium in the outside medium was necessary for this formation and that the egg contents flowed out when the eggs were torn in calcium-free fluid. This suggests that the limiting membrane of the protoplasm is produced by the formation of a protein gel and that this only occurs when calcium salts are present in the external medium..

HEILBRUNN's measurements of the viscosity of invertebrate eggs showed that in these the viscosity was only a few times greater than that of water and he concluded that the protoplasm was of the nature of a suspensoid sol. On the other hand in many cells, and notably in muscle cells, a considerable portion of the cell contents are organised as a rigid or semi-rigid structure.

Many simple drugs, e.g. narcotics, cyanides, potassium salts, produce similar effects both on cells in which the protoplasm is fluid and on those in which it is partly rigid and therefore any theory which explains their action must apply equally to both cases. This point is important because some theories which are applicable to rigid systems are inapplicable to cells with fluid protoplasm.

---

[1] Trans. Far. Soc. **1937**.
[2] MARSLAND, D.: J. Cell. Comp. Physiol. **4**, 9 (1934).
[3] CHAMBERS, R.: Harvey Lectures **22**, 41 (1926).

There is a general agreement that cells are protein structures and hence it is of interest to consider the manner in which chemicals can act upon proteins. This subject has been dealt with by MEYER (1929)[1] from whose article many of the following suggestions have been borrowed.

Proteins are built up of polypeptides chains with the type structure

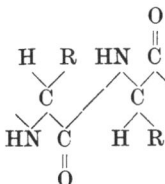

The dimensions of such chains are about 3.5 A in diameter and 100 A or more in length. The protein molecule is composed of hundreds of such chains. When a protein is in solution the molecules appear to be in the form of balls 20 A or more in diameter and presumably the chains have no definite orientation (BERNAL and CROWFOOT, 1934[2]). On the other hand proteins can form films about 10 A thick, and MOSS and RIDEAL (1935)[3] calculated that one molecule of myosin in the form of a film covered about 2000 sq. A. GORTER (1937)[4] has shown that various proteins at air-water surfaces occupy about 10,000 sq. A per molecule. The protein molecule can therefore assume the form of either a ball, a thread or a thin film.

When proteins are in the form of a gel the polypeptide chains are orientated as a lattice, and one of the most striking features of such gels is their power to imbibe a large quantity of water which is held between the chains. For example 100 g. dry gelatine can imbibe 850 g. water.

Proteins and in particular protein gels react with chemicals in an extremely complex manner, for the latter may be fixed by a protein gel in at least three different ways. In the case of substances with large molecules these may be too big to penetrate the gel but may be adsorbed on the surface. In the cases of substances with molecules small enough to penetrate the lattice, these may be loosely combined with a Neben-valenz or may form a firm chemical combination with a Haupt-valenz. The structure of the gel may be profoundly altered by some simple chemical combination. For example formaldehyde is believed to coagulate protein in virtue of its —$CH_2$— group which probably bridges the gaps between peptide chains and binds them together.

The number of reactive groups per molecule of protein is relatively large, for example COHN (1925)[5] found that each molecule of serum albumen combined with 50 molecules of hydrochloric acid. From such experiments he calculated that a molecule of egg albumin contained 27 basic and 27 acidic combining groups whilst the corresponding figures for casein were 115 and 265.

These properties of proteins are of importance in relation to two problems regarding the structure of the living cell, namely the nature of the cell surface and the condition of the water and small soluble molecules inside the cell.

The cell interior contains a solution of inorganic salts which usually is very different in composition from the fluid surrounding the cell. The simplest explanation is to postulate a semi-permeable cell membrane, but the peculiar

[1] MEYER, K. H.: Biochem. Z. 208, 1 (1929).
[2] BERNAL, J. D., and D. CROWFOOT: Nature (Lond.) 133, 794 (1934).
[3] MOSS, S. A., and E. K. RIDEAL: Nature (Lond.) 136, 260 (1935).
[4] GORTER, E.: Trans. Farad. Soc. 1937.
[5] COHN, E. J.: Physiologic. Rev. 5, 349 (1925).

properties of proteins make possible an alternative hypothesis that the internal solution is held in a protein lattice, and that the differences in composition of the fluids within and without the cell are dependent on the Donnan equilibrium.

(2) **The Cell Surface.** OSTERHOUT (1933, 1937)[1] reviewed the long controversy that has waged regarding the nature of the cell surface. STILES (1937)[2] pointed out that the views regarding the cell surface varied from the usual belief that the cell surface was an organised layer possessed of a special structure, which regulated the permeability of the cell to chemicals, to the belief of MARTIN H. FISCHER who regarded the plasmatic membrane as a figment of the imagination. The chief objection to the assumption of an organised cell surface is that no such structure can be observed under the microscope. On the other hand naked protoplasm brought into contact with water does not mix with it but tends to round up into a sphere. Moreover in micro-dissection experiments on amoebae the process of formation of a limiting surface can be observed at the injured point. The chief arguments in favour of an organised surface membrane are however derived from observations on the permeability of cells to chemicals.

(3) **Cell Permeability.** Evidence regarding cell permeability is derived from both plant and animal cells; these two types differ widely in their structure, and the evidence obtained in the two cases is different in nature, but it is obvious that any general theory of cell permeability ought to cover both classes.

The typical plant cell consists of a layer of protoplasm which is supported by a rigid internal vacuole. In large aquatic plant cells (e.g. *Valonia*) it is easy to analyse the content of the vacuole and its electrolytic content has been shown to be completely different from that of the water in which the cells live. The protoplasm of such cells therefore obviously possesses selective permeability and it usually is assumed that this selective permeability is dependent on special properties of the outermost and innermost layers of protoplasm (STILES, 1937[2]). Such cells are peculiarly well suited for the accurate measurement of rates of diffusion and COLLANDER (1937)[3] has shown in the case of *Chara* that these depend partly on the molecular volume, but that when molecules of similar size are compared there is a clear relation between the permeability and the oil/water distribution coefficient of non-electrolytes. An important point about these plant cells is that they consist of a layer of protoplasm with a watery phase on both sides and various electrolytes or non-electrolytes (e.g. cresyl blue, IRWIN, 1925[4]) when added to the external phase appear in the internal phase at 10 or more fold the external concentration. Such a process of concentration cannot be effected without the performance of work. Hence these cells provide a simple and clear proof that living cells can perform this type of work.

Animal cells do not possess a large central vacuole and in this case the movement of chemical substances can only be studied by the comparison of the chemical composition of the protoplasm with that of the surrounding fluid. One striking fact in the case of mammalian cells is that the Na/K ratio in the cell and in the surrounding fluids is completely different. GORTER (1937)[5] calculated the following ionic concentrations (in mille equivalents/litre) in the case of mammalian muscle.

|       | Muscle water | Serum water |
|-------|--------------|-------------|
| Na . . . | 48 | 154 |
| K . . . . | 112 | 5 |

[1] OSTERHOUT, W. J. V.: Erg. Physiol. **35**, 967 (1933) — Trans. Farad. Soc. **33** (1937).
[2] STILES, W.: Trans. Farad. Soc. **33** (1937).
[3] COLLANDER, R.: Trans. Farad. Soc. **33** (1937).
[4] IRWIN, M.: J. gen. Physiol. **8**, 147 (1925—26).
[5] GORTER, E.: Trans. Farad. Soc. **33** (1937).

The experiments of HILL and KUPALOV (1930)[1] showed that only a negligibly small fraction of the potassium within the muscle fibres of frogs could be osmotically inactive. Moreover measurements by BOZLER and COLE (1935)[2] on the internal conductivity of frogs' muscles showed that there were no unionised potassium compounds within the fibres.

A cell such as a muscle fibre has therefore the following outstanding characteristics:

(a) The osmotic pressures inside and outside the cell are equal. The salt content of the cells is known and all the salts of the cells must be free to exert osmotic pressure.

(b) The ionic composition of cell protoplasm and tissue fluids is completely different. In particular the cells contain far more potassium than sodium and the reverse is true of the tissue fluids.

These facts prove that the cell interior must be separated from the surrounding fluid by a barrier that is relatively impermeable to ions as small as those of potassium and sodium. It is simplest to call this barrier a cell membrane.

It is moreover obvious that the nature of the cell membrane must differ widely in different forms of cells. For example the protozoa which live in fresh water maintain an internal osmotic pressure much higher than that of the surrounding fluid whereas a red blood corpuscle cannot resist any difference in osmotic pressure.

The differential permeability of cells is a problem of great complexity, but one point deserves special mention, namely that in some cases we are dealing with differences in the rate of penetration rather than with an absolute difference between permeability and impermeability. For example in the case of the action of potassium on the frog's heart the concentration inside the cell (0.05 molar) is about 25 times the concentration in frog's plasma (0.002 molar) and hence we may say that the cell surface is impermeable to the potassium ion. This conclusion is supported by the fact that a 50 per cent. reduction in the activity of a frog's ventricle strip suspended in air is produced by the addition of a quantity of potassium chloride only sufficient to raise the concentration in the strip by 0.004 molar, and the same effect is produced if the strip is bathed in a large volume of fluid containing 0.009 molar potassium chloride (CLARK, 1926[3]). These effects are intelligible if one assumes that the potassium ion does not penetrate the cells and hence the potassium chloride added to the moist strip raises the potassium concentration in the intercellular spaces from 0.002 molar to about 0.01 molar. On the other hand, if the frog's heart is bathed in potassium-free RINGER's fluid it loses about one third of its potassium content in 2 hours, and hence slow diffusion of potassium from the heart cells is possible (CLARK, 1922[4]). Similarly although acids can diffuse out of cells fairly freely yet a sudden alteration in the $p_H$ of the surrounding fluid can alter cell functions without changing the $p_H$ of the cell (CLARK, 1913[5]).

According to the view outlined the cell is a protein sol bounded by a surface and the latter shows a marked selective permeability which imposes a considerable delay in the diffusion even of small ions or molecules to which it is permeable.

By means of a free use of the Donnan equilibrium and by the assumption of inert membranes which differentiate between the ionic volumes of potassium

[1] HILL, A. V., and P. S. KUPALOV: Proc. roy. Soc. B. **106**, 445 (1930).
[2] BOZLER, E., and K. S. COLE: J. Cell. Comp. Physiol. **6**, 229 (1935).
[3] CLARK, A. J.: J. Pharmacol. Baltimore **29**, 311 (1926).
[4] CLARK, A. J.: J. Pharmacol. Baltimore **18**, 423 (1922).
[5] CLARK, A. J.: J. Physiol. **46**, 20 (1913).

and of sodium it might be possible to account for the difference between the ionic composition of the protoplasm of animal cells and of the surrounding fluids and this avoid the assumption of a plasmatic membrane. This exercise of ingenuity seems however pointless since it leaves unexplained the power of the plant cell to concentrate ions within its internal valuole. In this case the cell transfers chemicals from one watery phase to another against a concentration gradient.

**(4) Structure of Plasmatic Membrane.** A number of authors have recently advanced hypotheses regarding the probable structure of the plasmatic membrane. The selective permeability of cells almost forces the assumption that the cell surface is composed of a lipine-protein mosaic.

CLOWES (1916)[1] suggested that the surface was a fat/water emulsion. THEORELL (1930)[2] suggested that cholesterin and phosphatides in cells were bound to the globulins and especially to the euglobulins. HEILBRUNN (1936)[3] showed that in frog's muscle and heart muscle treatment with ammonia caused a great increase in free fat and suggested that this was due to liberation of the lipins from combination with proteins. DANIELLI and HARVEY (1934)[4] made experiments on mackerel eggs and suggested that the cell surface was a mixture of proteins and of lipoids. ADAM (1935)[5] showed that proteins at an air/water interface spread into a layer about 5 A thick, that each molecule covered 1000 to 10,000 sq. A and that the protein became denatured in this process. This denaturation is however not an essential characteristic of the spreading of proteins in films for GORTER and MAASKANT (1937)[6] have shown that pepsin and trypsin can be recovered from a water surface without having lost more than 20 p.c. of their activity.

DANIELLI and DAVSON (1934)[7] concluded that the cell surface consisted of a film of lipoid covering the protoplasm and that there was a protein film outside the lipoid film.

DANIELLI (1937)[8] has elaborated the following hypothesis regarding the cell surface:

"The simplest possible concept of the cell surface which is compatible with permeability data, surface tension data and wetting properties, consists of a lipoid layer at least two molecules thick, with a layer of protein molecules adsorbed at each oil-water interface. At the external surface of the membrane there must be an excess of acidic groups $\cdots$ Owing to the excess of acidic groups at the interface, the surface will in general be more acid than the bulk phases. The maximum possible value of this difference with a cell in Ringer solution or sea water at $p_H$ 7.5 is two units of $p_H$. $\cdots$ Owing to the oriented dipoles of the oil and protein molecules, at each oil-water boundary there will be a potential of the order of 200 millivolts. $\cdots$ The potential drop at an interface is practically complete over a range of 5 A units or less, so the potential gradient at each interface is of the order of $10^7$ to $10^9$ volts/cm. $\cdots$ At each oil-water interface there will be a network of cross-linked polypeptide chains. The pore-size of this sieve will be greatly affected by e.g. surface $p_H$ changes and the salts of heavy metals. In this case drugs may affect the behaviour of the cell without entering or penetrating the lipoid layer of the cell wall."

RIDEAL (1937)[9] and SCHULMAN (1937)[10] studied the properties of mixed films. They found that composite films (e.g. protein and cholesterol) were more stable

[1] CLOWES, G. H. A.: J. physic. Chem. **20**, 407 (1916).
[2] THEORELL, H.: Biochem. Z. **223**, 1 (1930).
[3] HEILBRUNN, L. V.: Biol. Bull. Mar. biol. Labor. Wood's Hole **71**, 299 (1936).
[4] DANIELLI, J. F., and E. N. HARVEY: J. Cell. Comp. Physiol. **5**, 483 (1934).
[5] ADAM, N. K.: Nature (Lond.) **136**, 499 (1935).
[6] GORTER, E., and L. MAASKANT: Proc. kon. Akad. Wetensch. **40**, 77 (1937).
[7] DANIELLI, J. F., and H. DAVSON: J. Cell. Comp. Physiol. **5**, 495 (1934).
[8] DANIELLI, J. F.: Proc. roy. Soc. B. **121**, 605 (1937).
[9] RIDEAL, E. K.: Trans. Farad. Soc. **33** (1937).
[10] SCHULMAN, J. H.: Trans. Farad. Soc. **33** (1937).

than films of either component. This work suggests the probability of the cell surface being composed of mixed films of protein, cholesterol and lipines such as sphingo-myelin.

This hypothesis appears to meet the needs of pharmacology better than any other hypothesis previously put forward. RIDEAL has, for example, shown that the actions of many haemolytic agents can be accounted for by the effect they produce on the stability of mixed films of this type.

WRINCH (1936)[1] has outlined an attractive theory of the mode of organisation of the protein framework of the cell surface. She points out that proteins consist of condensations of optically active amino (and imino) acids. She postulates a hexagonal cyclol structure of laminae, orientated, owing to the optical activity of the component parts, so that all the side chains are on one surface. She suggests that the surface with the free side chains could function as a kind of template on which complex biosyntheses could be carried out. This hypothesis provides an explanation for many outstanding features of the selective action of drugs. The interference produced by a drug in the biochemical activities of cells would depend upon the manner in which it fitted the template, and in particular such a hypothesis explains the remarkable relation between optical activity and pharmacological action seen in the case of many drugs.

WRINCH considers particularly the remarkable pharmacological actions produced by the phenanthrene derivatives and suggests that this is dependent on the manner in which these complex structures fix the template of the cell surface. The great advantage of the theory of a surface composed of a mixture of proteins and lipines is that it explains how cell surfaces can be affected both by substances which presumably act on proteins, e.g. the active substances in haemolytic sera, and also by substances characterised by high lipoid solubility.

The following considerations are also of importance in relation to the problems of quantitative pharmacology. Enzyme activity is believed to be due to active groups fixed on to protein molecules. The speed of action of many cellular enzymes suggests that these are situated close to the surface of the cells. Hence it is difficult to account for the enzyme activity of cells without assuming the presence of proteins at the cell surface.

Similarly the modern theories of humoral transmission are only intelligible on the assumption that drugs such as acetylcholine react very rapidly with active patches on the cell surface. The nature of these active patches or receptors is unknown but in view of their very highly specific nature it seems probable that they are part of protein molecules.

For these and many other reasons it appears to the writer that the simplest form of cell surface that will account for a reasonable proportion of the phenomena observed is a mosaic of lipines and proteins. RIDEAL's scheme of a mixed film of interlocking molecules of proteins, cholesterol and lipines promises to account for a larger proportion of the observed phenomena than does any previous hypothesis.

(5) Cell Organisation. The manner in which the living cell is organised is the fundamental unsolved problem of biology. The alteration of cellular functions by drugs is an important method by which the functions of cells can be analysed, but in order to discuss the results of quantitative pharmacology it is convenient to have some tentative hypothesis regarding the nature of cellular function.

The chief aim of the present monograph is to discover how far the actions of drugs on cells can be interpreted by the known laws of physical chemistry, and this excludes the adoption of "vitalist" hypotheses which attribute to living

---

[1] WRINCH, D. M.: Nature (Lond.) **138**, 651 (1936).

matter properties unknown to physical chemistry. On the other hand it is completely unscientific to assume that physical chemistry is a completed science in which there are no new facts to discover. The history of biology shows the danger of any such perverted "mechanist" attitude. Repeated attempts were made, before the discovery of osmotic pressure and of the properties of matter in the colloidal state, to interpret the properties of living matter by the then known laws of physical chemistry. If biologists had recognised frankly that these laws were then inadequate to explain the phenomena they observed, the advance of physical chemistry would have been greatly accelerated.

The writer considers it to be important to interpret as many biological phenomena as possible by the laws known to regulate reactions in simpler systems, and equally important to recognise the phenomena which these laws in their present form do not explain.

The outstanding properties of living cells have been summarised by Hopkins (1924)[1] as follows:

"The characteristic of a living unit—whether it be the cell or another system—is that it is heterogeneous. There is no such thing as living matter in a specific sense. The special attribute of such systems from a chemical standpoint is that these reactions are organised, not that the molecules concerned are fundamentally different in kind from those the chemists meet elsewhere."

It will be generally agreed that the cell is a complex heterogeneous system, and many phenomena such as mitosis, etc. show that the living cell is organised in some manner of which we have at present little comprehension.

The assumption that the cell is a complex heterogeneous system organised in some manner, immediately encounters the difficulty that in many cells the protoplasm is obviously in a fluid condition. This is not the case in all cells, but no theory of cell organisation is of any value unless it covers the cases where the protoplasm is fluid and shows streaming movements. The conception of the interior of any cell as an unorganised fluid raises however almost impossible difficulties for both the biochemist and the pharmacologist. For example the modern theory of the glycolysis of carbohydrates postulates a most intricate process which proceeds in many stages and which is effected by means of several enzymes, coenzymes and organic phosphate compounds. Moreover the occurrence of glycolysis in most cells is checked by the presence of oxygen. Glycolysis is only one of many complex processes that proceed simultaneously within the cell, and these processes can be modified in a varied manner by different drugs.

Peters (1930)[2] stated the outlook of a biochemist on this problem as follows:

"The theories which have been advanced to account in chemical and physical terms for the fact that processes in the cell are continuously directed are insufficient. The fact that the cell contents are often quite fluid can be reconciled with the fact that the living cell shows a continuous directive power by the view that protein surfaces in the cell constitute a mosaic, controlled by their attachment to the central mosaic. These constitute a fluid anatomy of the cell, and the central mosaic behaves as a kind of central nervous system. The groups responsible for this appear to be terminal groups of the proteins, —COOH and basic groups and —CONH linkages. By change of reaction and varying adsorption, the activity of such groups can be controlled. Within this matrix, it is possible to picture the dynamic chains of chemical reaction taking place, controlled inside the cell not by ordinary considerations of mass action, but by the exigencies of the matrix."

Needham (1936)[3] has recently reviewed modern research on the forms of organisation known to occur in liquids in the paracrystalline state. In this connection the pioneer researches of Hardy on lubricants are of particular

[1] Hopkins, F. G.: Lancet 1, 1247 (1924).
[2] Peters, R. A.: J. State Med. 37, 1 (1930).
[3] Needham, J.: Order and Life. Cambridge: Univ. Press 1936.

interest. HARDY and NOTTAGE (1928)[1] showed that orientation effects could be transmitted from a metal surface and influence a surrounding film to a depth of several micra. It appears to the writer that it is essential to postulate for the cell some form of fluid organisation of the type outlined above, in order to form any picture of the manner in which the activities of enzymes in cells are coordinated and of the manner in which drugs produce alterations in cellular function.

The author feels that he owes an apology for introducing somewhat vague speculations. It is however very difficult for the human mind to function without some form of working hypothesis. The adoption of the conceptions outlined regarding the structure of the cell surface does help to suggest a means by which minute quantities of drugs can produce a highly selective action. Furthermore the author feels that it is very difficult to explain such actions unless one adopts the hypothesis that cellular activities are dependent on receptor groups arranged in some pattern on the cell surface and that the drugs produce their effect by combining with these receptors. This hypothesis is of course very similar to that put forward by EHRLICH a quarter of a century ago.

The present monograph has been planned with a view to testing the possibility of this belief by a consideration of the evidence available. Quantitative pharmacology is such an undeveloped subject that it is hopeless to expect formal proof for any hypothesis, and equally hopeless to expect any hypothesis to explain all the facts observed. The author has found however that the hypothesis outlined above explains a considerable proportion of the known experimental facts.

## Chapter 3
## General Characteristics of the Cell-Drug System.

**Dimensions of Molecules and Cells.** The sizes of certain molecules, visible organisms, and ultra-microscopic viruses and phages are shown in Tables 1, 2 and 3. The measurements in these three tables are, for convenience, given in different units, but these can readily be transposed. (1 micron = 1000 millimicra, 1 mμ = 10 A., 1 cubic micron = $10^9$ cubic millimicra and 1 cu.mμ = 1000 cubic A.)

The sizes of viruses and phages appear now to be established with

Table 1. Dimensions of Cells.

| Cell | Linear dimensions in micra | Surface in sq.micra | Volume in cubic micra |
|---|---|---|---|
| Small coccus . . . . . . | 0.8 | 2.0 | 0.25 |
| B. coli . . . . . . . . . | 3×1.2 | 12.0 | 3.4 |
| Trypanosoma rhodesiense . | 25×5 [2] | 100 | 30 |
| Yeast cells . . . . . . . | 4—7 | 50—150 | 33—180 |
| Human erythrocyte . . . | 9×2.5 | 120 | 120 |
| Arbacia eggs . . . . . . | 74 | 17,200 | 212,000 |
| Muscle cell in frog's ventricle . . . . . . | 131×9 | 1,900 | 2,600 |
| Uterine muscle of virgin rat | 30×2 | 90 | 30 |

some certainty. The figures shown in Table 3 are quoted from ELFORD (1937)[3] and were obtained by ultra-filtration. They agree with the results of other workers who have used this method. HERZBERG (1936)[4] has collected such figures from various sources. LEVADITI and his co-workers (1936)[5] using ultrafiltration found that the size of viruses ranged from 320 to 3 millimicra, and the size of phages from 120 to 8 millimicra.

[1] HARDY, W. B., and M. NOTTAGE: Proc. roy. Soc. A. **118**, 209 (1928).
[2] REINER, L., C. S. LEONARD and S. S. CHAO: Arch. int. Pharmacodyn. **43**, 186 (1932).
[3] ELFORD, W. J.: Trans. Farad. Soc. **33** (1937).
[4] HERZBERG, K.: Klin. Wschr. **15**, 1665 (1936).
[5] LEVADITI, C., M. PAIC, J. VOET and D. KRASSNOFF: C. r. Soc. Biol. Paris **122**, 354 (1936).

The results obtained by SVEDBERG with the ultracentrifuge also agree fairly well with the results obtained with ultrafiltration.

The figures given in Table 3 show that the viruses and phages form a continuous series as regards size, and range from forms as large as the smallest visible organisms to forms smaller than the largest protein molecules. The conclusion that the smallest viruses resemble protein molecules as regards size, is confirmed by the discovery that the tobacco mosaic virus can be isolated as a crystalline protein (STANLEY, 1935[7]).

Table 2. Dimensions of Molecules.

|  | Molecular weight | Volume in cubic A. |
|---|---|---|
| Phenol. . . . . . . . | 94 | 100[1] |
| Sodium oleate . . . . | 304 | 616[2] |
| Castor oil . . . . . | 929 | 1600[3] |
| Egg albumen. . . . . | 36,400[4] | 39,000[2] |
| Haemoglobin. . . . . | $2 \times 36,400$[4] | 80,000[5] |
| Serum globulin . . . . | $4 \times 36,400$ |  |
| Haemocyanins . . . . | from    400,000 to $24 \times 400,000$[4] |  |

Table 3. Dimensions of Viruses and Phages.
(ELFORD, 1937[6].)

|  | Diameter in millimicra | Volume in cubic millimicra estimated as spheres |
|---|---|---|
| Visible organisms |  |  |
| B. prodigiosus . . . . . . | 750 |  |
| B. pleuropneumoniae . . . | 150 |  |
| Spirochaeta pallida . . . . | 200 |  |
| Viruses |  |  |
| Large:— psittacosis. . . . | 250 | 2,200,000 |
| Small:— foot and mouth disease. . . . . . . . | 10 | 523 |
| Phages |  |  |
| Largest . . . . . . . . | 60 | 32,000 |
| Smallest . . . . . . . . | 10 | 523 |
| Proteins |  |  |
| Haemocyanin (Helix) . . . | 22 | 1,500 |
| Serum albumen. . . . . . | 5 | 18 |
| Oxyhaemoglobin . . . . . | 5 | 18 |
| Egg albumen. . . . . . . | 4 | 9 |

The viruses and phages are more difficult to study than are visible organisms and knowledge of their properties is correspondingly scanty. In general they appear to be more rather than less resistant to drug action than are visible organisms. These remarkable ultramicroscopic forms cannot be ignored when theories of drug action are postulated, but at present our knowledge of how they are affected by drugs is too limited to form a satisfactory basis for dicussion.

A comparison of the sizes of ordinary drugs and of visible cells shows at once that in this case the difference in magnitude is very great. For example the molecular volume of phenol is about 100 cu.A. whilst the volume of a human red blood corpuscle is about $100 \times 10^{12}$ cu.A. This is the relation between a microgram and a ton (1000 kg.). Even a small coccus, with a volume of 0.25 cu.$\mu$., is very much larger than a molecule of a protein such as haemoglobin, which has a volume of 80,000 cu.A. or $8 \times 10^{-8}$ cubic micron (KUNITZ, ANSON and NORTHROP 1934[5]).

The number of molecules of phenol needed to cover a red blood corpuscle with a monomolecular layer is of the order of $10^8$, and the corresponding figure

[1] LANDOLT-BÖRNSTEIN: Physikalisch-chemische Tabellen 1, 119. 5. Aufl. Berlin: Julius Springer 1923.
[2] NOUY, P. L. DU: Surface Equilibria of Biological and Organic Colloids. Amer. chem. Soc. Monogr. 1926.
[3] LANGMUIR, I.: Amer. chem. Soc. Abstr. 11, 2422 (1917).
[4] SVEDBERG, T., and I.-B. ERIKSSON: Tab. Biol. Period. 5, 351 (1936).
[5] KUNITZ, M., M. L. ANSON and J. H. NORTHROP: J. gen. Physiol. 17, 365 (1934).
[6] ELFORD, W. J.: Trans. Farad. Soc. 33 (1937).
[7] STANLEY, W. M.: Science (N. Y.) 81, 644 (1935).

in the case of a protein covering a coccus is $10^5$. In the case of a red blood corpuscle the amount of drug required to cover it with a monomolecular layer has a volume of about $1/_{1000}$ the volume of the cell, whilst in the case of the coccus the corresponding drug volume is about $1/_{100}$ the cell volume.

**The Number of Molecules in Single Cells.** A small coccus with a volume of 0.25 cu.micra contains about 2 per cent. of nitrogen, which is equivalent to about 12 per cent. of protein. If the protein has a molecular weight of 66,000 then each coccus contains more than $10^5$ molecules of protein. In the case of most of the common molecules such as inorganic salts there will be a large number per coccus. The only important exception is the hydrogen ion, for in this case, if the interior is at $p_H$ 7,0, there will be only 2 free hydrogen ions per coccus. PETERS (1930)[1] calculated that in the case of an organism 0.2 micron in diameter there would be only one free hydrogen ion when the contents were neutral. CAMERON (1929)[2] calculated the number of molecules and ions present in a red blood corpuscle and found that the numbers lay between $10^8$ and $10^{10}$.

In general it may be said that in the case of ultramicroscopic viruses the number of molecules per cell must be too small to permit the application of the ordinary laws of physical chemistry, which are based on mass action. In the case of visible cells on the other hand the number of most varieties of molecules per cell must be large, although the hydrogen ions form an important exception, hence it would appear that cells, which are not smaller than ordinary bacilli, may be regarded as entities containing a sufficient number of molecules to permit the application of the ordinary laws of mass action.

PETERS (1930)[1] concluded however that the laws of mass action as derived from homogeneous solutions were unlikely to apply to molecules inside a cell because "when once a molecule enters the surface film, which it may do merely by the forces of diffusion, it becomes subject mainly to surface forces and therefore to forces which are different in kind".

If we assume that the cell protoplasm is bounded by a semipermeable surface with specific receptors arranged in some form of mosaic then it follows that drugs may exert their action on cells in several manners. The simplest condition is when the drug is not adsorbed but reacts with a receptor on the cell surface. In this case the course of the reaction will depend on the concentration of drug in the solution. If a drug is adsorbed however three phases are present namely the general bulk of the solution, the adsorbed layer and the cell surface. In the case of drugs which are adsorbed but do not produce an action until they have penetrated the cell four phases are involved, namely the solution, the adsorbed layer, the surface of the cell and the cell interior.

It is unreasonable to hope for clear cut physico-chemical explanations of more than a fraction of the phenomena observed in systems of this complexity and the general principle followed by the writer has been to pay chief attention to the cases which appear to follow the simplest laws.

**The Number of Enzyme Molecules per Cell.** The molecular weights of enzymes in the cases which have been estimated lie between 30,000 and 300,000. HALDANE (1930)[3] calculated that one yeast cell contained 15,000—150,000 molecules of saccharase. He concluded that this was an exceptional case, that a cell of *Aspergillus niger* probably contained less than 1,000 molecules of saccharase and that the number of molecules per cell in the case of rare enzymes might be very small.

[1] PETERS, R. A.: J. State Med. **37**, 1 (1930).
[2] CAMERON, A. T.: Trans. roy. Soc. Canada, Sect. **5**, 151 (1929).
[3] HALDANE, J. B. S.: Enzymes. London: Longman, Green and Co. 1930.

WARBURG and CHRISTIAN (1933)[1] found 24 $\gamma$ of yellow pigment per gram of yeast cells. If the molecular weight of the pigment is taken as 30,000 and the volume of the yeast cell as 200 cu.$\mu$. there are 80,000 molecules of pigment per cell. Even if all these enzymes were arranged on the cell surface this quantity would cover less than $1/_{1000}$ of the surface. ZEILE (1933)[2] calculated from the results of WARBURG and KUBOWITZ (1929)[3] that there were about 2,000,000 molecules of respiratory ferment per yeast cell.

These figures agree in indicating that in most cases the number of molecules of an enzyme in a cell is large. This fact is of importance in relation to calculations regarding the amount of drug needed to paralyse any particular enzyme activity of a cell.

**Lethal Doses of Drugs per Cell.** Quantitative estimations of the amount of drugs fixed by bacteria, trypanosomes and red blood corpuscles show that the number of molecules fixed per cell is very large.

KRUSE and FISCHER (1935)[4] found that silver salts in a concentration of 1 in $10^8$ killed staphycococci when these were present in a concentration of $10^7$ per c.c. If all the silver present were fixed this would correspond to $10^7$ molecules of silver per coccus. LEITNER (1929)[5] gave figures which indicated that B. coli was killed by about $6 \times 10^5$ molecules per bacillus.

Quantitative estimations of the fixation by spirogyra of silver from dilute solutions (3 $\gamma$ per litre) showed that the algae contained 60 $\gamma$ Ag per g. dry weight. This would correspond to more than 10,000 atoms of silver per cu.micron of filament (FREUNDLICH and SÖLLNER, 1928[6]).

In the case of drugs of low toxicity such as phenol the concentration in bacteria when a lethal action is produced lies between 1 and 0.1 per cent. and this corresponds to more than 1,000,000 molecules per coccus. Estimations of the amount of trypanocides fixed by trypanosomes show figures of the order of millions of molecules per organism. REINER, LEONARD and CHAO (1932)[7] found that each trypanosome fixed $6 \times 10^6$ molecules of arsenious acid.

In the case of red blood corpuscles the amount of drug fixed per cell when haemolysis is produced is even larger. The following estimates have been made: $10^7$ molecules of silver or of mercury (MENINGHETTI, 1922[8]); $10^8$ molecules of saponin or of sodium oleate (PONDER, 1930[9]); $10^9$ molecules of acid or of alkali (CHRISTOPHERS, 1929[10]).

These results indicate that the amount of saponin or of sodium oleate that must be fixed by the red blood corpuscle in order to produce haemolysis is similar to the quantity needed to cover the surface of the red blood corpuscle with a monomolecular layer. GORTER (1937)[11] made quantitative studies on this subject and concluded that this quantity was needed to produce haemolysis, and that fixation of amounts too small to cover the red blood corpuscle did not produce haemolysis although it sensitised the cell to other haemolytic agents.

---

[1] WARBURG, O., and N. CHRISTIAN: Biochem. Z. **266**, 377 (1933).
[2] ZEILE, K.: Erg. Physiol. **35**, 498 (1933).
[3] WARBURG, O., and F. KUBOWITZ: Biochem. Z. **214**, 5 (1929).
[4] KRUSE, W., and M. FISCHER: Arch. f. Hyg. **113**, 46 (1935).
[5] LEITNER, N.: Klin. Wschr. **8**, 1952 (1929).
[6] FREUNDLICH, H., and K. SÖLLNER: Biochem. Z. **203**, 1 (1928).
[7] REINER, L., C. S. LEONARD and S. S. CHAO: Arch. internat. Pharmacodynamie **43**, 186 (1932).
[8] MENINGHETTI, E.: Biochem. Z. **131**, 38 (1922).
[9] PONDER, E.: Proc. roy. Soc. B. **106**, 543 (1930).
[10] CHRISTOPHERS, S. R.: Indian J. med. Res. **17**, 54 (1929).
[11] GORTER, E.: Trans. Farad. Soc. **33** (1937).

In general the evidence available agrees in showing that the amount of drug required to produce a lethal action on a cell as small as a coccus is at least of the order of thousands of molecules per cell, and in the case of larger cells it is at least of the order of millions of molecules per cell.

In the case of bacterial antibodies the minimum figures obtained for the number of molecules fixed per cell are considerable lower than in the case of ordinary drugs. MARRACK (1934)[1] gives certain quantitative figures for the amount of antibody globulin necessary to produce agglutination of bacteria. Agglutinin solutions can be prepared which contain less than 0.002 per cent. protein but which will agglutinate B. typhosus at a dilution of 1 in 1000. If the globulin has a molecular weight of 146,000 and is all fixed by the bacteria and there are $10^9$ bacteria per c.c. then each bacterium must fix 100 molecules of globulin. The relative volumes of the protein fixed and of the bacteria will be about as 1 is to $10^5$. OTTENBERG and STEENBUCK (1923)[2] have calculated that the amount of antibody fixed cannot cover more than $1/_{50}$ of the surface of the bodies of the bacteria.

**Effective Doses of Drugs per Cell.** The following estimates have been made of the amount of certain powerful drugs which are fixed by isolated tissues when a recognisable effect is produced.

STRAUB's (1910)[3] experimental results showed that the amount of ouabain fixed by the heart of a frog when a lethal action was produced corresponded to a concentration of 2 parts per million in the tissue. Various other workers have obtained similar results with other cardiac glucosides in both the frog and the cat (CLARK, 1933[4]). The author has calculated (CLARK, 1933[5]) that this quantity would not cover more than about 3 per cent. of the surface of the heart cells.

In the case of acetylcholine the author (CLARK, 1933[5]) found that the amount fixed by the frog's heart when 50 per cent. inhibition was produced was only 2 parts per 100 million. These experiments were carried out on non-eserinised hearts and therefore this is a maximum figure which makes no allowance for destruction of the drug. The author obtained figures of a similar order for the amount of adrenaline fixed by mammalian plain muscle. In this case also the figure is a maximum one which does not allow for destruction by oxidation.

These figures indicate that the amount of drug needed to be fixed by cells, in order to produce a marked response, is very small and in particular that it is too small to form a monomolecular layer over the cell surfaces.

These drugs, if they act on cell surfaces, must therefore produce their effect by uniting with specific receptors which form only a small fraction (probably less than 0.1 per cent.) of the total cell surface. On the other hand the number of molecules of drug per cell is relatively large; for instance a concentration of 1 in 1000 million of acetylcholine in the frog's ventricular muscle implies about 10,000 molecules per cell. ARMSTRONG (1935)[6] found that $2.3 \times 10^{-5} \gamma$ acetylcholine caused diastolic arrest of the heart of the Fundulus embryo, when administered by micro-injection. The egg volume was 4 cmm. and hence the drug concentration in the egg was about 2 parts per 100 million. The total dose in this case contained $6 \times 10^{10}$ molecules.

[1] MARRACK, J. R.: Med. Res. Counc. Spec. Rep. **194**, 115 (1934).
[2] OTTENBERG, R., and F. A. STEENBUCK: Proc. Soc. exper. Biol. a. Med. **21**, 203 (1923).
[3] STRAUB, W.: Biochem. Z. **28**, 392 (1910).
[4] CLARK, A. J.: The Mode of Action of Drugs on Cells, p. 16. London: Arnold and Co. 1933.
[5] CLARK, A. J.: Ibid. p. 17.
[6] ARMSTRONG, P. B.: J. of Physiol. **84**, 20 (1935).

**Minimum Active Doses of Drugs per Organism.** The progress of vitamin chemistry and of endocrinology has accustomed us to think of doses in terms of micrograms. The smallest recognised unit of dosage known to the author is that of auxine which is $2 \times 10^{-11}$ g. or $2 \times 10^{-5} \gamma$ (ERXLEBEN, 1935[1]). This unit contains however between $10^{10}$ and $10^{11}$ molecules.

The unit of vitamin D ($0.02 \gamma$ per kilo rat per diem) is larger than this. The number of cells per kilo in the body of man has been calculated as $3 \times 10^{11}$ (average cell size 2700 cu.μ.). A dose of $0.02 \gamma$ calciferol per kilo would provide about 20 molecules per cell.

The smallest doses recorded as producing a recognisable effect when injected intravenously into mammals (cats) are $2 \times 10^{-6} \gamma$ acetylcholine per kilo (HUNT, 1918[2]), $5 \times 10^{-6} \gamma$ adrenaline per kilo (DALE and RICHARDS, 1918[3]), and $10^{-3} \gamma$ histamine per kilo (ELLINGER, 1930[4]). The two former doses would contain about $10^{10}$ molecules and would produce concentrations in the blood of the order of 1 part in $10^{13}$. GREMELS (1936)[5] found with the dog's heart-lung preparation that a single dose of $1 \gamma$ adrenaline, or the addition of $0.3 \gamma$ per min. to the perfusion fluid caused a 10 per cent. increase in the oxygen consumption, whilst a well marked diminution in this was caused by the addition of $1.7 \times 10^{-5} \gamma$ per min. of acetylcholine.

**Minimum Active Dilutions of Drugs.** The high dilution at which drugs can produce a recognisable effect on living cells is one of the most striking phenomena in pharmacology, and has provoked many wild hypotheses regarding drug action. Quantitative measures of drug uptake have in the case of the heavy metals shown that the so-called "oligodynamic action" is due to selective adsorption, that the concentration of metal in the cell is relatively high, and that there is no need to postulate modes of action unknown to physical chemistry.

In the case of several hormones the minimum concentrations that will produce a specific response in sensitive cells lie between 1 in $10^9$ and of 1 in $10^{10}$. Figures of this order have been found for acetylcholine acting on the frog's heart or on eserinised leech muscle; adrenaline acting on the isolated gut of the rabbit or guinea pig (ACHUTIN, 1933[6]); histamine acting on the isolated guinea pig's gut (WATANABE, 1930[7]), and on the perfused rabbit's ear (ROTHLIN, 1920[8]). In the case of the posterior pituitary hormone, KROGH (1926)[9] found that this produced dilatation of the melanophores of the frog at a dilution of not more than 1 part in $10^{12}$. It may be said therefore that a number of common drugs produce recognisable pharmacological response on standard preparations at dilutions between 1 part in $10^9$ and 1 part in $10^{12}$. AHLGREN (1924, 1926)[10] found that adrenaline and thyroxine both produced a well marked effect on the rate of reduction of methylene blue by tissues at a concentration of 1 in $10^{16}$. This has been confirmed by other workers (VON EULER, 1930, 1933[11]), although some

[1] ERXLEBEN, H.: Erg. Physiol. **37**, 186 (1935).

[2] HUNT, REID: Amer. J. Physiol. **45**, 197 (1918).

[3] DALE, H. H., and A. N. RICHARDS: J. of Physiol. **52**, 110 (1918).

[4] ELLINGER, FR.: Quoted from W. FELDBERG and E. SCHILF: Histamin. Berlin: Julius Springer 1930.

[5] GREMELS, H.: Arch. f. exper. Path. **182**, 1 (1936).

[6] ACHUTIN, N.: Arch. f. exper. Path. **171**, 668 (1933).

[7] WATANABE: Quoted from W. FELDBERG and E. SCHILF: Histamin, p. 175. Berlin: Julius Springer 1930.        [8] ROTHLIN, E.: Biochem. Z. **111**, 299 (1920).

[9] KROGH, A.: J. Pharmacol. Baltimore **29**, 177 (1926).

[10] AHLGREN, G. A.: Klin. Wschr. **1**, 667 (1924) — Skand. Arch. Physiol. (Berl. u. Lpz.) **47**, 271 (1926).

[11] EULER, U. VON: Skand. Arch. Physiol. (Berl. u. Lpz.) **59**, 123 (1930) — Klin. Wschr. **12**, 671 (1933).

workers have failed to confirm the effect (KISCH and LEIBWITZ, 1930[1]; MYRHMAN, 1932[2]; v. VEREBELY, 1932[3]; BÜNGELER, 1933[4]).

The writer expressed doubt regarding the validity of this result (CLARK, 1933[5]) but AHLGREN (1934)[6] has pointed out that his results have been confirmed by other workers, and that the failures to confirm his results may be attributed to faulty technique. He regards the production of stimulation of metabolism by thyroxine at a dilution of 1 in $10^{16}$ as a fact established with fair certainty. This conclusion also has been supported by HAARMANN (1936)[7].

These dilutions are less surprising if the number of molecules present are considered for 1 c.c. of a solution at a dilution of 1 in $10^{16}$ will in the case of adrenaline contain 300,000 molecules, and in the case of thyroxine 100,000 molecules.

The literature contains reports of drugs producing actions at concentrations considerably lower than those quoted, but in most cases these have not been confirmed and since the possibility of experimental error becomes very great when high dilutions are employed, only those results which are generally accepted are worth discussion.

**Intracellular Administration of Drugs.** The intracellular method of administration of drugs elaborated by CHAMBERS is obviously of very great importance for the determination of the mode of action of drugs, because the injection of a drug into the interior of a cell eliminates a very large number of unknown variables. The only alternative method which gives comparable results is the study of the distribution of dyes which are visible after they have penetrated the cell, a method which was used with great success by EHRLICH.

The most striking fact proved by micro-injection experiments is that the action of a drug applied to the outside of the cell may be completely different from its action when applied inside the cell. Many drugs paralyse cells when present in the surrounding medium, but do not produce this effect when administered as a micro-injection.

BRINLEY (1928)[8] showed that *Amoeba proteus* was killed in about 24 hours by immersion in N/3000 HCN, but micro-injection of N/100 HCN produced no more effect than the injection of a similar amount of distilled water. Moreover amoebae which had been injected with HCN were killed by immersion in HCN in the same manner as normal amoebae. These facts indicate that HCN acts on the surface of the amoeba, and also that in this case the action of the drug is not a "potential action". Similarly narcotics paralyse *Amoeba dubia* when applied externally but do not produce narcosis when injected (HILLER, 1927[9]; MARSLAND, 1934[10]).

BRINLEY (1928)[11] also showed that $H_2S$ acted as a poison externally, but did not produce poisoning on injection into amoebae.

The simplest explanation of these experiments is that there is a limiting cell membrane, and that many functions of the cell are regulated by receptors located

[1] KISCH, B., and J. LEIBWITZ: Biochem. Z. **220**, 97 (1930).
[2] MYRHMAN, G.: Klin. Wschr. **11**, 2139 (1932).
[3] VEREBELY, T. VON: Klin. Wschr. **11**, 1705 (1932).
[4] BÜNGELER, W.: Klin. Wschr. **12**, 933 (1933).
[5] CLARK, A.J.: The Mode of Action of Drugs on Cells. p. 25. London: Arnold and Co. 1933.
[6] AHLGREN, G.: Hygiensk Revy **1934**.
[7] HAARMANN, W.: Arch. f. exper. Path. **180**, 167 (1936).
[8] BRINLEY, F. J.: Proc. Soc. exper. Biol. a. Med. **25**, 305 (1928) — J. gen. Physiol. **12**, 201 (1928).
[9] HILLER, S.: Proc. Soc. exper. Biol. a. Med. **24**, 427, 938 (1927).
[10] MARSLAND, D.: J. Cell. Comp. Physiol. **4**, 9 (1934).
[11] BRINLEY, F. J.: Amer. J. Physiol. **85**, 355 (1928).

on the outside of this membrane. Unfortunately however these experiments are open to the general criticism that the amount of drug introduced into the cell is so small that it may be inactivated by combination with the cell contents, whereas when the drug is applied to the outside of the cell the volume of the solution is very large in comparison with the volume of the cell and hence although the concentration of the drug may be very low, yet the amount of drug in the cell solution system is much larger than when the drug is administered by micro-injection.

The action of dyes on cells is not open to this criticism and certain experiments by Cook (1926)[1] on the action of methylene blue appear to the author to show fairly conclusively that this dye acts on receptors situated on the outside of the cell surface. Methylene blue produces an atropine-like action on the frog's ventricle which can be measured quantitatively by its inhibition of the action of acetylcholine. Methylene blue in low concentration produces a deep staining of the frog's ventricle; the staining is produced slowly and is not reduced by prolonged washing out. Cook found that low concentrations of methylene blue abolished the action of acetylcholine before visible staining was produced. On the other hand if the heart were dyed with methylene blue then, on washing out with dye-free fluid, the atropine-like effect was rapidly abolished, although the heart remained deeply coloured with the dye. Addition of a fresh solution of methylene blue produced the atropine effect on a deeply dyed heart.

These results indicate that the dye produced an atropine-like effect on the surface of the heart cells and that this effect was freely reversible. At the same time the dye entered the cells and stained the ventricle but the dye thus fixed did not produce any atropine-like action.

This simple experiment shows that in this case:

(1) The bulk of the dye taken up by the heart cells entered the cells and produced no pharmacological action.

(2) The pharmacological action was due to some reversible compound formed between the dye in solution and receptors which probably were on the heart surface.

(3) There was no immediate relation between the pharmacological effect and the visible dyeing of the heart either as regards amount of dye taken up or as regards rate of uptake.

(4) There was no evidence of any potential action since the dye applied outside the cell acted when the interior of the cell was dyed deeply.

The effects of potassium ions on the frog's heart provide another example in which it is certain that the action of potassium salts outside and inside the cell is completely different. The example of potassium illustrates the general principle that the ionic content of the cell is completely different from that of the tissue fluids around the cell. It also is found that alterations of the ionic content of the tissue fluid produce changes in the function of cells such as those of the frog's heart very rapidly, and these phenomena can only be explained by assuming that ionic changes alter the surface layer of the cell.

These facts make it necessary to assume that the cell surface contains receptors which are accessible to drugs outside the cell but inaccessible to the same drugs when these are inside the cell, and that the action of the drug depends upon its combination with these receptors and not upon any general action on the cell interior. Moreover there is no necessary relation between the amount of drug taken up by the cell and the amount of action produced upon the cell.

---

[1] Cook, R. P.: J. of Physiol. **62**, 160 (1926).

**Types of Action of Drugs on Cells.** The hypothesis outlined suggests two very distinct types of drug action.

(a) Specific action on receptors of cell surface.

(b) Action on cell structure.

In the first case drugs may be expected to act rapidly by occupying the cell receptors. The rate of action will be determined by the rate of diffusion and there is likely to be a simple relation between the drug concentration and the amount of action produced. The action of acetylcholine and adrenaline on cells is an example of this type of action.

In the second case the action is likely to be much more complex and to include the following stages:

(a) Adsorption of drug on cell surface. This will be a rapid action and will produce a high concentration of drug on the cell surface.

(b) Diffusion of drug through the cell membrane into the cell interior. This is likely to be a slow process.

(c) Chemical changes in cell structure, such as aggregation of proteins, caused by the entrance of drug into cell.

(d) Response of cell (e.g. by death) to chemical changes.

The action of phenol on bacteria is an example of this latter type of action. In this case it is obvious that the time relations of the action of the drug are likely to be extremely complex. Furthermore the relation between concentration and action is likely to be obscure, because it will depend firstly on the intensity of adsorption of the drug on the surface, and secondly on the relation between surface concentration and concentration in the interior.

This type of action, namely rapid adsorption on a surface followed by slow diffusion into the interior is frequently met with in inorganic systems (e.g. adsorption of oxygen by charcoal) and the term sorption has been introduced to cover the whole process.

The general theory of drug action adopted by the writer is therefore as follows. Many drugs (e.g. phenol or formalin) produce non-specific toxic effects presumably by entering the cell and deranging the protein structure. Furthermore a certain number of drugs produce a selective toxic effect on nuclear processes. Colchicine is the typical example of such substances. In this case the drug must presumably enter the cell before it produces its special action on the nucleus.

In the case of most drugs which act at high dilutions the evidence indicates that they act on the cell surface. This class includes most of the hormones and many of the specific enzyme poisons.

Certain drugs of this latter class, e.g. acetyl choline and adrenaline, are of special interest not only on account of their physiological importance but also because the care with which their actions have been studied has resulted in the accumulation of exceptionally full quantitative evidence regarding their pharmacological action. This class of drugs therefore deserves special attention on account of its peculiar interest.

**Discussion.** The minimum active doses and minimum active concentrations of certain drugs are surprisingly small, but when the number of molecules involved is considered it is evident that these results do not conflict with the ordinary laws of physical chemistry. It has been shown in several cases that the amount of drug fixed is too small to cover more than a very small proportion of the cell surfaces with a monomolecular layer. This fact, together with the fact that the drugs act in such extraordinarily high dilutions are difficult to explain except on the assumption that the drugs react with specific receptors on the cell surfaces, and by occupying these receptors modify the functions of the cell in much the same manner as an enzyme poison can modify the functions of an enzyme by reacting with the active group of the enzyme, although this active group may only constitute a small fraction of the total enzyme molecule.

If the cells be regarded as a large and complex machine, there is no difficulty in finding analogies for the derangement of its action by small quantities of drug. The effect of a drop of water in the carburettor of a motor car is a familiar analogy, and another perhaps better simile is the possible effect on a chemical factory of a minute amount of a catalyst poison which has interfered with some essential process. It may be noted that the results quoted in this section have no relation to the claims of homoeopathy, for HAHNEMANN claimed that drugs produced effects when given in the 30th potency. This corresponded in the original nomenclature to a concentration of 1 part in $10^{60}$, which works out at 1 molecule in a sphere of astronomical dimensions. In the alternative nomenclature of 1 potency equalling a dilution of 1 in 10, the 30th potency means 1 part in $10^{30}$, which, in the case of a drug with a molecular weight of 100, corresponds to 1 molecule in about 100,000 litres. It is obvious that is a sample of a few c.c. of such a mixture is taken, the odds against the presence in the sample of a single molecule of the drug are at least a million to one. Hence the claims of the homoeopathist conflict more immediately with the laws of mathematics, physics and chemistry than with the biological sciences. It does not appear necessary for pharmacologists to discuss the evidence adduced by the homoeopathists until the latter have succeeded in convincing the physicists that they have demonstrated the existence of a new form of subdivision of matter. It may be mentioned that the existence of such recognised subdivisions of the atom as electrons etc. does not help the homoeopathic claims in a significant manner because, to explain the results obtained by HAHNEMANN, it is necessary to assume that a molecule can be divided into millions of sub-units.

## Chapter 4
### Reactions between Drugs and Active Proteins.

**Symplex Compounds.** The great complexity of living cells is one of the chief difficulties in the analysis of the action of drugs. Many of the functions of cells are carried out by means of proteins carrying active groups and since these proteins are acted upon by many drugs, the study of the reactions between active proteins and drugs provides valuable information regarding the more complex problem of the action of drugs on cells.

WILLSTÄTTER and ROHDEWALD (1934)[1] have suggested the name of symplex compounds to describe firstly the compounds formed by the combination of a prosthetic group with component of high molecular weight and secondly compounds formed from two or more components of high molecular weight. Enzymes, antibodies and haemoglobin are examples of the first group and combinations of antigen and antibody or toxin and antitoxin are examples of the second group.

The following substances of biochemical importance are included in this general class. (a) Haemoglobin, cytochrome; (b) Enzymes; (c) Antibodies. Von EULER has also suggested the name hormozyme to describe hormones which contain polypeptides or proteins. Insulin, oxytocin and vasopressin belong to this class, and it is possible that the true form of the thyroid active principle may be a combination between thyroxin and a protein carrier.

[1] WILLSTÄTTER, R., and M. ROHDEWALD: Hoppe-Seylers Z. **225**, 103 (1934).

In some cases (haemoglobin, cytochrome etc.) the prosthetic group contains a special element namely iron, and this facilitates quantitative estimations in these cases. In most cases the activity of the prosthetic groups appears to depend upon some special configuration or pattern, and not upon the presence of any special element.

WILLSTÄTTER's general theory as to the structure of enzymes is as follows (WILLSTÄTTER and ROHDEWALD, 1934[1]):

„Nach unserer Vorstellung setzt sich ein Enzym aus einer aktiven Gruppe und einem kolloiden Träger zusammen, so daß durch ihre Synergie, nämlich durch die Wechselwirkung ihrer Affinitätsfelder, das katalytische Reaktionsvermögen der spezifischen Gruppe entweder hervorgerufen oder gesteigert wird."

In most cases the activity of the prosthetic group is destroyed by the denaturation of the protein carrier, but in some cases (e.g. antibodies) the prosthetic groups are heat stable and can be activated by introducing a fresh carrier (complement). WILLSTÄTTER's hypothesis as to the general nature of symplex compounds suggests that their activity can be altered by drugs in two distinct manners: (a) specific poisoning of the active group. (b) non-specific denaturation of the carrier. Actions of these two types can be demonstrated in many cases and are highly probable in other cases.

The study of the action of poisons on symplex compounds is a favourable introduction to the study of quantitative pharmacology. Many important drugs are known to act in vivo by poisoning a cellular ferment and in such cases it is possible to compare the action of a drug on living cells and on the much simpler system represented by a solution of purified ferment.

The group of substances mentioned above varies greatly in their complexity, but the uptake of oxygen by haemoglobin and the inhibition of this action by carbon monoxide is an effect which is exceptionally favourable for quantitative study, and has been studied very intensively, hence it is a favourable subject on which to commence the study of the action of drugs on living systems.

**Combination of Haemoglobin with Oxygen and Carbon Monoxide.** The properties of haemoglobin have been described in great detail by BARCROFT (1928)[2]. Pure haemoglobin in watery solution has a molecular weight of 66,000 and each molecule carries 4 haem molecules which act as oxygen acceptors. Each molecule of haem contains one atom of ferrous iron and its molecular weight is about 630, hence the prosthetic groups only constitute about 4 per cent. of the whole molecule, whilst the iron content is 0.336 per cent. The haemoglobin of every species is slightly different, but these differences are not of importance for the present discussion. Haemoglobin can be inactivated in two ways, firstly by non-specific agents (e.g. strong alkalies or acids), which produce denaturation of the protein (globin), and secondly by specific agents (e.g. carbon monoxide) which unite with and inactivate the prosthetic groups.

The effects observed are however more complex than this simple scheme indicates because changes in the globin alter the properties of the haem and vice versa. The iron in haemoglobin (ferrous haem + native globin) is not oxidised to the ferric state by exposure to air but each atom forms a freely reversible combination with two atoms of oxygen, and the oxygen carrying powers of haemoglobin depend on this peculiarity. When the globin is denatured this property is lost, the iron is oxidised on exposure to air, and the compound becomes ferric haem + denatured globin.

---

[1] WILLSTÄTTER, R., and M. ROHDEWALD: Hoppe-Seylers Z. **229**, 241 (1934).
[2] BARCROFT, J.: Respiratory Functions of the Blood. Part II, Haemoglobin. Cambridge: Univ. Press 1928.

In this state each atom of iron combines firmly with one atom of oxygen and the oxygen carrying power is lost. Hence the functional activity of the prosthetic group is dependent on the state of the protein carrier. Conversely the combination of the iron with carbon monoxide may alter non-specific properties of the haemoglobin. For example HARTRIDGE (1912)[1] showed that the rate of heat precipitation of oxyhaemoglobin at 64° C. was about the same as the rate of heat precipitation of carboxyhaemoglobin at 74° C. Another familiar fact is that the dissociation curve of haemoglobin is altered by any alteration in its physico-chemical state.

The uptake of oxygen at various pressures by a solution of pure haemoglobin in distilled water follows a simple law of mass action. Under ordinary experimental conditions the oxygen is present in such great excess that its concentration does not alter, and only the change of state of the haemoglobin need be considered. The simplest condition is when one molecule of oxygen unites with one haem group and each haem group can associate or dissociate with oxygen independently. If $x$ = oxygen pressure and $y$ = percentage of total haem groups that are oxidised, then the following general formula can be applied: $Kx = \dfrac{y}{100 - y}$.
With this formula the relation between oxygen concentration ($x$) and oxy-haemoglobin ($y$) follows a rectangular hyperbola. The curve obtained with weak solutions of pure haemoglobin in distilled water closely follows this formula.

The state of aggregation of haemoglobin under these conditions has however been determined and the molecular weight is 67,000 and each molecule carries 4 haem groups, each of which combined with one molecule of oxygen. Hence the reaction is: $Hb + 4O_2 = HbO_8$. If this reaction were followed, that is to say if all 4 haem groups had to be oxidised simultaneously, then the reaction would follow the formula: $Kx^4 = \dfrac{y}{100 - y}$. The course of the reaction is totally different from this and hence it is necessary to assume that the 4 haem groups in the molecule of haemoglobin can be oxidised independently. This assumption however raises another difficulty because the uptake of oxygen by blood or even by haemoglobin dissolved in saline follows a course that approximates to the formula: $Kx^{2.5} = \dfrac{y}{100 - y}$. This can be explained by supposing that 2 or 3 haem groups need to take up oxygen simultaneously, but there is very little justification for making such an assumption. ADAIR (1925)[2] suggested that the shape of the dissociation curve of haemoglobin was due to the pigment forming intermediate and partly saturated compounds with oxygen and carbon monoxide. ROUGHTON (1934)[3] has advanced experimental evidence in favour of the view that in the case of carbon monoxide a series of compounds are formed of the type $HbCO$, $Hb(CO)_2$, $Hb(CO)_3$, $Hb(CO)_4$.

The curves relating carbon monoxide pressure and formation of HbCO show the same diversity as do those relating oxygen pressure and formation of HbO. BARCROFT (1928)[4] quotes results which show that fresh solutions of haemoglobin give sigmoid curves which follow the formula $Kx^n = \dfrac{y}{100 - y}$ ($n = 1.5$), but that solutions of haemoglobin which have been kept for some days give curves which approximate to a rectangular hyperbola $\left(Kx = \dfrac{y}{100 - y}\right)$.

[1] HARTRIDGE, H.: J. of Physiol. **44**, 34 (1912).
[2] ADAIR, G. S.: J. of biol. Chem. **73**, 533 (1925).
[3] ROUGHTON, F. J. W.: Proc. roy. Soc. B. **115**, 451, 464 and 473 (1934).
[4] BARCROFT, J.: Respiratory Functions of the Blood. Part. II, Haemoglobin. Cambridge: Univ. Press 1928.

The dissociation curves of haemoglobin with oxygen or carbon monoxide are of interest in the first place because the simplest curve obtained, namely HÜFNER's rectangular hyperbola, follows the formula $Kx = \dfrac{y}{100 - y}$, and this expresses the concentration-action relation obtained with many enzyme poisons and important drugs. A closer study of haemoglobin shows however that this curve is an artefact which is only obtained when the haemoglobin has been partially denatured by rough handling, prolonged keeping etc.

When haemoglobin is studied under conditions approximating to the normal the dissociation curve is much more complex, and the simplest interpretation of the shape obtained is to assume that saturation is a chain process which occurs in four stages, the velocity of reaction being slightly different at each stage.

There is no drug action which can be studied by methods which in any way approach the accuracy of the modern methods used to measure the reactions of haemoglobin. The fact that the application of accurate methods has proved this apparently simple system to be in fact highly complex is an indication of the degree of complexity which it is reasonable to expect in the case of drugs acting on cells.

**Antagonism of Oxygen and Carbon Monoxide.** A mixture of 1 part of carbon monoxide in 245 parts of oxygen produces 50 per cent. each of carboxyhaemoglobin and oxyhaemoglobin. The analyses of HARTRIDGE and ROUGHTON (1923, 1925, 1927)[1] have shown that the reaction $CO + Hb = HbCO$ is much slower than the reaction $O_2 + Hb = HbO$, and that the greater affinity of haemoglobin for CO than for oxygen depends on the fact that HbCO decomposes much more slowly than does HbO. HARTRIDGE and ROUGHTON (1927)[2] have shown that under conditions of temperature and reaction such as exist in the body a certain degree of union between oxygen and haemoglobin occurs in 0.001 sec. whereas the same amount of union with carbon monoxide and haemoglobin would take 0.01 sec.

The reverse process of dissociation of oxyhaemoglobin would take at least 0.05 sec. and in the case of carboxyhaemoglobin not less than 3 min. The time ranges of the various processes are as follows (ROUGHTON, 1934[3]).

$$O_2 + Hb \rightarrow O_2Hb \qquad 0.1 - 0.001 \text{ sec.}$$
$$CO + Hb \rightarrow COHb \qquad 1.0 - 0.01 \text{ sec.}$$
$$O_2Hb \rightarrow O_2 + Hb \qquad 30 - 0.1 \text{ sec.}$$
$$COHb \rightarrow CO + Hb \qquad 600 - 10 \text{ sec.}$$

The influence of temperature on the kinetics of the combination of oxygen and carbon monoxide with haemoglobin is remarkable on account of the complexity of the results obtained.

The following figures are taken from BARCROFT's work (1928)[4].

$$\begin{array}{ll} & Q/10 \\ Hb + O_2 \rightarrow HbO_2 & 1 - 1.5 \\ Hb + CO \rightarrow HbCO & 1.4 - 2 \\ HbO_2 \rightarrow Hb + O_2 & 4 \\ HbCO \rightarrow Hb + CO & 3 - 6 \end{array}$$

[1] HARTRIDGE, H., and F. J. W. ROUGHTON: Proc. roy. Soc. B. **94**, 336 (1923); A. **104**, 395 (1923); A. **107**, 654 (1925) — J. of Physiol. **62**, 232 (1927).

[2] HARTRIDGE, H., and F. J. W. ROUGHTON: J. of Physiol. **62**, 232 (1927).

[3] ROUGHTON, F. J. W.: Proc. roy. Soc. B. **115**, 451, 464 and 473 (1934).

[4] BARCROFT, J.: Respiratory Functions of the Blood. Part II, Haemoglobin. Cambridge: Univ. Press 1928.

Similarly these different processes are affected differently by changes in the hydrogen ion concentration. In consequence of these facts the partition of haemoglobin between oxygen and carbon monoxide differs for different conditions of temperature and of hydrogen ion concentration. Most of the results obtained can however be expressed approximately by the formula

$$\frac{[O_2]}{[CO]} \times \frac{[HbCO]}{[HbO_2]} = \text{constant.}$$

A curious paradox is however observed when the pressure of CO and $O_2$ is so low that the whole of the haemoglobin is not combined. DOUGLAS, HALDANE and HALDANE (1913)[1] showed in the case of haemoglobin exposed to a CO pressure of 0.067 mm. Hg. that the amount of carboxyhaemoglobin formed was twice as great in the presence of 4 per cent. oxygen as when no oxygen was present. This paradox can be explained by application of the formulae given above: it depends on the fact that the dissociation curves of $HbO_2$ and HbCO follow different courses. This peculiar effect is mentioned here because it is the simplest example known to the writer of a reaction following the "ARNDT-SCHULZ law". In this case a high concentration of oxygen prevents the formation of HbCO but if haemoglobin is exposed to a low concentration of carbon monoxide, then a low concentration of oxygen may increase the formation of HbCO. Hence oxygen may be said to stimulate in low concentrations and to inhibit in high concentrations. This diphasic action can be explained on physico-chemical grounds and although our present knowledge is inadequate to explain most of the diphasic actions met with in more complex systems, yet there seems no reason to consider them as peculiarly mysterious.

The reactions between haemoglobin and oxygen or carbon monoxide are in every way more favourable for quantitative study than are any reactions between drugs and cells, since the haemoglobin-gas system is far simpler than any cell, and the course of the reaction can be measured with great exactitude.

The peculiar characteristics of the reactions between haemoglobin and gases are their simplicity and the accuracy with which they have been measured. The intricacies that have been revealed by the accurate study of this system therefore indicate the probable complexity both of the action of drugs on cells and of the antagonism of drugs.

**Discussion.** In this simple system so favourable for quantitative measurement the following facts are observed.

The concentration-action relations obey the laws of mass action under certain conditions, but these conditions cannot occur in the living organism, and as soon as the conditions approximate to those which do occur in the living organism the concentration-action relation assumes a form which cannot be interpreted by simple physico-chemical laws. The study of the temperature coefficients of a single reaction $Hb + O_2 \leftrightarrows HbO_2$, shows that the association has a temperature coefficient typical of physical processes whilst the dissociation has a temperature coefficient typical of chemical processes. This fact suggests that a study of temperature coefficients of processes that are far more complex and obscure, such as are the reactions between drugs and cells, is unlikely to give any certain evidence regarding the nature of the process studied. Finally the fact that the equilibrium attained by the system $CO + O_2 + Hb$ is altered by either a change in temperature or by a change in $p_H$ reaction, helps us to understand why the phenomena observed with drug antagonism are usually obscure.

---

[1] DOUGLAS, C. G., J. B. S. HALDANE and J. S. HALDANE: J. of Physiol. **44**, 275 (1913).

The general characteristic of the results obtained by the study of haemoglobin reactions appears to the writer as follows. The uptake by haemoglobin of $O_2$ or CO and the antagonism between these gases can be expressed approximately by surprisingly simple formulae. As soon as accurate methods of analysis are applied however this apparent simplicity at once disappears and the processes that actually occur are shown to be highly intricate.

The most accurate methods available for the study of the action of drugs on enzymes and cells are of a much lower order of accuracy than were the original studies of haemoglobin dissociation, which today are regarded as crude approximations. The writer has no wish to adopt a nihilist attitude regarding the possibility of interpreting the nature of drug action, but it is only by a consideration of the known complexity of relatively simple systems which have been investigated thoroughly, that it is possible to form a rational estimate of the probable complexity of reactions which involve living cells.

It is very important to recognise frankly that, measured by the standards of physical chemistry, all quantitative estimations of drug action are only rough approximations, and the simple formulae advanced to express the data probably provide no indication of the complexity of the reactions which are really occurring.

## Chapter 5
## The Action of Drugs on Catalysts and Enzymes.

The study of this subject is of interest because the action of poisons on certain enzymes can be studied both in solution and in the cell, and thus provides a particularly favourable introduction to the study of the action of drugs on cell functions. Moreover some important drugs are known to produce their pharmacological action by inactivating either enzymes or co-enzymes (e.g. arsenious acid, physostigmine, iodoacetic acid).

Some enzyme poisons inhibit the action of enzymes both in purified solution and in living cells, and a comparison of these actions is an obviously favourable method of approach to the general study of the mode of action of drugs on cells. One great advantage of such a study is that we know the nature of the action on the cell that is being measured, whereas in the case of drugs such as acetylcholine or adrenali.. we know nothing about the nature of the receptors with which it is presumed that they unite. The action of enzyme poisons on cells is however likely to be complex because the poison does not merely inhibit the activity of an enzyme, but deranges a complex balance of enzymatic activity. For this and other reasons the quantitative relations of enzyme poisoning is likely to be much more obscure in vivo than in vitro.

**Poisoning of Inorganic Catalysts.** Inorganic catalysts show numerous resemblances to enzymes and this is particularly true as regards the action of poisons on these two groups of substances. It is therefore worth noting certain striking features shown in catalyst poisoning.

In the first place these catalysts can be poisoned by drugs in very high dilutions. This sensitivity to poisons is indeed one of the chief troubles in the commercial use of chemical processes depending on catalysts. Quantitative study of catalyst poisoning has shown that the activity of a catalyst can be abolished by an amount of drug far too small to cover the whole of its surface. The catalytic activity must therefore be due to active centres which only represent a small fraction of the total surface of the catalyst.

TAYLOR (1925)[1] suggested that these active centres were isolated atoms with high residual fields, and other workers have shown that these centres occur along the lines of cracks and imperfections on surfaces. It has also been shown that on a single surface there may be centres showing different types of activity. A poison may act on one type of centre only and may thus abolish one catalytic action and leave another unimpaired.

Another interesting consequence of the existence of these active centres is that there may be no direct relation between the amount of poison fixed by a surface and the amount of action it produces, because the action is produced by the poison acting on the active centres but the poison may also be fixed by the remaining inert surface. For example PEASE and STEWART (1925)[2] found that a copper surface could adsorb firmly 5 c.c. of carbon monoxide but that the adsorption of as little as 0.05 c.c. was sufficient to reduce the catalytic activity of the surface by 90 per cent. Different gases may be adsorbed at different points on a metal surface. For instance PEASE (1923)[3] found that traces of mercury poisoned adsorbent copper surfaces and reduced the adsorption of ethylene to 86 p.c. but that of hydrogen to 20 p.c. of the value obtained with the clean copper surface. The same quantity of mercury reduced the catalytic efficiency of the surface to less than $1/_{200}$ part of the original value.

Even such simple systems as inorganic catalysts provide interesting examples of specificity of drug fixation. For example methylene blue is adsorbed by diamond but not by graphite whilst succinic acid is adsorbed by graphite and not by diamond. These differences must be due to the difference in the lattice pattern of the atoms in the graphite and diamond; the pattern fits one compound and not the other (NELLENSTEYN, 1925[4]).

The action of drugs on catalysts is not limited to inhibition because in some cases substances which are not themselves good catalysts will greatly increase the catalytic activity of surfaces.

Inorganic catalysts as a class and in particular polished metal surfaces are systems far simpler in every respect than the simplest form of living cell. It is instructive to consider the complexities that are met when the actions of drugs on these simple catalysts are measured accurately, because such a study provides a hint as to what must be expected when more complex systems are studied.

The following are the chief points that have been established regarding the actions of catalyst poisons.

The activity of a metal surface is due to the presence of certain active patches which only constitute a very small fraction of the total surface. These active patches differ qualitatively both as regards their catalytic action and as regards their sensitivity to drugs. Poisons act in very high dilutions and can exert a highly selective action since one type of catalytic activity may be abolished and others may be unaffected. Moreover there is no simple relation between the amount of poison fixed by a surface and the amount of inhibition which it produces. In some cases it can be proved that the whole inhibitor action produced by a poison is due to only a very small fraction of the total quantity of poison that is fixed.

Finally as regards the kinetics of drug action it can be shown that in the case of many catalysts (e.g. charcoal) the fixation of a gas such as oxygen is

[1] TAYLOR, H. S.: Proc. roy. Soc. A. **108**, 105 (1925).
[2] PEASE, R. N., and L. STEWART: J. amer. chem. Soc. **47**, 1235 (1925).
[3] PEASE, R. N.: J. amer. chem. Soc. **45**, 1196, 2235, 2296 (1923).
[4] NELLENSTEYN, F. J.: Chem. Weekblad. **22**, 291 (1925). Quoted from W. E. GARNER: Trans. Farad. Soc. **22**, 433 (1926).

a complex chain process. The fixation of the gas is the first event but this is followed by a series of slow complex changes. Hence the kinetics of such a process are extremely difficult to interpret. A consideration of the difficulties encountered in the study of the action of drugs on a simple inorganic catalyst raises a natural doubt as to the value of any attempt to interpret the action of drugs on cells by physico-chemical laws. In actual fact however the actions of many drugs on cells appear to follow laws not more complex than do the action of poisons on catalysts. This is satisfactory provided that the apparent simplicity is not due solely to lack of accuracy in measurement. The chief general rule that the author has found to hold in regard to heterogeneous reactions is that their known complexity varies according to the care and accuracy with which they have been studied, and since colloidal chemists usually choose the simplest system available for study the paradox results that the simpler the system the more complex are the laws which are known to govern its behaviour.

**General Characters of Enzymes.** Inorganic catalysts are so different in character from the lyophilic colloids which compose the living cell, that any similarities which may be observed between the two systems must be regarded merely as interesting analogies. It is for example improbable that active atoms of the type constituting the active centres on metallic surfaces could exist on any but rigid surfaces. The actions of drugs on enzymes have however a more direct interest, because most of the activities of living cells are carried out by enzyme systems.

The nature of enzyme structure is only partly known but WILLSTÄTTER's hypothesis that it consists of an active group anchored to a colloidal carrier is widely accepted. The specific properties of the active group probably depend on the arrangement of molecules in some special pattern, and this pattern can be deranged by changes in the carrier. Recent reviews of modern conceptions of enzyme structure have been given by OPPENHEIMER (1935)[1], by JOSEPHSON (1935)[2] and by LANGENBECK (1933)[3] and other authors in the Ergebnisse d. Enzymforschung. According to the hypothesis generally adopted enzyme poisons may either act directly on the active group or may affect the active group by denaturation of the protein carrier.

PACE (1931)[4] pointed out that non-specific toxic agencies such as heat, oxidation or irradiation produced similar effects on a number of different enzymes and that probably the core or carrier was similar in these cases. Such procedures probably change the carrier in some way that destroys the delicately balanced orientation of the active groups.

A study of the enzyme poisoning led EULER and JOSEPHSON (JOSEPHSON, 1935[2]) to postulate the "Zwei-affinitäts" theory according to which the substrate must unite with two points on the enzyme. For example MYRBÄCK (1926)[5] found that iodine immediately inhibited the activity of saccharase, whatever the quantity of iodine present, but that full inactivation was produced much more slowly. A complex structure for the prosthetic group was assumed in order to account for this and for other similar facts. EULER and JOSEPHSON suggested that the prosthetic groups contained one or a few active groups which reacted with the substrate and that these active groups were made capable of carrying out the reaction by the presence of a larger number of activating groups.

[1] OPPENHEIMER, C.: Die Fermente. Suppl. **1935**, 221.
[2] JOSEPHSON, K.: Oppenheimers Handb. Biochem., 2. Aufl., Ergänzbd. **1**, 669 (1935).
[3] LANGENBECK, W.: Erg. Physiol. **35**, 470 (1933) — Erg. Enzymforsch. **2**, 317 (1933).
[4] PACE, J.: Biochemic. J. **25**, 485 (1931).
[5] MYRBÄCK, K.: Hoppe-Seylers Z. **159**, 1 (1926).

This conception allows of three modes of action of drugs on enzymes: (a) on the active groups, (b) on the activating groups, and (c) on the protein carrier. The fact that modern conceptions of enzyme structure are largely based on a study of the mode of action of poisons is a gratifying tribute to the importance of pharmacology, but as in the case of the study of the nature of the cell surface, this fact must be remembered when seeking evidence to establish the nature of drug action, for otherwise it is very easy to argue in a circle.

**Enzyme Activity.** Two outstanding features of enzyme activity are that these substances produce effects at extraordinary low concentrations and secondly that their speed of action is very great. For example a solution of pepsin containing less than $10^{-7}$ g. of nitrogen per c.c. has a powerful effect on the coagulation of milk. Certain figures for the rate of action of purified enzyme are shown in Table 4.

Table 4. Activity of Enzymes.

| Enzyme-substrate system | No. of molecules of substrate split per sec. per active centre of enzyme | Author |
|---|---|---|
| Horse liver catalase acting on $H_2O_2$ at $0°$ C and M/100 substrate conc. | 54,200 | HALDANE (1931)[1] using results of ZEILE and HELLSTRÖM (1930)[2] |
| Peroxidase in $H_2O_2$ . . . . . . . | 100,000 | KUHN, HAND and FLORKIN (1931)[3]; |
| Invertase on sucrose at $10°$ C and optimum $p_H$. . . . . . . . . | 200 | LANGENBECK (1933)[4] |
| Same preparation at $37°$ C . . . . | 7,000 | KUHN and BRAUN (1926)[5] |
| Pepsin on protein, carboxyl groups liberated . . . . . . . . . . | 0,1 to 16 | MOELWYN-HUGHES (1933)[6] NORTHROP (1932)[7] LANGENBECK (1933)[4] |
| Choline-esterase on butyryl choline at $30°$ C . . . . . . . . . . | 3,500 | EASSON and STEDMAN (1936)[8] |

These calculations show that the rates of action vary over a very wide range in the case of different enzymes, but that in several cases more than 1000 substrate molecules are split per second by each enzyme molecule. Rates of activity of similar magnitude have been found in the case of respiratory pigments. MILLIKAN (1936)[9] found that the half saturation time in the case of muscle haemoglobin and oxygen was 0.000,4 sec. Rates of action of this magnitude make it easy to understand why minute quantities of enzyme poison can produce easily measurable effects on enzyme activity. For example, in the case of peroxidase $10^{11}$ molecules of enzyme would liberate 1 c.c. of oxygen in an hour, and this activity would be inhibited by the fixation of $10^{11}$ molecules of an enzyme poison. In the case of a poison with a molecular weight between 100 and 500 the weight of $10^{11}$ molecules would be of the order of 0.000,1 microgram.

**General Characters of the Poisoning of Enzymes.** Any procedure which precipitates proteins is likely to inactivate enzymes, and the process of inactivation will follow a course similar to the precipitation of proteins. These

[1] HALDANE, J. B. S.: Proc. roy. Soc. B. **108**, 559 (1931).
[2] ZEILE, K., and H. HELLSTRÖM: Hoppe-Seylers Z. **192**, 171 (1930).
[3] KUHN, R., M. B. HAND and M. FLORKIN: Hoppe-Seylers Z. **201**, 255 (1931).
[4] LANGENBECK, W.: Erg. Enzymforsch. **2**, 317 (1933).
[5] KUHN, R., and L. BRAUN: Ber. dtsch. chem. Ges. **59**, 2370 (1926).
[6] MOELWYN HUGHES, E. A.: Erg. Enzymforsch. **2**, 1 (1933).
[7] NORTHROP, J. H.: Erg. Enzymforsch. **1**, 302 (1932).
[8] EASSON, L. H., and E. STEDMAN: Proc. roy. Soc. B. **121**, 142 (1936).
[9] MILLIKAN, G. A.: Proc. roy. Soc. B. **120**, 366 (1936).

non-specific actions of drugs on enzymes are of much less interest than the action of specific poisons, which act on enzymes at very low concentrations and produce a reversible effect.

The actions of poisons on enzymes show certain features of interest. Some poisons such as heavy metals act at very high dilutions, and the action of poisons is in many cases highly selective, for a single poison may act powerfully on one enzyme and have no effect on another enzyme, and on the other hand an enzyme may be poisoned by one substance but be unaffected by another closely related substance. For instance RONA, AIRILA and LASNITZKI (1922)[1] found that quinine inhibited serum lipase at the low concentration of 2 parts in $10^7$, whereas liver lipase was not affected by quinine at 2000 times this concentration. Similarly sodium fluoride had little effect on pancreatic lipase but produced a powerful inhibitory action on liver lipase and on serum lipase (RONA and PAVLOVIC, 1923[2]). These are striking examples of the differences shown in the response to poisons by closely related lipases, and similar differences have been noted by many other workers In the second place RONA and his coworkers showed that the relative sensitivity of two enzymes might be completely different when different drugs were applied. For example whilst serum lipase was 2000 times more sensitive to quinine than was liver lipase, yet liver lipase was much more sensitive to atoxyl (RONA and PAVLOVIC, 1922[3]). RONA, AIRILA and LASNITZKI (1922)[2] also found that a single enzyme showed a high specificity as regards the action of poisons, when tested with a series of related compounds. For example maltase was poisoned by methyl arsinoxide at a low concentration but atoxyl and arsenious acid produced little effect at much higher concentrations.

In some cases a drug may inhibit some enzymes and activate others. For example cyanides inhibit oxidase and peptidase but activate cathepsin and papain (TAUBER, 1935[4]) and also urease (BERSIN, 1935[5]). The last mentioned effect may be due to the cyanide inactivating traces of heavy metals since these are very powerful inhibitors of urease (JACOBY, 1927[6]).

Many curious phenomena met with in enzyme poisoning have not yet been explained. As a general rule the more highly an enzyme is purified the more readily it is inhibited by drugs, but there are certain exceptions to this rule. For example crude saccharase is inhibited by alcohol whereas purified preparations are not affected.

A wide variety of diphasic effects have been recorded with enzyme poisons. In some cases poisons first stimulate and then inhibit enzymes whilst in other cases an initial inhibition is followed by an activity greater than the initial activity: these effects will be discussed later.

The activity of enzymes is dependent in most cases on the reaction of the surrounding fluid, and the researches of EULER and of MYRBÄCK (1919)[7] showed in the case of saccharase that this could be explained on simple physico-chemical laws.

Similarly the action of enzyme poisons is in many cases dependent on the reaction. MYRBÄCK (1926)[8] showed that the concentration of silver needed to

---

[1] RONA, P., Y. AIRILA and A. LASNITZKI: Biochem. Z. **130**, 582 (1922).
[2] RONA, P., and R. PAVLOVIC: Biochem. Z. **134**, 108 (1923).
[3] RONA, P., and R. PAVLOVIC: Biochem. Z. **130**, 225 (1922).
[4] TAUBER, H.: Erg. Enzymforsch. **4**, 42 (1935).
[5] BERSIN, T.: Erg. Enzymforsch. **4**, 68 (1935).
[6] JACOBY, M.: Biochem. Z. **181**, 194 (1927).
[7] EULER, H. VON, and K. MYRBÄCK: Hoppe-Seylers Z. **107**, 269 (1919).
[8] MYRBÄCK, K.: Hoppe-Seylers Z. **158**, 160 (1926).

produce 50 p.c. inhibition of saccharase was 25 times greater at $p_H$ 4.2 than at $p_H$ 6.1, whereas the activity of mercury was decreased as the $p_H$ was increased. He showed that these results could be explained fully by the assumption that silver reacted with an acid radicle and mercury with a basic radicle in the enzyme. RONA and BLOCH (1921)[1] found that the activity of quinine on urease was increased 9 times by raising the $p_H$ from 4 to 8.

The action of many drugs on cells is altered by changes in reaction and this often is quoted as evidence of changes in the power of the drug to penetrate the cells. These examples show however that in the case of drugs acting on enzymes the effect of change of reaction may be due simply to changes in the degree of dissociation of acid or basic groups in the enzyme.

As regards the minimum effective concentrations of enzyme poisons, the examples given in Table 5 show that these can act in dilutions similar to the minimum dilutions of drugs which produce actions on living cells.

Table 5. Concentrations of Enzyme Poisons.

| Drug | Ferment | Minimum conc. producing demonstrable action | Author |
|---|---|---|---|
| Atoxyl . . . . . . | Liver lipase | 2 in 10⁹ | RONA, AIRILA and LASNITZKI (1922)[2] |
| Quinine . . . . . . | Serum lipase | 2 in 10⁷ | RONA, AIRILA and LASNITZKI (1922)[2] |
| Silver nitrate . . . | Urease | 1 in 10⁷ | SUMNER and MYRBÄCK (1930)[3] |

**Diphasic Actions of Enzyme Poisons.** Diphasic actions of drugs on tissues are frequently observed, and their occurrence led to the postulation of the "ARNDT-SCHULZ law", which states that drugs which paralyse at high concentrations stimulate at low concentrations. It is true that such effects are often observed but there is no necessity to postulate any mysterious property of living tissues, because similar effects are frequently observed with enzyme solutions. For example SOBOTKA and GLICK (1934)[4] found that octyl alcohol $1.6 \times 10^{-5}$ molar increased the rate of tributyrin hydrolysis by liver esterase, but at concentrations of $6.8 \times 10^{-5}$ molar and over it produced increasing inhibition. They explained this effect by supposing that the active portion of the ferment comprised only a small proportion of the total surface and that the octyl alcohol competed with the substrate, hence at low concentrations its dominant action was to prevent fixation of the substrate by inactive areas.

MICHAELIS and STERN (1931)[5] measured the action of iron salts on kathepsin from calves spleen. They found in some cases only augmentation, in other cases only inhibition and in some cases augmentation followed by inhibition.

Zinc was similarly found to have a diphasic action on peptidase (LINDERSTROM-LANG, 1934[6]). KREBS (1930)[7] and SUMNER and MYRBÄCK (1930)[3] showed that many pure ferments were extremely sensitive to metal poisoning. For example ordinary metal-distilled water reduced the activity of urease by 80 p.c. in 3 min. Under such conditions low concentrations of KCN actually augmented ferment

[1] RONA, P., and E. BLOCH: Biochem. Z. **118**, 185 (1921).
[2] RONA, P., V. AIRILA and A. LASNITZKI: Biochem. Z. **130**, 582 (1922).
[3] SUMNER, J. B., and K. MYRBÄCK: Hoppe-Seylers Z. **189**, 218 (1930).
[4] SOBOTKA, H., and D. GLICK: J. of biol. Chem. **105**, 199 (1934).
[5] MICHAELIS, L., and K. G. STERN: Biochem. Z. **240**, 193 (1931).
[6] LINDERSTROM-LANG, K.: Hoppe-Seylers Z. **224**, 121 (1934).
[7] KREBS, H. A.: Biochem. Z. **220**, 289, 296 (1930).

action by inactivating the poisonous metal, although in some cases higher concentrations of cyanide inhibited the enzyme activity, hence, in this case the diphasic action has a very simple chemical explanation.

Another complication of enzyme poisoning is that self-regeneration is frequently observed. The poison rapidly produces a marked inhibition and this is followed by a spontaneous recovery of enzyme activity which may result in the final activity of the poisoned enzyme being greater than that of the control. These effects can be explained in part as being due to deflection of the enzyme poison, which first unites with the active groups and then is deflected to combine with inert portions of the protein carrier. It is however difficult to explain why the regeneration process should sometimes proceed until the activity is considerably above the normal.

The fact that inexplicable aberrant results, of which a few examples have been given, are frequently observed in the relatively simple system of an inorganic poison acting on an enzyme, indicates that it is quite unreasonable to hope to find explanations for all the effects observed when drugs act on living cells. These aberrant effects are of special interest because they are also found when drugs act on living cells. The fact that drugs frequently produce diphasic actions on cells is the basis of the "ARNDT-SCHULZ law", the potential and the phasic theories of drug action. Since these phasic effects are also found with purified enzymes it is evident that their occurrence is not dependent on the organisation of the living cell, and no explanation of phasic actions can be regarded as satisfactory which does not explain their occurrence both with enzymes and with living cells.

**The Rate of Action of Enzyme Poisons.** Studies on this subject show that in many cases the enzyme poisoning is a complex process, in which a rapid action is followed by a slower process. JACOBY (1933)[1] found that the poisoning of urease by copper was at first reversible but later became irreversible. The reversibility was affected by the reaction: the action of copper was least reversible at $p_H$ 7—8, whilst the action of mercury was least reversible in acid solution. These results indicated a double action of the metals: (a) an initial combination with the active groups which produced a reversible inhibition; (b) a slow denaturation of the protein molecule which was irreversible.

In many cases specific enzyme poisons produce their full action in a minute or two, e.g. metals act on purified urease in less than 3 min. (SUMNER and MYR-BÄCK, 1930[2]), whilst quinine produces full action on invertase in a time too short to be measured (RONA and BLOCH, 1921[3]). In other cases the action is slower, for example atoxyl takes 15 to 30 minutes to produce its full action on serum lipase (RONA and BACH, 1920[4]), but in this case it is probable that the pentavalent atoxyl is reduced to a trivalent form before it produces its effect.

In some cases the influence of concentration on rate of action is very erratic. For example RONA and BACH (1921)[5] found in the case of poisoning of invertase by nitrophenol that increasing the concentration by 25 p.c. reduced the time until half action was produced from 30 min. to 5 min.

**Relation between Concentration of Poison and Inhibition of Enzyme.** The literature regarding ferment poisons provides a large mass of quantitative data, from which concentration-action curves can be constructed. Unfortunately the

[1] JACOBY, M.: Biochem. Z. **262**, 181 (1933).
[2] SUMNER, J. B., and K. MYRBÄCK: Hoppe-Seylers Z. **189**, 218 (1930).
[3] RONA, P., and E. BLOCH: Biochem. Z. **118**, 185 (1921).
[4] RONA, P., and E. BACH: Biochem. Z. **111**, 115, 166 (1920).
[5] RONA, P., and E. BACH: Biochem. Z. **118**, 232 (1921).

results are frequently contradictory, since different workers in some cases have found different relations with the same systems. This is not surprising because differences in the degree of purity of the enzyme and differences in the amount of enzyme poison added are likely to affect the concentration-action relation. For example in the case of a heavy metal the most favourable method for determining the concentration-action relation is to use a low concentration of purified enzyme, so that the metal concentration is not greatly changed by the amount fixed. If on the other hand an unpurified enzyme is used and the quantity of metal is relatively small, then extensive deviation of the metal is likely to occur and the concentration-action relation is likely to be distorted.

Another point is that concentration-action relations can only be deduced from experiments in which the effects observed cover a considerable proportion of the total possible range of action. Fortunately RONA and

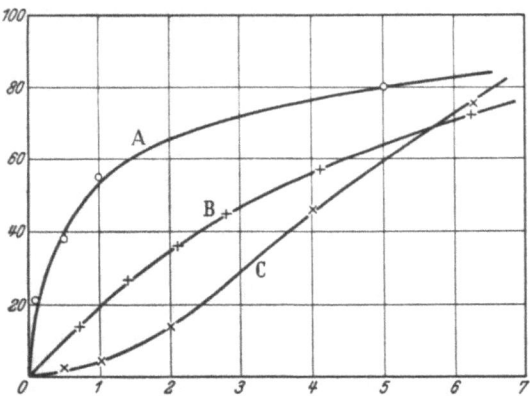

Fig. 1. Concentration-action curves of enzyme poisons. Abscissa: — concentration; ordinate: — per cent. inhibition. *A* Action of mercury perchloride on urease. Conc. in mg. × 10. (JACOBY, 1927[1].) *B* Action of ethyl alcohol on invertase. Molar conc. (MEYERHOF, 1914[2].) *C* Action of m-nitro-phenol on invertase. Molar conc. × 50. (RONA and BACH, 1921[3].)

his coworkers and EULER and MYRBÄCK, have made extensive series of experiments with a wide variety of enzymes and poisons and hence there is a large amount of data available which is suitable for comparison.

There is a fair agreement that there at least three distinct types of curves relating drug concentration and amount of action on ferments. Examples of these curves are shown in fig. 1. They are as follows:

(a) Cases in which the relation between drug concentration and amount of action is certainly not linear, but in which the curves may follow one of the three types:—

$$\text{action} = k. \log. \text{conc. (exponential curve)}$$
$$= k. (\text{conc.})^n \text{ (adsorption curve)}$$
$$\text{conc.} = k. \frac{\text{p.c. action}}{100 - \text{p.c. action}} \text{ (hyperbola)}$$

(b) Cases in which the relation between concentration and action is nearly linear. The narcotics are the most important class showing this relation; but it has been described in the case of other drugs.

(c) All-on-none action. Examples of this are the actions of m-nitrophenol on invertase (RONA and REINECKE, 1921[4]) and of dinitro-α-naphthol on the oxygen uptake of muscle pulp (v. EULER, 1932[5]).

The possible physico-chemical explanations of these three types of curves will be described later.

Fig. 1 shows the striking differences in the shapes of the concentration-action curves obtained in the case of different drugs. Table 6 shows that curves ap-

[1] JACOBY, M.: Biochem. Z. **181**, 194 (1927).
[2] MEYERHOF, O.: Pflügers Arch. **157**, 251, 307 (1914).
[3] RONA, P., and E. BACH: Biochem. Z. **118**, 232 (1921).
[4] RONA, P., and D. REINECKE: Biochem. Z. **118**, 232 (1921).
[5] EULER, H. VON: Arch. int. Pharmacodyn. **44**, 464 (1932).

proximating in shape to curve *A* in fig. 1 have been obtained in a considerable variety of drug-ferment systems. In some cases however simple linear concentration-action relations have been described with enzyme poisons similar to those included in Table 6 e. g. methyl-arsin oxide on maltase (RONA, AIRILA and LASNITZKI, 1922[1]); silver nitrate and aniline on amylase (OLSSON, 1921[2]); calomel on amylase (OLSSON, 1921[3]).

Table 6. Enzyme poisons which show exponential relations between concentration and action.

| System | Author |
|---|---|
| Atropine, cocaine and pilocarpine on yeast invertase . . . . . . . . . . . . . . . . | RONA, EWEYK and TANNENBAUM (1924)[4] |
| Cocaine on serum lipase . . . . . . . . . . | RONA and AMMON (1926)[5] |
| Quinine on invertase. . . . . . . . . . . . | RONA and BLOCH (1921)[6] |
| Quinine on serum lipase . . . . . . . . . . | RONA and REINECKE (1921)[7] |
| Quinine on stomach lipase . . . . . . . . . | RONA and TAKATA (1923)[8] |
| Quinine on pancreatic lipase . . . . . . . . | RONA and PAVLOVIC (1923)[9] |
| Aniline on saccharase . . . . . . . . . . . | EULER and GRAUBERG (1920)[10] MYRBÄCK (1926)[11] |
| Cyanides on protease. . . . . . . . . . . . | LINDERSTORM-LANG (1934)[12] |
| Heavy metals (various) on blood catalase . . . | BLEYER (1925)[13] |
| Mercury on urease. . . . . . . . . . . . . | JACOBY (1927, 1933)[14] |
| Mercury on saccharase . . . . . . . . . . . | EULER and MYRBÄCK (1919)[15]; MYRBÄCK (1926)[11] |
| Mercury on amylase . . . . . . . . . . . . | OLSSON (1921)[3] |
| Silver on urease . . . . . . . . . . . . . . | SUMNER and MYRBÄCK (1930)[17] |
| Silver on saccharase . . . . . . . . . . . . | MYRBÄCK (1926)[11] |
| Copper on amylase . . . . . . . . . . . . | OLSSON (1921)[3] |
| Zinc on peptidase . . . . . . . . . . . . . | LINDERSTORM-LANG (1934)[12] |
| Atoxyl on serum lipase . . . . . . . . . . . | RONA and BACH (1920)[18] |
| Atoxyl on liver lipase . . . . . . . . . . . | RONA and PAVLOVIC (1922)[19] |
| Atoxyl on kidney lipase . . . . . . . . . . . | RONA and HAAS (1923)[20] |

Enzymology is a comparatively young science which is at present developing rapidly, and hence much of the existing evidence is uncertain or contradictory. The author has endeavoured to select evidence on which hypotheses are based from the work of recognised authorities on the subject, but it is important to remember that the accuracy of the measurements of actions of drugs on enzymes approximates to the standards of pharmacology rather than those of inorganic chemistry.

[1] RONA, P., V. AIRILA and A. LASNITZKI: Biochem. Z. **130**, 582 (1922).
[2] OLSSON, U.: Hoppe-Seylers Z. **114**, 51 (1921).
[3] OLSSON, U.: Hoppe-Seylers Z. **117**, 91 (1921).
[4] RONA, P., C. VAN EWEYK and M. TENNENBAUM: Biochem. Z. **144**, 490 (1924).
[5] RONA, P., and R. AMMON: Biochem. Z. **181**, 49 (1926).
[6] RONA, P., and E. BLOCH: Biochem. Z. **118**, 185 (1921).
[7] RONA, P., and D. REINECKE: Biochem. Z. **118**, 213 (1921).
[8] RONA, P., and M. TAKATA: Biochem. Z. **134**, 118 (1923).
[9] RONA, P., and R. PAVLOVIC: Biochem. Z. **134**, 108 (1923).
[10] EULER, H. VON, and O. GRAUBERG: Fermentforsch. **4**, 29 (1920).
[11] MYRBÄCK, K.: Hoppe-Seylers Z. **158**, 160 (1926).
[12] LINDERSTORM-LANG, K.: Hoppe-Seylers Z. **224**, 121 (1934).
[13] BLEYER, L.: Biochem. Z. **161**, 91 (1925).
[14] JACOBY, M.: Biochem. Z. **181**, 194 (1927); **259**, 211 (1933).
[15] EULER, H. VON, and K. MYRBÄCK: Hoppe-Seylers Z. **107**, 269 (1919).
[16] MYRBÄCK, K.: Hoppe-Seylers Z. **158**, 160 (1926).
[17] SUMNER, J. B., and K. MYRBÄCK: Hoppe-Seylers Z. **189**, 218 (1930).
[18] RONA, P., and E. BACH: Biochem. Z. **111**, 115, 166 (1920).
[19] RONA, P., and R. PAVLOVIC: Biochem. Z. **130**, 225 (1922).
[20] RONA, P., and H. E. HAAS: Biochem. Z. **141**, 222 (1923).

**Discussion.** This brief review of the mode of action of enzyme poisons shows that these actions are highly complex. A considerable proportion of the phenomena can be explained on the assumption that the poison forms a reversible compound with an active group in the enzyme. This hypothesis suffices to explain such phenomena as the remarkable selective action of enzyme poisons, their power to act at high dilutions and the great effect produced by alterations in the reaction.

There are however many effects such as diphasic actions, self regeneration etc. which cannot be explained in any simple manner, and it has been found necessary to postulate the existence of accessory activating groups, with which the poison also can combine.

The fact that relatively simple systems of purified enzymes and enzyme poisons present many unsolved problems indicates the probable complexity likely to be encountered in the case of drugs acting on living cells, which are far more complex than any enzymes.

## Chapter 6

## Action of Heavy Metals on Enzymes in vitro and in vivo.

The poisoning of enzymes by heavy metals is a subject of special interest because it shows many analogies with the so-called "oligodynamic" action of heavy metals on living cells. Furthermore the heavy metals are particularly favourable drugs for quantitative measurement, and since their action on enzymes has been studied intensively the evidence provides an instructive basis for the consideration of their action on living cells.

**Action of Heavy Metals on Saccharase.** This reaction has been investigated by many authors and the information obtained has provided a considerable amount of information regarding the structure of the enzyme. Silver and mercury salts poison pure saccharase at very high dilutions, e.g. 1 part of metal in $10^9$ parts of solution. This fact has made it possible to estimate the amount of metal combining with each molecule of enzyme. EULER and MYRBÄCK (1919)[1] found that about 80 p.c. inhibition of saccharase was produced when there was one gram molecule of mercuric chloride (271 g.) present for every gram molecule of saccharase (30,000). Similarly SUMNER and MYRBÄCK (1930)[2] found that purified urease was inactivated when one gram atom of silver combined with 40,000 g. urease. These authors also showed that urease could fix ten times as much silver as was needed to inactivate the enzyme.

These results indicate that the molecule of enzyme can be inactivated by a single atom of metal. This supports the view that the activity of the enzyme is due to a particular chemical group, and that the metal combines with this group in preference to other groups on the enzyme molecule. This conclusion agrees with the results of EULER and JOSEPHSON (1923)[3] who calculated that 1 mol iodine produced inhibition of 20,000 g. enzyme. This relation suggests that 1 mol iodine combines with 1 mol of enzyme and inactivates some particular group.

MYRBÄCK (1926)[1] made exact observations on the poisoning of saccharase by silver and mercury. He found that silver combined with a carboxyl group in saccharase to form a feebly dissociated salt. He described the reaction as follows:

[1] EULER, H. VON, and K. MYRBÄCK: Hoppe-Seylers Z. **107**, 269 (1919).
[2] SUMNER, J. B., and K. MYRBÄCK: Hoppe-Seylers Z. **189**, 218 (1930).
[3] EULER, H. VON, and K. JOSEPHSON: Hoppe-Seylers Z. **127**, 97 (1923).

„Es wird also das vom Ampholyten abdissoziierte H-Ion durch ein fester gebundenes Ag-Ion ersetzt, und da das H-Ion für die katalytische Wirkung unentbehrlich ist, so erfolgt Inaktivierung. Da die bindende (basische) Gruppe dabei nicht betätigt ist, so muß diese Reaktion von der Substratkonzentration unabhängig sein, was der Versuch erweist. Die Vergiftung ist völlig reversibel, z. B. durch H$_2$S, die Kurve Inaktivierungsgrad—Giftmenge ist eine Dissoziationskurve. Es herrscht das Gleichgewicht

$$\frac{[Ag][E^1]}{[AgE]} = K_{Ag}."$$

The value of $K_{Ag}$ was found to be $10^{-7.4}$.

MYRBÄCK found that mercury combined with a basic group in saccharase to form an inert compound. This effect also could be reversed by H$_2$S. In this case the binding group was affected and hence the reaction was influenced by the concentration of substrate.

The conclusions outlined above were based largely on the manner in which the enzyme poisoning was influenced by changes in the reaction. MYRBÄCK (1926)[1] concluded:

„Die Inaktivierung eines Enzyms, z. B. durch ein Hg-Salz, mußte als eine Reaktion zwischen einem organischen Stoff und Quecksilber (oder Salz) aufgefaßt werden, die sich von anderen in der organischen Chemie vorkommenden Reaktionen mit Quecksilber nur in der Hinsicht unterscheiden konnte, daß die Affinität möglicherweise größer war."

In particular he deprecated calling the enzyme poisoning an oligodynamic effect, and the regarding of it as something outside of the ordinary laws of chemistry.

These results agree in showing that the action of a heavy metal on a purified enzyme is due to the combination of the heavy metal with an active group. The results also show that even when highly purified enzymes are used the metal can combine with portions of the enzyme other than the active group and hence there is no simple relation between the amount of metal fixed and the amount of inhibition. Deviation of this character is likely to be much greater in the case of heavy metals acting on partly purified enzymes and still greater when the heavy metals act on enzymes in cells. The experimental evidence available indicates that in the last mentioned case the deviation is so great that it obscures the quantitative relation between the concentration of poison and the inhibition produced.

EULER and WALLES (1924)[2] found that the quantity of metal fixed by yeast cells from a concentration of 1 part of silver in $10^5$ was equal to 4 per cent. of the dry weight of the cells, and they calculated that this was 200 times the quantity necessary to inactivate the saccharase. Hence the "deflection" or "deviation" of the metal by inert material which was observed in the case of purified enzymes was much more marked in the case of yeast cells.

Figures relating the amount of silver added and the inhibition of saccharase present in yeast cells can be extracted from the figures of EULER and WALLES. These results are shown in fig. 2 together with the concentration-action relation observed with purified saccharase. In the latter case the relation is in accordance with the theory that the enzyme and metal react according to a simple law of mass action. In the case of silver acting on yeast cells this relation disappears and the relation between concentration and action suggests an all-or-none effect. JOACHIMOGLU (1922)[3] obtained a similar all-or-none effect in the case of mercuric chloride inhibiting the carbon dioxide production of yeast cells. The measurements of the fixation of silver by the cells show that this is a continuous process; at first the metal produces no certain effect on the enzyme activity, but after a concentration has been reached which is sufficient to interfere with the enzyme

[1] MYRBÄCK, K.: Hoppe-Seylers Z. **158**, 160 (1926).
[2] EULER, H. von, and E. WALLES: Hoppe-Seylers Z. **132**, 167 (1924).
[3] JOACHIMOGLU, G.: Biochem. Z. **130**, 239 (1922).

activity, a small additional increase is sufficient to produce nearly complete inactivation. The result closely resembles the action of phenol in killing yeast cells (fig. 9, p. 55).

This result therefore shows that a concentration-action relation which may be clear in the case of a poison acting on a purified enzyme in solution may be obscured when the same poison acts on the same enzyme in living cells.

EULER and WALLES also noted several other striking irregularities in the action of metals on the enzyme activity of yeast. In most cases self regeneration was noted. The fixation of the metal by the cells was a very rapid process and more than 95 p.c. of the total fixation occurred in the first minute. The inactivation also reached its maximum in a minute or two, but after this a considerable recovery occurred, for example in one case the activity after 4 hours was 4 times as great as it was shortly after the introduction of the metal. This effect is obviously a serious complication of quantitative studies. They also found that low concentrations of metal frequently produced activation (ARNDT-SCHULZ effect); this effect, which is shown in fig. 2, was not found in the case of silver acting on saccharase solutions and the authors were unable to suggest any explanation for this difference.

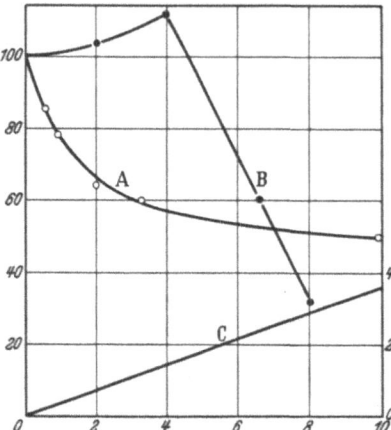

Fig. 2. Inactivation of invertase by silver *in vitro* and *in vivo*. Ordinates:— (left) per cent. activity:— (right) amount of silver fixed as per cent. dry weight of yeast. (curve C). Abscissa:— conc. of silver salts. *A* Inhibition of purified saccharase by silver nitrate. Conc. in arbitrary units. (MYRBÄCK, 1926[1].) *B* Inhibition of enzymatic activity of yeast cells. Conc. mg. Ag per 40 cc. (EULER and WALLES, 1924[2].) *C* Amount of silver fixed by yeast cells. Conc. as in B. (EULER and WALLES, 1924[2].)

**Concentration-action Relations of Heavy Metals and Enzymes.** The relation between concentrations of heavy metals and the amount of inhibition of enzyme activity produced has been measured by a number of workers, but unfortunately the results are conflicting. In some cases a linear relation between concentration and amount of action has been obtained (e.g. silver nitrate on amylase, OLSSON, [1921][3]; mercuric chloride on kathepsin from calves' spleen, MICHAELIS and STERN [1931][4]). In other cases an all-or-none effect has been observed, e.g. silver nitrate on urease (JACOBY, 1933[5]); zinc on invertase (ZLATAROFF et al., 1931[6]).

In several cases a linear relation has been found between the logarithm of the concentration of the metal and the amount of inhibition produced, and in a considerable number of cases the relation between metal concentration and inhibition approximates to a hyperbola. References to the latter results are given in Table 6. The cases in which the results most closely approximate to a hyperbola are as follows. Mercuric chloride on saccharase (EULER and MYRBÄCK, 1919[7]); silver nitrate on malt amylase (OLSSON, 1923[8]); mercuric and cupric chloride on urease (JACOBY, 1933[5]); various metals on blood catalase (BLEYER, 1925[9]).

[1] MYRBÄCK, K.: Hoppe-Seylers Z. **158**, 160 (1926).
[2] EULER, H. VON, and E. WALLES: Hoppe-Seylers Z. **132**, 167 (1924).
[3] OLSSON, U.: Hoppe-Seylers Z. **114**, 51 (1921).
[4] MICHAELIS, L., and K. G. STERN: Biochem. Z. **240**, 193 (1931).
[5] JACOBY, M: Biochem. Z. **259**, 211 (1933).
[6] ZLATAROFF, A. S., M. ANDREITSCHEWA and D. KALTSCHEWA: Biochem. Z. **231**, 123 (1931).
[7] EULER, H. VON, and K. MYRBÄCK: Hoppe-Seylers Z. **107**, 269 (1919).
[8] OLSSON, U.: Hoppe-Seylers Z. **126**, 29 (1923).
[9] BLEYER, L.: Biochem. Z. **161**, 91 (1925).

This diversity of results is not surprising when the possible experimental errors are considered. Even in the case of highly purified enzymes the amount of metal required to produce full inhibition is only a small fraction of the amount of metal that the enzyme can fix. With ordinary enzyme preparations the amount of metal deflected by combination with inert material must be very large in proportion to the amount producing the specific action. The relation between metal concentration and enzyme inhibition is therefore likely to be influenced by both the total quantity of metal added and the degree of purification of the enzyme. If MYRBÄCK's equation is accepted, then a wide variety of relations may result with varying conditions. If the enzyme is highly purified and present in small amount, then the quantity of metal fixed will be small in comparison to the amount present and the concentration-action relation will approximate to a hyperbola. If the metal and purified enzyme are present in approximately equivalent quantities, then the relations will resemble those found with a bimolecular reaction, but the results are likely to be distorted on account of the amount of metal deflected. If the enzyme is not highly purified and the amount of metal is relatively small, then the relation between concentration and

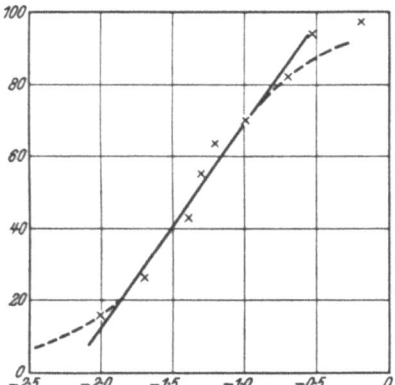

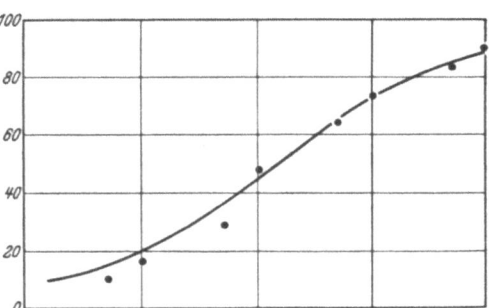

Fig. 3. Inhibition of urease by mercuric nitrate. Abscissa: — log. of conc. $(x)$ in mg. per 10 cc. Ordinate: — per cent. inhibition $(y)$. Broken curve drawn to formula

$$kx = \frac{y}{100 - y}.$$ (JACOBY, 1933[1].)

Fig. 4. Action of silver nitrate on blood catalase. Abscissa: — log. m. molar conc. $(x)$. Ordinate: — per cent. inhibition $(y)$. Curve drawn to formula

$$kx^{\frac{1}{2}} = \frac{y}{100 - y}.$$ (BLEYER, 1925[1].)

action is likely to be dominated by deflection. With low concentrations nearly all the metal is deflected and little effect is produced, but when the quantity of metal added rises above a certain value inhibition of enzyme activity commences and a comparatively small further increase in concentration is sufficient to produce a powerful inhibition.

The relations found between metal concentration and enzyme inhibition are so varied that it is unsafe to use them as a basis for argument. In some cases however curves have been obtained which are hyperbolae. Fig. 3 shows the action of mercuric nitrate on purified urease and the results are fitted by the formula $Kx = \dfrac{y}{100 - y}$ but all, except the extreme results, can equally well be interpreted as expressing a linear relation between log. concentration and action.

Fig. 4 shows the action of silver nitrate on blood catalase and in this case the results can be interpreted either as a hyperbola $\left(Kx^{\frac{1}{2}} = \dfrac{y}{100 - y}\right)$ or as a

[1] JACOBY, M.: Biochem. Z. **259**, 211 (1933).
[2] BLEYER, L.: Biochem. Z. **161**, 91 (1925).

linear relation between log. concentration and effect. The chief point of interest about these figures is that they show a graded action extending over ranges of concentration which are nearly 100 fold in fig. 3 and 10,000 fold in fig. 4. MYRBÄCK's theory of the mode of action of metals provides a reasonable physico-chemical explanation for this range of action.

**The Action of Metals on Living Cells.** The poisoning of enzymes by metals shows the following outstanding characteristics: (1) The metals act in very low concentrations; (2) Metals produce a graded action over a wide range of concentration; (3) The relation between concentration and amount of action can in some cases be interpreted as an expression of simple reaction between metals and enzymes.

The toxic action of heavy metals on all forms of living cells is a very well known phenomenon and it is of interest to consider how far the effects observed can be correlated with the phenomena of enzyme poisoning.

**Relation between Metal Concentration and Action on Cells.** The study of enzyme solutions shows that the relation between concentration of metal and enzyme inhibition is distorted by the presence of organic impurities which deflect the metal. It is therefore not surprising that the relation between metal concentration and amount of inhibition of enzyme activity in cells (fig. 2) shows a curve which is not suggestive of any particular physico-chemical process.

In view of the fact that heavy metals can combine with such a wide variety of organic material, it would be a very fortunate chance if any clear quantitative relation could be found between the metal present and the amount of enzyme inhibition. The general effect of heavy metals on living cells tends to approximate to an all-or-none-action. The living cell surface appears to be able to resist the entrance of drug, but after a certain degree of injury has been produced this resistance is broken down, the amount of drug entering the cell increases rapidly and death occurs. The shape of the curve in fig. 2 suggests this type of effect.

**Minimum Lethal Concentrations of Heavy Metals.** Heavy metals produce lethal actions on living cells at very low dilutions, and a striking feature of this action is that it occurs with a wide variety of cell populations such as plants, micro-organisms, mammalian tissues etc. NÄGELI (1893)[1] found that spirogyra was killed by copper salts at a dilution of 1 in 77 million. LOCKE (1895)[2] found that concentrations of copper of about 1 in 10 million were toxic to *tubifex* and to tadpoles. Similar toxic effects have been observed with plants, for example BRENCHLEY (1927)[3] found that the growth of barley seedlings in distilled water was inhibited by 1 part of copper salts per million.

The action of traces of heavy metals in killing bacteria and in killing isolated vertebrate tissues is common knowledge. This general lethal action of traces of heavy metals was considered so remarkable when first discovered that it was given the special name of "Oligodynamic action" and a number of fanciful suggestions have since been advanced to explain its nature. Full references to the extensive literature on this subject are given by FULMER and BUCHANAN (1930)[4] and by HEUBNER (1934)[5]. There is however no particular mystery about this action of heavy metals because quantitative analyses have shown that living organisms can adsorb metals from very high dilutions, and that a considerable

[1] NÄGELI, C. VON: Denkschr. schweiz. Naturforsch.-Ges. **33**, 1 (1893).
[2] LOCKE, F. S.: J. of Physiol. **18**, 319 (1895).
[3] BRENCHLEY, W. M.: Inorganic Plant Poisons, 2nd Ed. Cambridge: Univ. Press 1927.
[4] FULMER, E. I., and R. E. BUCHANAN: Physiology and Biochemistry of Bacteria. London: Bailliere, Tyndall and Cox 1930.
[5] HEUBNER, W.: Heffters Handb. exper. Pharmakol. **3**, 621 (1934).

amount of metal is fixed by the organism when a lethal action is produced. LOCKE actually noted in 1895 that when minnows were killed by copper distilled water they at the same time detoxicated the water. DRESCHEL (1921)[1] calculated the amount of copper that was fixed by spirogyra filaments. He showed that these filaments were killed by a concentration of 1 part of copper in $10^8$, but that the amount of copper fixed was equal to 0.02 p.c. of the weight of the spirogyra filaments. FREUNDLICH and SÖLLNER (1928)[2] found that spirogyra was killed by 3 $\gamma$ Ag per litre (3 parts in $10^9$) but that the algae contained about 60 $\gamma$ Ag per g. dry substance. The process of adsorption in both these cases caused the concentration in the filaments to be about 1000 times greater than the concentration in the water.

EICHHOLTZ (1934)[3] quoted various other quantitative results which are in harmony with those mentioned and concluded:

„Bei gewichtmäßiger Beobachtung ist danach die oligodynamische Kupferwirkung ihres Zaubers entkleidet."

Quantitative measurements of the fixation of mercuric chloride by yeast (HERZOG and BETZEL, 1911)[4] and of silver nitrate by yeast and B. coli (LIESE and MENDEL, 1923)[5] indicate that when death occurs there is a considerable concentration of metal in the cell. In other cases however measurements of the total amount of metal present in solutions which kill cells show that the concentration of metal in the cells must be relatively small. LEITNER (1929)[6] found that the minimum lethal concentration of $AgNO_3$ for B. coli was $5 \times 10^{-8}$ molar, and his figures show that the amount fixed per cell cannot have been more than $6 \times 10^5$ molecules, which would give a concentration in the cells of about 1 part in 30,000.

The amounts of heavy metals fixed by cells are much larger than the amounts calculated in the case of many organic drugs (e.g. adrenaline, acetylcholine and strophanthin). The remarkable feature about this action of metals is the selective adsorption of the metal by the cell. This adsorption is not a highly specific effect because traces of metal can be removed from distilled water by a number of adsorbents such as charcoal or proteins. Owing to this fact, the toxicity of heavy metals is greatly reduced by the addition of serum or other organic matter to the solutions. For example GLÜCK (1933)[7] found that silver nitrate killed B. coli in tap water at a dilution of 1 in $10^8$, but in broth or serum a concentration of 1 in 50,000 was required. The disinfectant activity of mercuric chloride can be modified in a similar manner.

Although heavy metals have a very wide spread lethal action on living tissues yet there are striking exceptions to this general rule. An extreme example of immunity to metals is provided by moulds such as *Penicillium glaucum* which is said to be able to grow in a 14 p.c. solution of copper sulphate.

The action of heavy metals and of other disinfectants on viruses does not differ markedly from their action on visible bacteria, but such wide variations in action (GYE and LEDINGHAM, 1930[8]) are observed in both cases

[1] DRESCHEL, O.: Zbl. Bakter. I Orig. **53**, 2, 288 (1921).
[2] FREUNDLICH, H., and K. SÖLLNER: Biochem. Z. **203**, 1 (1928).
[3] EICHHOLTZ, F.: Heffters Handb. exp. Pharmakol. **3**, 1928 (1934).
[4] HERZOG, R. A., and R. BETZEL: Hoppe-Seylers Z. **74**, 221 (1911).
[5] LIESE, W., and B. MENDEL: Z. Hyg. **100**, 454 (1923).
[6] LEITNER, N.: Klin. Wschr. **8**, 1952 (1929).
[7] GLÜCK, G.: Arch. f. Hyg. **110**, 38 (1933).
[8] GYE, W. E., and J. C. G. LEDINGHAM: Med. Res. Council, System of Bacteriology **7**, 1 (1930).

that it is difficult to make any generalised statement. Bacteriophage shows however an extraordinary power of resistance to heavy metals and to many other forms of disinfectant. KRUEGER (1936)[1] quotes the following facts. Phage can survive exposure to $HgCl_2$ for 3 days at 0.5 p.c. and for months at 0.01 p.c. Exposure to 2.8 p.c. $HgCl_2$ inactivates phage rapidly but after 216 hours exposure the phage can be reactivated by washing with hydrogen sulphide. The resistance of phage to other disinfectants is in general similar to that of anthrax spores. The lower limit of size of phages is smaller than that of some protein molecules and hence the resistance of phage to chemicals cannot be due to any protective membrane. Too little is known about the nature of phage for the significance of this remarkable phenomenon to be understood. Phage however possesses many of the properties usually considered to be specific attributes of living organisms, and it is of interest to note that such properties can in this case survive chemical treatment of an extremely drastic nature.

**Relative Toxicity of Metals.** MATTHEWS (1903)[2] pointed out that as a general rule the metals which produced a strong toxic action on cells were those which had a low electrolytic solution pressure and the same generalisation holds for the action of metals upon enzymes. The metals listed in LANDOLT-BORNSTEIN's tables (1923)[3] which have low electrolytic solution pressures, show the following sequence when arranged in ascending order according to the magnitude of this pressure:—

$$Au^{\cdots}, \quad Pb^{\cdots\cdots}, \quad Hg^{\cdot\cdot}, \quad Tl^{\cdots}, \quad Pd^{\cdot\cdot}, \quad Co^{\cdots}, \quad Au^{\cdot}, \quad As^{\cdots}, \quad Bi^{\cdots},$$

$$Cu^{\cdot\cdot}, \quad Sb^{\cdots}, \quad Hg^{\cdot}, \quad Ag^{\cdot}, \quad Cu^{\cdot}, \quad Fe^{\cdots}, \quad Sn^{\cdot\cdot}, \quad Pb^{\cdot\cdot} \quad \text{etc.}$$

The most important metallic enzyme poisons, disinfectants and chemotherapeutic agents occur in the first fourteen places of this list, but it is impossible to show any exact correlation between electrolytic solution pressure and toxic action.

For example silver, copper and mercury are three metals particularly distinguished for their power to kill organisms in low concentration but only one of these (Hg) is near the commencement of the list. The inhibitory action of metals on enzymes is a simpler effect than their action on living cells for quantitative study, but in this case also there is no real correlation between toxicity and electrolytic solution pressure since different orders in the activity of metals are obtained with different ferments. Tables 7 and 8 show that the metals which have the most powerful action on both enzymes and cells are those with low electrolytic solution tensions. There are however striking irregularities since copper is a powerful poison to paramoecium and to Fundulus eggs but has a weak action on bacteria.

Gold, mercury, silver and copper inhibit a wide variety of enzymes but the action of iron and zinc is much more variable. These latter metals inhibit papain enzyme (KREBS, 1930[4]), but augment the action of other enzymes: e.g. calf liver kathepsin (MICHAELIS and STERN, 1931[5]); tissue proteinase (STERN, 1931[6]).

---

[1] KRUEGER, A. P.: Physiologic. Rev. **16**, 129 (1936).
[2] MATTHEWS, A. P.: Amer. J. Physiol. **10**, 290 (1903).
[3] LANDOLT-BÖRNSTEIN: Physikalisch-chemische Tabellen **2**, 1028. 5. Aufl. Berlin: Julius Springer 1923.
[4] KREBS, H. A.: Biochem. Z. **220**, 289, 296 (1930).
[5] MICHAELIS, L., and K. G. STERN: Biochem. Z. **240**, 193 (1931).
[6] STERN, K. G.: Biochem. Z. **234**, 116 (1931).

Table 7. Molar concentrations at which metals inhibit enzyme activity.

| | (I)<br>50 p. c. inhibition of papain (KREBS 1930[1]) | (II)<br>Minimum active conc. on urease (JACOBY 1933[2]) | (III)<br>50 p. c. inhibition blood catalase (BLEYER 1925[3]) |
|---|---|---|---|
| Hg·· | $5 \times 10^{-6}$ | $3 \times 10^{-5}$ | $5 \times 10^{-5}$ |
| Ag· | $5 \times 10^{-6}$ | $1.7 \times 10^{-3}$ | $1.6 \times 10^{-4}$ |
| Au··· | $1.3 \times 10^{-6}$ | — | — |
| Cu·· | $1.3 \times 10^{-5}$ | $3 \times 10^{-4}$ | — |
| Zn·· | $4.6 \times 10^{-5}$ | — | — |
| Pb·· | $10^{-5}$ no action | — | $4 \times 10^{-5}$ |
| Fe·· | $10^{-5}$ no action | $9 \times 10^{-1}$ | — |
| Bi | — | — | $5 \times 10^{-5}$ |
| Mo | — | — | $1.6 \times 10^{-4}$ |
| La | — | — | $7 \times 10^{-4}$ |
| Ce | — | — | $2 \times 10^{-3}$ |

Table 8. Toxicities of heavy metals for cells.

| (I)<br>Usual order of toxicity of metals to bacteria (EISENBERG 1919[4]) | (II)<br>Molar conc. inhibiting B. coli in peptone broth (WINSLOW and HOTCHKISS 1921[5]) | (III)<br>Equiv. conc. killing Paramoecium (WOODRUFF and BUNTZEL 1910[6]) | (IV)<br>Equiv. conc. killing Fundulus eggs (MATTHEWS 1903[7]) |
|---|---|---|---|
| $AgNO_3$ | $HgCl_2$ 0.00001 | $AgNO_3$ 0.00033 | $AgNO_3$ 0.00001 |
| $HgCl_2$ | $CdCl_2$ 0.0001 | $HgCl_2$ 0.00035 | $HgCl_2$ 0.00002 |
| | $CuCl_2$ | $PbCl_2$ 0.0005 | $AuCl_3$ 0.00005 |
| $PtCl_4$ | $AlCl_3$ 0.0005 | $FeCl_2$ 0.0006 | $CuCl_2$ 0.00006 |
| $AuCl_3$ | $PbCl_2$ 0.0005 | $CdCl_2$ 0.0045 | $Pb(CH_3COO)_2$ 0.0002 |
| $COCl_2$ | $COCl_2$ 0.0005 | $CuCl_2$ 0.0045 | $FeCl_3$ 0.00025 |
| $CdCl_2$ | $FeCl_3$ 0.001 | | $ZnCl_2$ 0.0012 |
| $NiCl_2$ | $CuCl_2$ 0.001 | | |
| $CuCl_2$ | $ZnCl_2$ 0.001 | | |
| $PbCl_2$ | | | |

**Course of Reaction between Metals and Cells.** The action of metals on enzymes has been shown to be a double effect, firstly a rapid fixation and reversible inhibition, which is due to a combination with the prosthetic group and secondly a slow irreversible injury which is probably due to denaturation of the protein carrier. The action of metals on cells is more complex but two stages can be distinguished. Firstly a rapid adsorption of the metal on the surface, which may inhibit the activity of enzymes, but which is reversible by washing with sulphuretted hydrogen. Secondly a slow process of penetration which produces irreversible effects and finally results in the destruction of the cell.

In consequence of this two stage action there is no direct relation between the rate of fixation of the metal and the rate of its acting on the cell. The fact that mercuric chloride was rapidly fixed by bacteria but that its disinfectant action could be stopped at this stage by washing with sulphuretted hydrogen was noted by CHICK (1908)[8] and has been since confirmed repeatedly (HAHN, 1922[9]). Particularly striking evidence has been obtained in the case of metals acting on bacterial spores. MÜLLER (1920)[10] found that anthrax spores when

[1] KREBS: H. A.: Biochem. Z. **220**, 289, 296 (1930).
[2] JACOBY, M.: Biochem. Z. **259**, 211 (1933).
[3] BLEYER, L.: Biochem. Z. **161**, 91 (1925).
[4] EISENBERG, P.: Zbl. Bakter. I Orig. **82**, 69 (1919).
[5] WINSLOW, C. E. A., and M. HOTCHKISS: Proc. Soc. exper. Biol. a. Med. **19**, 314 (1921).
[6] WOODRUFF, L. L., and H. H. BUNTZEL: Amer. J. Physiol. **25**, 190 (1910).
[7] MATTHEWS, A. P.: Amer. J. Physiol. **10**, 290 (1903).
[8] CHICK, H.: J. of Hyg. **8**, 92 (1908).    [9] HAHN, M.: Z. Hyg. **98**, 569 (1922).
[10] MÜLLER, A.: Arch. f. Hyg. **89**, 363 (1920).

exposed to 3 p.c. HgCl$_2$ were still viable if washed with sulphuretted hydrogen after 7 days exposure. PICHLER and WÖBER (1922)[1] measured the rate of adsorption by anthrax spores of metal from a solution containing about 0.5 p.c. copper and found that more than half the total adsorption occurred in a minute and three quarters within an hour.

SÜPFLE (1923)[2] studied the action of mercuric chloride on anthrax spores. Microscopic examination showed an all-or-none effect since some spores were unstained and other spores were deeply stained. LIESE and MENDEL (1923)[3] found in the case of silver salts that with sublethal concentrations no metal penetrated the bacteria but that higher concentrations penetrated the bacteria and produced death. The evidence on this subject has been collected recently by REICHEL (1935)[4]. Bacteria are cells with a relatively thick cellulose wall and delay in penetration of heavy metals through such a structure is not surprising. Yeast cells and animal cells have no such cell wall but nevertheless also show the phenomenon of rapid adsorption of heavy metals followed by slow secondary changes.

In the case of Arbacia eggs, HOADLEY (1930)[5] concluded that low concentrations of mercuric chloride entered the cells and were dissolved in the pigment granules and that higher concentrations caused coagulation of the proteins. His figures show that at least 20 min. immersion was required for a solution of M/150,000 HgCl$_2$ to produce its full effect.

The experiments already described by EULER and WALLES (1924)[6] on yeast cells show that metals are adsorbed quickly, and that the specific effect of enzyme inhibition also is rapidly produced, but that this initial effect is followed by a redistribution of the metal throughout the cell, which usually results in a reduction of the enzyme inhibiting effect.

In the case of mercury acting on the glycolytic activity of mammalian cells (rat sarcoma) JOWETT and BROOKS (1928)[7] concluded that there was a rapid adsorption, which did not inhibit the enzyme, and that this was followed by a slow chemical reaction, which took hours to complete, and which caused inhibition of the enzyme.

The chemical processes involved in the inhibition of glycolysis by heavy metals in yeast and in mammalian tissues appear therefore to be similar, but the course of action appears completely different since in the case of yeast there is immediate full inhibition followed by partial recovery, whereas in the case of the rat sarcoma there is a slow progressive inhibition. These results agree in indicating an initial adsorption of metal followed by a diffusion of the metal into the cell, but in some cases the redistribution increases and in other cases it decreases the effect measured.

**Diphasic Actions of Metals on Cells.** Many workers have described complex diphasic effects of heavy metals on enzymes, and similar results have been recorded with living cells. HEUBNER (1934)[8] gives a number of references to these actions which are in many cases very complex. WARBURG (1910)[9] found

[1] PICHLER, F., and A. WÖBER: Biochem. Z. **132**, 420 (1922).
[2] SÜPFLE, K.: Arch. f. Hyg. **93**, 252 (1923).
[3] LIESE, W., and B. MENDEL: Z. Hyg. **100**, 454 (1923).
[4] REICHEL, H.: Medizinische Kolloidlehre, p. 758. Dresden: Steinkopff 1935.
[5] HOADLEY, L.: Biol. Bull. **58**, 123 (1930).
[6] EULER, H. VON, and E. WALLES: Hoppe-Seylers Z. **132**, 167 (1924).
[7] JOWETT, M., and J. BROOKS: Biochemic. J. **22**, 720 (1928).
[8] HEUBNER, W.: Heffters Handb. exper. Pharmakol. **3**, 670 (1934).
[9] WARBURG, O.: Hoppe-Seylers Z. **69**, 452 (1910).

for example that gold, silver and copper in concentrations of $10^{-5}$ molar all increased the oxygen uptake of sea urchin eggs but at the same time nearly completely inhibited cell division.

HOTCHKISS (1923)[1] described stimulation of bacterial growth by many heavy metals in low concentrations.

The diphasic effects produced by heavy metals on yeast has been the subject of extensive research and considerable controversy.

MEIER (1926)[2] showed that the effects of poisons on the respiration and fermentation of yeast were complex. In some cases (e.g. $HgCl_2$, chromate, oxyquinoline etc.) the fermentation was inhibited by lower concentrations than was the respiration, and hence the effect appeared to be purely inhibitory, whatever activity was measured. In other cases a cyanide-like effect was produced and the respiration was inhibited by concentrations too low to affect fermentation. In such cases a compensatory increase in fermentation occurred, and if the fermentation alone was measured the effect recorded was a stimulation with low concentrations followed by an inhibition with higher concentrations. This example illustrates the general principle that when a poison acts on a system as complex as a cell the results recorded are nearly certain to be very complex unless great care is taken in arranging the experimental conditions.

**Discussion.** At first sight the action of heavy metals on cells appears to be an exceptionally favourable subject for quantitative analysis. Unfortunately the detailed evidence available shows that these reactions are in reality extremely complex. The action of metals on purified enzymes indicates a simple chemical reaction between the metal and the enzyme but this simple relation becomes obscured when the action of metals on intracellular enzymes is studied.

The fundamental difficulty is as follows. Firstly, the metals unite with a wide variety of cellular constituents and the enzyme inhibition is produced by a very small proportion of the total metal fixed. Secondly, the fixation of the metal is a complex process, the first process is a simple adsorption, but after this an extensive redistribution occurs. The initial adsorption inhibits certain enzyme activities immediately and in these cases the subsequent redistribution of the metal, probably due to the metal penetrating the cell, may be accompanied by a considerable recovery in the enzyme activity. In other cases however the enzyme inhibition only begins after the metal has penetrated the cell.

Other measurable actions of metals are the haemolysis of red blood corpuscles and the death of bacteria and in both these cases an all-or-none effect is produced. In the case of bacteria the death of the cell is accompanied by a rise in the permeability of the cell to the metal, and consequently the amount of metal fixed is increased and this constitutes a further complication in the estimation of quantitative relations.

The lethal action of metals on organisms is presumably due to precipitation of proteins, and heavy metals such as Hg and silver have a general non-specific action as protein precipitants. Nevertheless the lethal action of metals on cells shows in many cases selective effects. The probable cause of these specific actions is selective adsorption, rather than any selective toxic action after the metal has entered the cell. The quantitative evidence regarding the amount of metal fixed by cells from dilute solutions, shows that this quantity is considerable. The remarkable fact about the so called oligodynamic action is that cells can adsorb relatively large quantities of metal from very high dilutions, the amount adsorbed is so large that the toxic action produced is not surprising.

[1] HOTCHKISS, M.: J. Bacter. **8**, 142 (1923).
[2] MEIER, R.: Biochem. Z. **174**, 384 (1926).

From the point of view of therapeutics the lethal action of metals on spiro-chaetes and trypanosomes is by far the most important action which they produce. This subject is however beset by all the difficulties outlined above and in addition presents a variety of special problems. For example, in many cases the drug introduced is activated either by the host or by the parasite, and moreover the parasites can acquire immunity to the drugs. In view both of the importance and of the peculiar difficulty of the subject of chemotherapy it has been thought wisest to defer its discussion until the end of this monograph.

## Chapter 7
## Action of Various Enzyme Poisons in vitro and in vivo.

There are a number of common enzyme poisons which have been studied extensively and which are of interest either because they show special forms of concentration-action relations or because they permit the comparison of the action of enzyme poisons on purified enzymes and on the living cell.

In the case of the heavy metals the concentration-action relations between metals and purified enzymes indicate the occurrence of a simple chemical reaction, but these relations are obscured when the metals act on enzymes present in living cells. A similar result is obtained with other important enzyme poisons (e.g. quinine), but in certain other cases (e.g. narcotics, cyanides and phenols) it is possible to show a relation between the concentration-action relations obtained with purified enzymes and with enzymes in cells.

**The Action of Dyes on Enzymes.** The inhibition of enzymes by dyes has been investigated by QUASTEL and co-workers (1931, 1932, 1936)[1] and their results confirm and amplify those obtained by MYRBÄCK with heavy metals. QUASTEL and YATES (1936)[2] found that inhibition of invertase was produced by many basic and acid dyes at fairly low concentrations ($10^{-4}$ to $10^{-3}$ molar). The action was reversible and was expressed by formula 1.

$$(1) \qquad \frac{1}{[D]} \cdot \frac{I}{1-I} = K .$$

($I$ = fractional inhibition, and $[D]$ = molar concentration.)

This formula is the same as that found by MYRBÄCK for the action of silver on invertase (cf. p. 41). It has been shown to express a reversible reaction between the drug (or dye) and the active group of the enzyme, provided that the drug is present in excess.

These workers also studied the effect of changes in $p_H$ on the action produced by basic or acid dyes. Increase in $p_H$ augmented the inhibition in the former case and reduced it in the latter case. When the $p_H$ was varied and the concentration of basic dye was constant the relation between $p_H$ and amount of inhibition followed formula 2.

$$(2) \qquad p_H - \log \frac{I}{1-I} = \text{constant} .$$

When both $p_H$ and dye concentration were varied, then the concentrations producing a constant effect (50 per cent inhibition) were found to follow formula 3.

$$(3) \qquad p_H - \log \frac{1}{[D]} = \text{constant} .$$

---

[1] QUASTEL, J. H., and A. H. M. WHEATLEY: Biochemic. J. **25**, 629 (1931). — QUASTEL, J. H.: Biochemic. J. **26**, 1685 (1932). — QUASTEL, J. H., and E. D. YATES: Enzymologia **1**, 60 (1936).

[2] QUASTEL, J. H., and E. D. YATES: Enzymologia **1**, 60 (1936).

Formula (3) can be derived from formulae (1) and (2).

These results provide a simple example of antagonism. Since $p_H = \log \frac{1}{[H]}$ hence formula (3) can be transposed to formulae (4) and (5).

(4) $$\log[D] - \log[H] = \text{constant},$$

(5) $$[D]/[H] = \text{constant}.$$

The special interest of this last result is that it approximates closely to the relations found between the action of acetylcholine on the frog's heart and its antagonism by atropine (cf. chapter 17).

In the case of acid dyes the effect of $p_H$ changes is more complex and the effect of $p_H$ change with a constant concentration of dye is expressed by the formula (6).

(6) $$p_H + \frac{1}{n} \cdot \log \frac{I}{1 - I} = \text{constant},$$

whilst the relation of $p_H$ and $[D]$ producing a constant effect (50 per cent.) inhibition) is expressed by formula (7).

(7) $$p_H + \frac{1}{n} \cdot \log \frac{1}{[D]} = \text{constant}.$$

QUASTEL and YATES explain these varied effects of dyes and $p_H$ changes on invertase by the assumption that the active group of invertase is a zwitterion ($E^{\pm}$) which forms an anion $HO \cdot E^-$ and a kation $HE^+$, and that only the zwitterion is enzymatically active. This hypothesis is supported by the fact that excess of sucrose diminishes the inhibitory activities of both acid and basic dyes, fructose antagonises the acid dyes more powerfully than the basic dyes and glucose has the greater action on the basic dyes.

A purified enzyme is much simpler than a living cell, but these investigations show that in the case of enzymes a whole range of complex antagonisms and synergisms can be demonstrated, which can only be explained on the assumption that the active group is complex in character. The general resemblance between these results and the results obtained when drugs act on simple cell systems such as the frog's heart, is very striking.

**Action of Quinine on Enzymes.** Quinine acts as a poison on a considerable number of ferments but RONA and REINECKE (1921)[1] have shown that it has in some cases a markedly selective action. For example quinine poisons the lipases of the serum, pancreas and stomach, but does not affect liver and kidney lipase. The action of quinine is dependent on the concentration of free base and is much greater in alkaline than in acid solution. The results obtained by RONA and his co-workers show two types of concentration-action relations for the inhibition of ferments by quinine:

(1) Linear relation between inhibition and logarithm of the concentration of quinine e.g. action on pancreatic lipase (RONA and PAVLOVIC, 1923[2]) and action on invertase (RONA and BLOCH, 1921[3]).

(2) Linear relation between the logarithms of the inhibition and of the concentration (RONA and REINECKE, 1921[1]), (RONA and TAKATA, 1923[4]).

Most of these results can be interpreted as representing portions of a hyperbola as is seen in fig. 5 which shows the figures obtained by RONA and BLOCH (1921)[3]

[1] RONA, P., and D. REINECKE: Biochem. Z. **118**, 213 (1921).
[2] RONA, P., and R. PAVLOVIC: Biochem. Z. **134**, 108 (1923).
[3] RONA, P., and E. BLOCH: Biochem. Z. **118**, 185 (1921).
[4] RONA, P., and M. TAKATA: Biochem. Z. **134**, 118 (1923).

for the inhibition of invertase by quinine. The action of quinine on ferments can therefore be interpreted as a simple monomolecular reaction in which the quinine base reacts with a specific group of the enzyme.

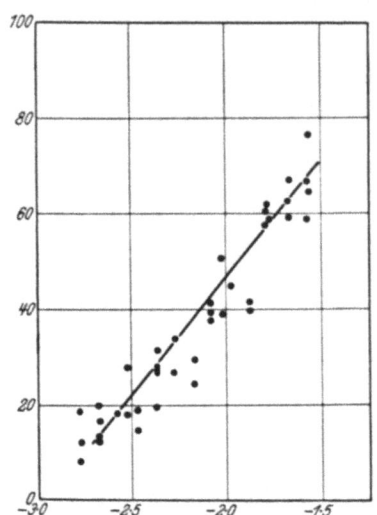

Fig. 5. Action of quinine on invertase. Abscissa:— log. molar conc. Ordinate:— per cent. inhibition. (RONA and BLOCH, 1921[1].)

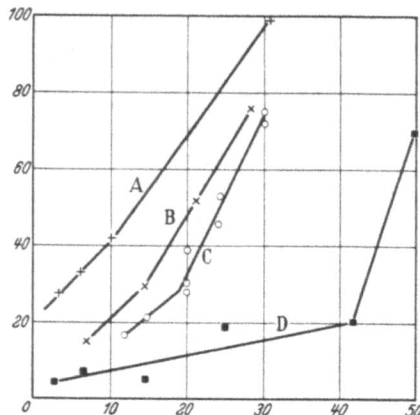

Fig. 6. Action of quinine on living cells. Abscissa:— conc. Ordinate:— per cent. inhibition. *A* Inhibition of carbon dioxide production of yeast at $p_H$ 6. Molar conc. × 100,000. (RONA and NICOLAI, 1927[2].) *B* Inhibition of respiration of goose erythrocytes. Molar conc. × 10,000. (RONA and BLOCH, 1922[3].) *C* Inhibition of yeast respiration. Molar conc. × 1000. (RONA and GRASSHEIM, 1923[4].) *D* Inhibition of carbon dioxide production of yeast. Molar conc. × 5,000. (JOACHIMOGLU, 1922[5].)

**Action of Quinine on Cells.** The action of quinine in inhibiting the oxygen consumption of yeast cells and of red blood corpuscles is shown in fig. 6.

The concentration-action relation approximates to an all-or-none effect. Little action is produced until a certain concentration is attained and a relatively small further increase in concentration is sufficient to cause complete inhibition. A similar result was obtained by MEIER (1927)[6] who measured the action of quinine on the oxygen uptake of goose erythrocytes.

On the other hand LIPSCHITZ and FREUND (1923)[7] who measured the action of quinine on the oxygen use of bacteria and of guinea pigs muscles obtained results which show an approximately linear relation between inhibition and logarithm of the concentration.

Quinine therefore resembles the heavy metals in that its mode of action on ferments in solution can be interpreted as a simple monomolecular reaction, but this simple relation is obscured when the action of quinine on the enzyme activity of living cells is studied.

**Action of Cyanide on Enzymes and Cells.** Cyanide is an enzyme poison which has a very marked selective action. Some enzymes are inhibited by cyanide at a concentration of $10^{-6}$ molar, whilst others are unaffected by concentrations 1000 times this strength. In the case of enzymes which are sensitive to metals but

[1] RONA, P., and E. BLOCH: Biochem. Z. **118**, 185 (1921).
[2] RONA, P., and H. W. NICOLAI: Biochem. Z. **189**, 331 (1927).
[3] RONA, P., and E. BLOCH: Biochem. Z. **128**, 169 (1922).
[4] RONA, P., and K. GRASSHEIM: Biochem. Z. **140**, 493 (1923).
[5] JOACHIMOGLU, G.: Biochem. Z. **130**, 239 (1922).
[6] MEIER, R.: Arch. f. exper. Path. **122**, 129 (1927).
[7] LIPSCHITZ, W. L., and H. FREUND: Arch. f. exper. Path. **99**, 226 (1923).

insensitive to cyanide the latter often stimulates enzyme activity; the probable reason for this is that the cyanide inactivates traces of metals present in the distilled water. JACOBY (1926)[1] has shown this effect in the case of purified urease.

WARBURG (1914)[2] showed the general similarity of the action of cyanide in inhibiting the oxidation of cystin by blood charcoal and its action in inhibiting the oxygen consumption of cells such as birds red blood corpuscles and sea urchin eggs. He measured (WARBURG, 1921[3]) the adsorption of cyanide by charcoal and his figures show an approximately linear relation between log. concentration and log. amount adsorbed per unit mass (FREUNDLICH's formula). He found however that the oxidation of cystin was reduced 50 p.c. by about $1/_{1000}$ of the concentration of cyanide needed to half saturate the charcoal surface. Hence he concluded that the inhibition of oxidation of cystin by charcoal was not a general adsorption effect, but a selective action probably due to inactivation of iron. He produced a variety of evidence in support of the view that the inhibition by cyanide of oxygen uptake of cells was due to the drug inactivating a heavy metal (probably iron) which was an essential constituent of the oxidase.

This conclusion was supported by the effect on oxygen uptake of the combination of cyanide with narcotic poisoning. Both these drugs reduced the oxygen consumption of both blood charcoal and of living cells, but the addition of narcotics reduced the intensity of action of cyanide. This effect is readily explained on the assumption that narcotics cover the active surfaces and hence interfere with the fixation of cyanide.

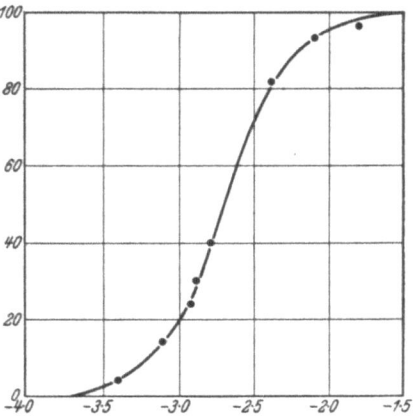

The hypothesis that cyanide acts on the surface of cells has received direct support from micro-injection experiments on amoebae. Cyanide paralyses amoebae when applied externally but produces no such effect when injected (BRINLEY, 1928[4]). There is therefore a wide variety of evidence supporting the theory that cyanide inactivates certain enzymes on the surface of cells, and that cyanide combines with these enzymes in concentrations much lower than it combines with or is adsorbed by the rest of the cell surface.

Fig. 7. Inhibition of peptidase by potassium cyanide. Abscissa:— log. molar conc. Ordinate:— per cent. inhibition. (LINDERSTROM-LANG, 1934[5].)

The action of cyanide is freely reversible in the case of both enzymes and cells, hence if cyanide reacts with an enzyme to form a reversible compound it is to be expected that when enzymes or cells are exposed to a solution of cyanide the concentration-action relation will follow the formula $Kx^n = \dfrac{y}{100 - y}$. LINDERSTROM-LANG (1934)[5] gives figures for the action of cyanide on peptidase which are fitted exactly by the formula $Kx^{\frac{1}{2}} = \dfrac{y}{100 - y}$, as is shown in fig. 7.

[1] JACOBY, M.: Biochem. Z. **181**, 194 (1927).
[2] WARBURG, O.: Erg. Physiol. **14**, 253 (1914).
[3] WARBURG, O.: Biochem. Z. **119**, 134 (1921).
[4] BRINLEY, F. J.: J. gen. Physiol. **12**, 201 (1928).
[5] LINDERSTROM-LANG, K.: Hoppe-Seylers Z. **224**, 121 (1934).

This type of curve is to be expected if one molecule of drug reacts with two receptors but unfortunately such an event seems impossible in the case of cyanide and hence no theoretical significance can be attached to the curve. LIPSCHITZ and GOTTSCHALK (1921)[1] studied the action of cyanide on the reduction of dinitrophenol by frogs muscle pulp. The results are not very clear but approximate to a linear relation between action and the logarithm of the concentration. Their results with earthworm muscle show this relation definitely (LIPSCHITZ and GOTTSCHALK, 1921[2]). These experiments of LIPSCHITZ and GOTTSCHALK agree with those of LINDERSTROM-LANG in suggesting that the concentration-action relation is a hyperbola, but the slope of the curve in the latter case is far steeper than in the former case. In the case of animal tissues a linear relation was found between cyanide concentration and inhibition of oxidation both by WARBURG (1911)[3] who measured the action of cyanide in inhibiting the oxygen uptake of birds red blood corpuscles and by MEYERHOF (1916)[4] who measured the action of cyanide in inhibiting the oxygen uptake of *nitro-somas*.

PICKFORD (1927)[5] found that the relation between cyanide concentration and depression of the mechanical activity of the frog's heart followed a similar curve but A. DALE (1937)[6] working with the I. A. A. poisoned frog's heart has found that a graded response is only shown over a relatively narrow range of concentrations.

The evidence regarding the general shape of the concentration-action relation in the case of cyanide action on enzymes in living cells is therefore conflicting. In several cases however results are recorded which show that there is not a simple linear relation between concentration and action. WARBURG (1910)[7] found that the oxygen consumption of fertilised eggs of *Strongylocentrotus* was reduced by 68 p.c. by $10^{-5}$ molar KCN, whilst ten times this concentration only reduced the oxygen consumption by 81 p.c.

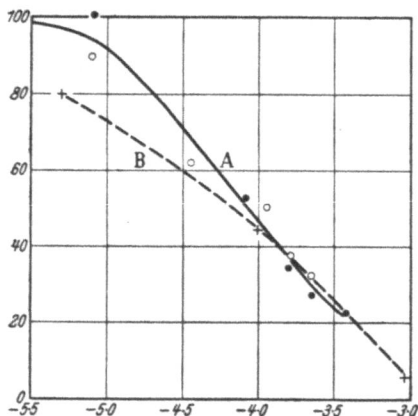

Fig. 8. Action of cyanide on living cells. Abscissa:— log. molar conc. Ordinate:— per cent. activity. *A* Uptake of oxygen by *Paramoecium caudatum*. (ALLEN, 1919[9].) *B* Assimilation of carbon dioxide by *Chlorella*. (WARBURG and UYESUGI, 1924[8].)

The figures of WARBURG and UYESUGI (1924)[8] show a linear relation between log. concentration cyanide and the amount of inhibition produced in the carbon dioxide assimilation of *Chlorella* (fig. 8, curve *B*), and also the inhibition of the destruction of hydrogen peroxide.

The figures obtained by ALLEN (1919)[9] for the inhibition by cyanide of the oxygen uptake of *Paramoecium caudatum* also show an approximately linear relation between log. concentration and inhibition as is shown in fig. 8, curve *A*.

[1] LIPSCHITZ, W., and A. GOTTSCHALK: Pflügers Arch. **191**, 1 (1921).
[2] LIPSCHITZ, W., and A. GOTTSCHALK: Pflügers Arch. **191**, 33 (1921).
[3] WARBURG, O.: Hoppe-Seylers Z. **76**, 331 (1911).
[4] MEYERHOF, O.: Pflügers Arch. **165**, 229 (1916).
[5] PICKFORD, L. M.: J. of Physiol. **63**, 19 (1927).
[6] DALE, A.: J. of Physiol. **89**, 316 (1937).
[7] WARBURG, O.: Hoppe-Seylers Z. **66**, 305 (1910) — Biochem. Z. **166**, 386 (1925).
[8] WARBURG, O., and T. UYESUGI: Biochem. Z. **146**, 486 (1924).
[9] ALLEN, G. D.: Amer. J. Physiol. **48**, 93 (1919).

The slope of the curves approximates to that shown by the central portion of the hyperbola which follows the formula $Kx = \dfrac{y}{100 - y}$.

These examples show that in the case of cyanide a characteristic relation, which suggests a reversible monomolecular reaction, is in some cases found to exist between the concentrations of cyanide and the amount of inhibition of pure enzymes, and this same relation occurs fairly frequently with a considerable variety of animal and vegetable cells.

Cyanides therefore are an example of a group of drugs whose mode of action seems fairly clear. The facts observed can be explained on the theory that the oxygen uptake of the cells is dependent on oxidases situated on the cell surface, and that cyanide forms a reversible compound with these oxidases.

The effect of cyanide in inhibiting the activity of the frog's heart cannot however be explained as being due solely to the inhibition of oxygen uptake because cyanide inhibits the activity of the normal frog's heart tissue in a few minutes, and this tissue can maintain anaerobic activity for hours under suitable conditions. It is probable that cyanide not only inhibits oxygen uptake but also inhibits glycolysis. It is interesting to note that the concentration-action relation of the inhibition of glycolysis appears to be similar to that of the inhibition of oxygen uptake.

**Diphasic Actions of Cyanide.** In many cases traces of cyanide increase the activity of enzymes and of cells, and this effect can be shown to be due to the cyanide inactivating the traces of heavy metals which are present in all distilled water which is condensed on metal surfaces.

Another apparent diphasic effect of cyanide depends on the fact that it inhibits respiration at much lower concentrations than those needed to affect glycolysis or fermentation. Consequently cyanide in low concentration in many cells causes a marked increase in glycolysis or fermentation whilst higher concentrations inhibit all cellular activity.

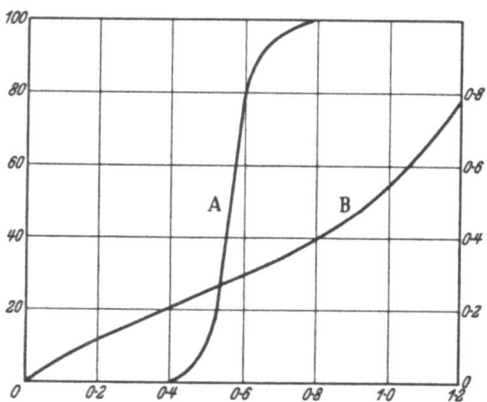

Fig. 9. Uptake of phenol by yeast and action produced. Abscissa:— per cent. conc. phenol. $A$ Per cent. mortality of yeast cells. (Left ordinate.) $B$ Per cent. conc. of phenol in cells. (Right ordinate.) (HERZOG and BETZEL, 1911[2].)

**Phenol Compounds.** RONA and BACH (1921)[1] found that p-nitrophenol acting on invertase showed a steep all-or-none effect, because the concentration needed to produce 84 p.c. inhibition was only 3 times that required to produce 16 p.c. inhibition. Similar results have been obtained in living cells. HERZOG and BETZEL (1911)[2] (fig. 9) showed that this was the case in the killing of yeast cells by phenol. MEIER (1927)[3] showed a similar all-or-none effect produced by phenol acting on the fermentation of yeast (fig. 10). KRAHL and CLOWES (1935)[4] showed the same type of action in the case of dichlorophenol acting on both the

[1] RONA, P., and E. BACH: Biochem. Z. **118**, 232 (1921).
[2] HERZOG, R. A., and R. BETZEL: Hoppe-Seylers Z. **74**, 221 (1911).
[3] MEIER, R.: Arch. f. exper. Path. **122**, 129 (1927).
[4] KRAHL, M. E., and G. H. A. CLOWES: Proc. Soc. exper. Biol. a. Med. **33**, 477 (1935).

respiration and the cell divisions of arbacia eggs (fig. 11). They obtained similar results with dinitrophenol and trichlorophenol.

These two latter cases also provide examples of complex drug actions. The phenol acting on the yeast caused a simple depression of respiration, but first

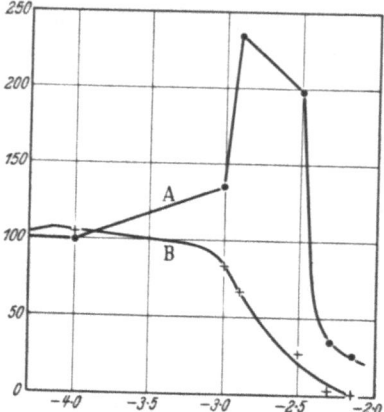

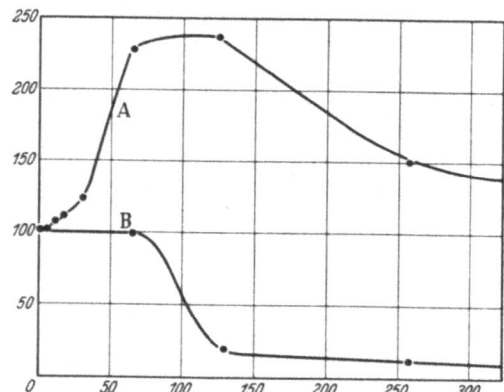

Fig. 10. Action of phenol on (A) fermentation and (B) respiration of *Torula*. Abscissa: — log. conc. Ordinate: — activity as per cent. normal. (MEIER, 1927[1].)

Fig. 11. Action of di-chloro-phenol on (A) oxygen consumption and (B) cell division of Arbacia eggs. Abscissa: — Molar conc. × 10[6]; ordinate: — activity as per cent. normal. (KRAHL and CLOWES, 1935[2].)

stimulated and then depressed fermentation. The stimulation of fermentation may reasonably be considered a secondary effect due to the interference with respiration. In the case of dichlorophenol acting on arbacia eggs, the respiration is first stimulated and then depressed, whilst the effect on cell division is purely inhibitory. The reason for the stimulation of oxygen consumption by substituted phenols is unknown.

The all-or-none lethal action of phenol can easily be explained by the fact that phenol has an all-or-none action in coagulating proteins (COOPER and SANDERS, 1927[3]), but the fact that stimulant actions of simple phenol compounds show this all-or-none effect is more difficult to explain.

The point of chief interest is that a similar concentration-action relation is found with proteins, enzymes and living cells.

**The Action of Narcotics.** The action of aliphatic narcotics has been studied intensively, for the last 40 years, and the literature is very extensive. Reviews of this literature have been given by WINTERSTEIN (1926)[4] and KOCHMANN (1923 and 1936)[5].

It is not possible to review here this extensive and controversial literature but there are certain salient facts regarding the action of narcotics that are of interest to the present discussion.

**Action of Narcotics on Enzymes.** The action of narcotics on enzymes is in some cases dependent on the degree of purification. For example MEYERHOF (1914)[6] found that invertase was inhibited by ethyl alcohol (fig. 12) whereas SCHÜRMEYER (1925)[7] found that saccharase, which has been purified until it was almost protein free, was not inhibited by ethyl alcohol.

[1] MEIER, R. Arch. f. exper. Path. **122**, 129 (1927).
[2] KRAHL, M. E., and G. H. A. CLOWES: Proc. Soc. exper. Biol. a. Med. **33**, 477 (1935).
[3] COOPER, E. A., and E. SAUNDERS: J. physic. Chem. **31**, 1 (1927).
[4] WINTERSTEIN, H.: Die Narkose. 2. Aufl. Berlin: Julius Springer 1926.
[5] KOCHMANN, M.: Heffters Handb. exper. Pharmakol. **1**, 449 (1923); Ergänzbd. **2**, 1 (1936).
[6] MEYERHOF, O.: Pflügers Arch. **157**, 251, 307 (1914).
[7] SCHÜRMEYER, A.: Pflügers Arch. **208**, 595; **210**, 753 (1925).

GLICK and KING (1932)[1] and SOBOTKA and GLICK (1934)[2] found that substances which lower surface tensions inhibit liver esterase but in low concentrations activate liver lipase. In the case of octyl alcohol acting on liver esterase low concentrations produce slight activation but higher concentrations cause inhibition.

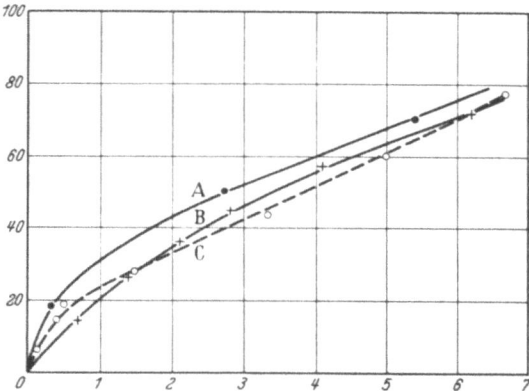

They accounted for this diphasic action on the theory that the surface alcohol competed with the substrate not only for the active patches on the enzyme but also for the inactive portions of the enzyme surface, and thus, in certain concentrations favoured the union of the substrate with the active portions of the enzyme surface. A considerable number of enzymes are poisoned by narcotics and a survey of the evidence shows two important facts namely that the action of aliphatic narcotics on enzymes follows the law of the homologous series and that the relation

Fig. 12. Concentration-action relations of alcohols. Abscissa:— molar conc.; ordinate:— per cent. inhibition. *A* Inhibition of catalytic activity of colloidal platinum by i-butyl alcohol (conc. × 10). (MEYERHOF, 1914[3].) *B* Inhibition of invertase by ethyl alcohol. (MEYERHOF, 1914[3].) *C* Inhibition of succino-dehydrogenase by n-propyl alcohol (conc. × 5). (GRÖNVALL, 1923[4].)

between concentration and amount of action approximates to the linear one. The law of the homologous series states that when the actions of the members of such a series are compared there is a regular increase in activity with each increase in the number of carbon atoms. WINTERSTEIN gives a large number of examples of this fact.

A few examples of the action of alcohols on ferments are given in Table 9

Table 9. Molar concentrations of normal alcohols producing 50 per cent. inhibition of enzyme activity.

| Alcohols | Pig liver lipase (KERNOT and HILLS 1933[5]) | | Succino-dehydrogenase (GRÖNVALL 1923[4]) | | Precipitation of liver nucleo-proteins at 40° C (BATELLI and STERN 1913[6]) | |
|---|---|---|---|---|---|---|
| | Conc. | Ratio | Conc. | Ratio | Conc. | Ratio |
| Methyl . . . . | | | 6 | | 7.24 | |
| | | 2.6 | | 2.7 | | 2.1 |
| Ethyl . . . . . | 0.69 | | 2.2 | | 3.50 | |
| | | 3.6 | | 2.7 | | 2.4 |
| Propyl. . . . . | 0.26 | | 0.8 | | 1.49 | |
| | | 2.4 | | 2.0 | | 2.4 |
| Butyl . . . . . | 0.073 | | 0.4 | | 0.63 | |
| | | 1.9 | | | | 2.4 |
| Amyl . . . . . | 0.030 | | — | | 0.26 | |
| | | 3.4 | | | | |
| Hexyl . . . . . | 0.017 | | — | | — | |
| | | 1,8 | | | | |
| Octyl . . . . . | 0.005 | | — | | — | |

[1] GLICK, D., and C. G. KING: J. of biol. Chem. **97**, 673 (1932).
[2] SOBOTKA, H., and D. GLICK: J. of biol. Chem. **105**, 199 (1934).
[3] MEYERHOF, O.: Pflügers Arch. **157**, 251, 307 (1914).
[4] GRÖNVALL, H.: Skand. Arch. Physiol. (Berl. u. Lpz.) **44**, 200 (1923).
[5] KERNOT, J. C., and H. W. HILLS: Hoppe-Seylers Z. **222**, 11 (1933).
[6] BATELLI, F., and L. STERN: Biochem. Z. **52**, 226 (1913).

to illustrate this well known fact. Exactly similar series have been obtained with other homologous series such as the urethanes.

The relation between concentration and amount of inhibition of ferments is illustrated in fig. 12. Curve $A$ shows the action of alcohol on an inorganic catalyst. This must be a simple adsorption process and the curve obtained suggests an adsorption curve. The other two curves approximate to a linear relation but are sligthly curved.

The difference between the curves is shown more clearly when they are plotted on a logarithmic scale (fig. 13). Curve $A$ approximates to a rectangular hyperbola, but the other two curves have a totally different shape.

The simplest explanation of the latter two curves is that they represent the lower half of an adsorption curve. If the alcohol produced full inhibition when it covered half the surface of the enzyme, then a curve of the shapes of $B$ and $C$ would be obtained. Curve $C$ has actually been drawn to the formula $Kx = \dfrac{y}{160 - y}$. In this case it is assumed that the surface is half saturated when 80 p.c. inhibition has been produced ($K = 0.71$). This assumption can be supported by analogies from inorganic catalyst since RIDEAL and WRIGHT (1925)[1] found that autoxidation of charcoal was completely inhibited by amyl alcohol when the amount adsorbed was only sufficient to cover 0.38 p.c. of the surface.

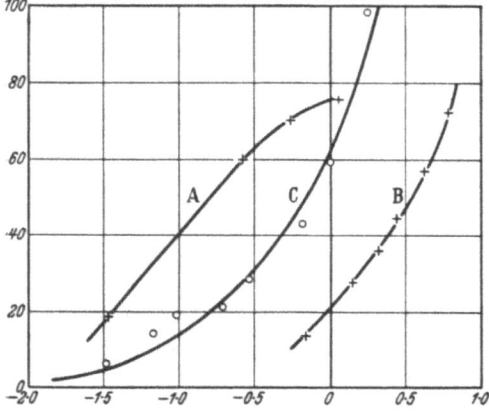

Fig. 13. Concentration-action relations of alcohols on logarithmic scale. Data from fig. 12. Abscissa:— log. molar conc. Ordinate:— per cent. inhibition.

These actions of alcohols on enzymes are of interest because they throw some light on the probable mode of action of narcotics on cells. The action of narcotics on cells has been interpreted as dependent on (a) differential lipoid solubility (OVERTON and MEYER) and (b) power of reducing surface tension (TRAUBE) and (c) adsorption and consequent blanketing of surfaces (WARBURG).

The ferments are lipoid-free and hence the first explanation will not hold in their case. The second and third explanations differ but little in practice because the lowering of surface tension of a water/air interspace is proportional to the intensity with which a substance is attracted to a water surface and this is likely to be similar for a water/air surface or for a water/solid surface. The fact that the law of homologous series holds for non-lipoid systems as well as for living cells shows that it does not simply depend on lipoid solubility, but if it is dependent on surface adsorption this is easily explained. The approximately linear relation between concentration and action of narcotics is usually considered evidence of their action depending on HENRY's law, but as has been shown this relation can also be explained as a portion of an adsorption curve.

Direct proof of the fact that narcotics coat surfaces is provided by the manner in which they protect surfaces from other poisons. WARBURG first showed this effect in the case of the action of cyanides on cystin oxidation by charcoal but it has also been shown in the case of other ferments.

---

[1] RIDEAL, E. K., and W. M. WRIGHT: J. chem. Soc. (Lond.) **127**, 1347 (1925).

RONA, AIRILA and LAS-NITZKI (1922)[1] studied the action of quinine and narcotics on invertase: and found that various alcohols and urethanes interfered with the inhibitory action of quinine.

LIPSCHITZ and GOTT-SCHALK (1921)[2] studied the action of narcotics on the reduction of di-nitro-phenol by minced frog's muscles. Their results agree with those of other workers in showing an approximately linear relation between concentration and action. They also showed that a narcotic such as ethyl urethane interfered with the action of quinine in the manner shown in Table 10 and had a similar effect on the action of cyanide as is shown in Table 11.

The results quoted agree in showing that the addition of a narcotic to an enzyme poison tends to interfere with the action of the poison, an effect which cannot be easily explained except by the hypothesis that the narcotic covers the enzyme surface and prevents fixation of the second drug.

**Action of Narcotics on Cells.** The outstanding features of narcotic action on enzymes are also found with living cells. In all cases where a series of related narcotics has been studied a regular increase of activity in proportion to the increase in the length of the carbon chain has been found. Fig. 14 shows the variation in the intensity of a few of the inhibitory actions produced by the normal alcohols (methyl-dodecyl) and also shows that the iso-capillary concentrations vary in the same manner. The curves show that the addition of each carbon atom increases the action on the surface tension 2.9 times and increases the action on biological systems 3.6 times.

Table 10. Action of quinine and urethane on the power of frog's muscle pulp to reduce di-nitro-phenol. (LIPSCHITZ and GOTTSCHALK, 1921[2].)

| Drug | Per cent. inhibition of enzyme action |
|---|---|
| (a) Quinine 0.0015 mol. . . . . . . . | 39,7 |
| (b) Ethyl urethane 0.45 mol. . . . . | 26.2 |
| (c) Quinine 0.0015 mol. and ethyl urethane 0.45 mol. . . . . . . | 44 |

Table 11. Action of cyanide and urethane on the power of frog's muscle pulp to reduce di-nitro-phenol. (LIPSCHITZ and GOTTSCHALK, 1921[2].)

| Drug | Per cent. inhibition of enzyme action |
|---|---|
| (a) Potassium cyanide 0.0046 mol. . . | 62 |
| (b) Ethyl urethane 0.678 mol. . . . . | 46 |
| (c) KCN 0.0046 mol. and ethyl urethane 0.678 mol. . . . . . . | 59 |

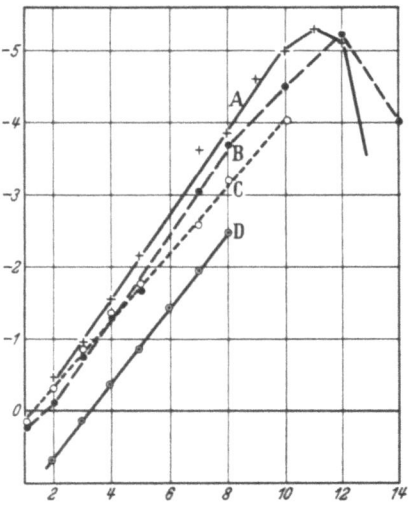

Fig. 14. Relations between length of carbon chain and activity of normal alcohols. Abscissa:— number of carbon atoms. Ordinate:— log. molar conc. which produces the action selected for comparison. *A* Narcosis of tadpoles. (MEYER and HEMMI, 1935[3].) *B* Inhibition (50 per cent.) of isolated frog's ventricle. (CLARK, 1930[4].) *C* Concentration reducing water/air surface tension to 63 dyne/cm. *D* Concentration lethal to *B. typhosus.* (TILLEY and SCHAFFER, 1926[5].)

Series of this type have been found with living systems varying from the depression of respiration of unicellular organisms to the depression of reflexes

[1] RONA, P., V. AIRILA and A. LASNITZKI: Biochem. Z. **130**, 582 (1922).
[2] LIPSCHITZ, W., and A. GOTTSCHALK: Pflügers Arch. **191**, 1 (1921).
[3] MEYER, K. H., and H. HEMMI: Biochem. Z. **277**, 39 (1935).
[4] CLARK, A. J.: Arch. int. Pharmacodyn. **38**, 101 (1930).
[5] TILLEY, F. W., and J. M. SCHAFFER: J. Bacter. **12**, 303 (1926).

in mammals. The evidence has been summarised by WINTERSTEIN (1926)[1]. Approximately linear relations between concentration of narcotics and amount of action have been found with a very wide range of systems, e.g. Respiration of nitrosomas, MEYERHOF (1917)[2]; of sea urchin eggs, MEYERHOF (1914)[3]; of frog's heart, CLARK and WHITE (1928)[4]. Reduction of nitrophenol by frog's muscle, LIPSCHITZ and GOTTSCHALK (1921)[5]. Mechanical response of frog's heart, CLARK (1930)[4]. Mammalian reflexes, STORM VAN LEEUWEN and LE HEUX (1919)[6].

The inhibition of the respiration of nitrobacter (MEYERHOF, 1916[7]) by ethyl alcohol is an exception to this rule since the concentration-action curves approximate to an all-or-none effect. In this case however the higher alcohols and also the urethanes gave approximately linear concentration-action curves and therefore the single atypical relation has no certain significance. Examination of the concentration-action curves which have been obtained on material best suited for accurate quantitative measurement shows that in most cases the relation is not linear but slightly curved. Fig. 15 shows results obtained by CLARK for depression of the frog's ventricle by ethyl alcohols together with the depression produced in the air/water surface tension and the amount of alcohol fixed by the tortoise ventricle.

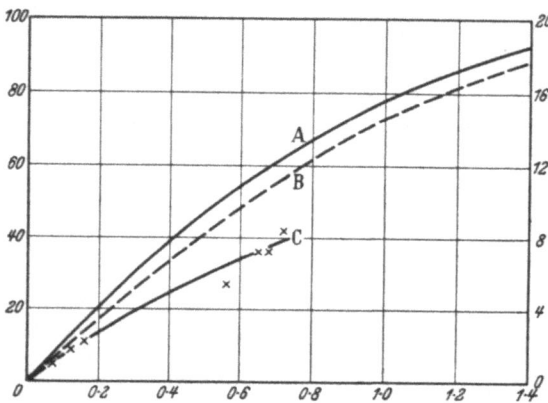

Fig. 15. Concentration-action relations of ethyl alcohol. Abscissa: — per cent. inhibition. Ordinates: — as below. *A* Lowering of air/water surface tension in dyne/cm. (right ordinate). *B* Per cent. inhibition of mechanical response of frog's ventricle (left ordinate). *C* Molar conc. (× 100) of ethyl alcohol taken up by isolated tortoise's heart (left ordinate). (ROBERTSON and CLARK, 1933[8].)

ROBERTSON and CLARK (1933)[8] have shown that the approximate linear relation between concentration and action produced by narcotics on cells can be accounted for in the same manner as the similar effects produced by narcotics on ferments, namely as a portion of an adsorption curve.

**Theories of Narcotic Action.** This problem has been summarised by WINTERSTEIN (1926)[9] and a recent important contribution has been made by MEYER and HEMMI (1935)[10] who support the theory that narcosis occurs when the narcotic attains a certain critical concentration in the cell lipoids. In the case of tadpoles they found that this concentration was 0.03 mol./litre.

The writer considers that the following points are of particular importance in relation to this problem.

The action of narcotics upon ferment activity in vitro and in vivo shows a very close resemblance, much closer than is found with most drugs (e.g. heavy

[1] WINTERSTEIN, H.: Die Narkose, p. 267ff. 2. Aufl. Berlin: Julius Springer 1926.
[2] MEYERHOF, O.: Pflügers Arch. **166**, 240 (1917).
[3] MEYERHOF, O.: Pflügers Arch. **137**, 307 (1914).
[4] CLARK, A. J., and A. C. WHITE: J. of Physiol. **66**, 185 (1928).
[5] LIPSCHITZ, W., and A. GOTTSCHALK: Pflügers Arch. **191**, 1 (1921).
[6] STORM VAN LEEUWEN, W., and J. W. LE HEUX: Pflügers Arch. **177**, 250 (1919).
[7] MEYERHOF, O.: Pflügers Arch. **164**, 353 (1916).
[8] ROBERTSON, J., and A. J. CLARK: Biochemic. J. **27**, 83 (1933).
[9] WINTERSTEIN, H.: Die Narkose, pp. 176—407. 2. Aufl. Berlin: Julius Springer 1926.
[10] MEYER, K. H., and H. HEMMI: Biochem. Z. **277**, 39 (1935).

metals). This makes it very probable that the mode of action is similar in the two cases, and the adsorption theory will account for this similarity. On the other hand it is difficult to explain the similarity of action on ferments in vitro and in vivo on the theory of differential solubility. The adsorption theory as set forth by WARBURG appears therefore to be preferable.

The fact of outstanding interest to the writer is that the mode of action of narcotics is still a matter of dispute, in spite of the facts that narcotics are in many respects exceptionally favourable subjects for the study of drug action and have been studied intensively with quantitative methods for the last 40 years.

The reason for this uncertainty is the deficiency of our knowledge of cell structure and cell function. The study of narcotic action actually has been used as a method for ascertaining the nature of the cell surface, but naturally this has not yielded much conclusive evidence.

**Discussion.** The comparison of the action of enzyme poisons on purified enzymes and on living cells shows that in some cases the concentration-action relations differ markedly in the two cases. With both heavy metals and quinine acting upon purified ferments there is an approximately linear relation between the log. of the concentration and the effect, but when these drugs are applied to cells an all-or-none effect is observed. This result suggests that the living cells have some defence mechanism which prevents the drug producing an effect until a critical concentration is attained, and that once this resistance is overcome a full inhibition is rapidly produced.

In the case of cyanides, phenols and narcotics there is however a marked resemblance between the concentration-action curves obtained with enzymes in vitro and living cells. This indicates that these drugs poison enzymes in cells in a manner similar to that in which they poison purified enzymes.

Cyanides, narcotics and phenols are the three groups of drugs which show the clearest relation between action on purified enzymes and action on cells. In the case of cyanides and of narcotics micro-injection experiments indicate that these act on the cell surface and not on the cell interior. The action of cyanides can be interpreted as a reversible chemical reaction between cyanide and a metal containing respiratory ferment. The action of narcotics can be interpreted as a simple blanketing effect produced by adsorption of the drugs on the cell surface. The action of phenol and of substituted phenols suggests some effect caused by alteration of the cell proteins which results in a fairly abrupt change when a certain threshold concentration has been reached. It will be shown later that a number of important drugs show concentration-action curves resembling those found with cyanide, and the simplest explanation of these resemblances is to assume that in all these cases the drug forms a reversible compound with a limited number of receptors on the cell surface.

Chapter 8

# Concentration-action Relations I.

The following three chapters (8, 9 and 10) give an account of the manner in which the actions of drugs on cells can be classified according to the relations observed between the concentration of the drug and the action produced. This relation has been chosen as the basis of classification for the following reasons.

The study of the poisoning of enzymes *in vitro* and *in vivo* shows that in many cases the poisoning of purified solutions of enzymes can be interpreted in a satisfactory manner as a relatively simple chemical reaction.

These studies show, however, that quantitative measurements of the amount of drug fixed give disappointing results. Even in the case of highly purified enzymes it is known that the amount of inhibition produced is not necessarily proportional to the amount of metal fixed, because the metal can unite with portions of the enzyme molecule other than the active groups. In the case of metals acting on enzymes within cells this deviation in greatly increased and only a small fraction of the metal fixed is responsible for the selective inhibition of the enzyme.

Quantitative measurements of the amount of enzyme poisons fixed by cells, therefore, only provide information regarding the maximum amount of poison that can be concerned with the production of any particular action, but the actual amount responsible for the effect is known in many cases to be only a small fraction of this maximum amount.

The study of the kinetics of drug action on ferments and on unicellular organisms also gives disappointing results, because of the difficulty in determining what process is causing the delay which is being measured.

Hence even in the case of relatively simple systems such as enzymes, the standard methods employed in physical chemistry for determining the nature of a reaction are of limited value, and it is to be expected that these methods will provide still more uncertain evidence in the case of living cells, which are far more complex systems than are purified enzymes.

The study of the relations between concentration of drug and amount of action produced when time is allowed for equilibrium to be attained does, however, provide information which, although indirect, is interesting and suggestive, because different drugs show widely different relations between concentration and action and a single drug often shows similar relations when acting on widely different systems.

## (1) Classification of Concentration-action Curves.

Enzyme poisons show at least three varieties of concentration-action curves, namely:—

(1) Curves attributable to mass action reactions, i.e. hyperbolae and linear relations between action and log. concentration.

(2) An approximately linear relation between concentration and action. This relation is nearly always shown by aliphatic narcotics and occasionally by other drugs.

(3) All-or-none effects.

These three types of relations have been found in a variety of biological relations. STORM VAN LEEUWEN and LE HEUX (1919)[1] pointed out that three types of relations existed between drug concentration or dosage and the effects produced on mammalian tissues.

(a) A simple linear relation, e.g. narcotics depressing reflexes.

(b) A linear relation between logarithm of dosage and effect, e.g. morphine depressing reflexes.

(c) A sigmoid relation indicating an all-or-none effect, e.g. action of histamine on isolated uterus.

The writer has shown (1933[2], fig. 31) that three similar types of curves can be obtained in a single tissue, namely the frog's heart. In this case the following relations occur:—

---

[1] STORM VAN LEEUWEN, W., and J. W. LE HEUX: Pflügers Arch. **177**, 250 (1919).
[2] CLARK, A. J.: The Mode of Action of Drugs on Cells. London: Arnold and Co. 1933.

(a) Linear—aliphatic narcotics,
(b) Hyperbola—acetylcholine,
(c) Sigmoid or all-or-none—potassium chloride.

The general aim of this article is to indicate the possible nature of the reactions that occur between drugs and cells, hence it is necessary to consider what physico-chemical processes are likely to be responsible for these processes.

**Relations Depending on Mass-action.** The actions of poisons on enzymes or on cells in many cases can be interpreted as the result of the poison forming a reversible combination with receptors on the enzyme or in the cell. The simplest conditions occur when one molecule of drug occupies one receptor, and the drug is present in excess so that its concentration does not change during the course of the reaction. HITCHCOCK (1926)[1] pointed out that under these conditions those equations applied, which LANGMUIR found to express the simplest case of the adsorption of gases by metal surfaces. These equations can be expressed as follows:—

If the total number of receptors $= 100$, and the percentage of receptors occupied $= y$, then the percentage of free receptors $= 100 - y$. If the concentration of drug in solution $= x$, and this is not altered significantly by the reaction, then:—

(1) The rate of combination varies as $x(100 - y)$.
(2) The rate of dissociation varies as $y$.
(3) Equilibrium occurs when $K_1 \cdot x(100 - y) = K_2 y$ or

$$K x = \frac{y}{100 - y}.$$

LANGMUIR (1917)[2] has shown that this simple relation may be modified in various ways. If two molecules of drug unite with one receptor then the rate of combination varies as $x^2$ and the equilibrium is expressed by the formula

$$K x^2 = \frac{y}{100 - y}.$$

If one molecule of the drug unites with two receptors which must be adjacent, then the rate of combination will vary as $(100 - y)^2$, and if two adjacent portions must be freed simultaneously to permit liberation of a molecule from the surface, then the rate of dissociation will vary as $y^2$.

Hence $$K x = \frac{y^2}{(100 - y)^2} \quad \text{or} \quad K x^{\frac{1}{2}} = \frac{y}{100 - y}.$$

The curve expressed by the formula $K x = \dfrac{y}{100 - y}$ is a hyperbola and has certain important characteristics. In the first place there is an approximate linear relation between $y$ and $\log x$, between the values $y = 16$ p.c. and $y = 84$ p.c.

With this formula the ratio between the values of $x$ for 16 p.c. ($C_{16}$) and 84 p.c. ($C_{84}$) action is $1/27$, and hence, when a linear relation is found between $y$ and log. $x$ over a considerable range of concentration, the slope of the line indicates whether or not the above mentioned formula will interpret the results. This fact is of importance because it is difficult to obtain accurate data outside the limits 16—84 p.c. action and logarithmic relations are extremely common in biological data. Measurement of the ratio between $C_{16}$ and $C_{84}$ will often decide whether or not the effect can be interpreted by a simple mass-action formula. A wide variety of slopes can, however, be interpreted by one or other

[1] HITCHCOCK, D. I. H.: J. amer. chem. Soc. **48**, 2870 (1926).
[2] LANGMUIR, I.: Amer. chem. Soc. Abstr. **11**, 2422 (1917).

of LANGMUIR's formulae which have been described above; for example when $\frac{y}{100-y} = Kx$, there is a ratio of $\frac{1}{27}$ between the values of $x$ for $y = 16$ and $y = 84$, but when the formula becomes $\frac{y}{100-y} = Kx^2$, the corresponding ratio is 5.2, and in cases where the formula is $\frac{y}{100-y} = Kx^{\frac{1}{2}}$, the ratio is 730.

In the second place the general formula given above shows a nearly linear relation between concentration and action between the values $y = 0$ and $y = 20$ p.c. of the maximum. Hence, if a drug produces its full effect when only a small fraction of the available receptors are saturated, then there will be a nearly linear relation between concentration and action. The writer believes that this is a probable explanation of the approximately linear relation so frequently found between the concentration of narcotics and their effects.

Experimental conditions can usually be arranged so that the drug is present in excess, and hence its concentration does not change significantly. If, however, the drug is not present in excess the relation between drug concentration and effect will be more complex. In most cases, however, it is either certain or strongly probable that only a small fraction of the drug fixed is responsible for the effect observed and hence relations of this latter type are difficult to interpret.

It will be seen that the mass-action or adsorption formulae are somewhat dangerous because they can provide an explanation for such a wide variety of relations, moreover the application of these formulae to biological data involves certain assumptions which are unproven. In the first place the formulae assume that the receptors in a cell resemble the surface of a polished metal, in that they are all equally accessible to the drug. In the second place the interpretation assumes that the amount of biological effect produced is directly proportional to the number of specific receptors occupied by the drug. Both these assumptions seem improbable and hence the fitting of data by these formulae does not provide any certain proof of the occurrence of any particular physico-chemical process. On the other hand it will be shown that numerous concentration-action relations in biological systems of varying degrees of complexity can be explained by these formulae and the general resemblance between the relations observed in these widely different systems suggests the probability of some physio-chemical process common to all cases.

**All-or-None Effects.** This term implies that a drug produces no effect until a certain concentration is attained and then a further and relatively small increase in concentration produces a maximum response. Since no cell populations are completely uniform a sharp all-or-none reaction is never obtained and the usual result seen is a sigmoid curve, of greater or less steepness. These all-or-none effects may be due to some peculiarity either of the drug or of the tissue. For example excess of potassium produces an all-or-none effect on tissues such as the frog's heart, which show a graded response to other drugs. On the other hand the guinea pig's uterus tends to respond in an all-or-none fashion to most drugs, including certain ones such as pilocarpine which produce a graded effect on other tissues.

In some cases the all-or-none effect can be attributed with certainty to some particular form of chemical action. For example the precipitation of protein by phenol shows an all-or-none relation between concentration and amount of action, and hence it is to be expected that a similar relation will be obtained when phenol acts on cells. In other cases, it is fairly certain that the all-or-none effect is due to the distortion of some chemical reaction. For example, the poisoning of purified ferments by heavy metals and by quinine shows a relation between concentration and action that can be attributed to a mass-action effect, but the poisoning of ferments in cells by these drugs shows a sigmoid relation between concentration and action. This latter relation may be due to the cell surface offering a resistance to the entrance of the metal and hence preventing any effect until a concentration sufficient to break down this resistance has been attained. If in any system where a chain of actions occurs between the drug and the tissue, any stage is a fairly sharp all-or-none effect, this form will be imposed on all subsequent stages.

All-or-none effects are of less interest than relations which show graded response over a wide range of drug concentrations because the former can be produced by a variety of causes, and the only information they give regarding the nature of the action of the drug is that a particular effect occurs when a certain critical concentration of drug has been attained. Moreover in the cases where these curves are due to some peculiarity of the tissue causing an all-or-none response to a chemical action, their shape expresses chiefly the individual variation of the population of cells upon which the drug acts.

### (2) Concentration-action Relations Attributable to Mass-action Laws.

The concentration-action relations which approximate to a rectangular hyperbola are of exceptional interest because this class includes a large proportion of the hormones and of the more powerful alkaloids; furthermore the action of the narcotics can be interpreted as following a portion of a hyperbola.

STORM VAN LEEUWEN and LE HEUX (1919)[1] pointed out that the relation between the dosage of morphine and the amount of depression of reflexes produced approximated to a linear relation between log. dosage and effect. A large number of other authors have found a similar relation with a variety of drugs and in most cases have merely quoted the effect as an example of WEBER's law. This statement does not, however, connect the drug action with any recognisable physico-chemical action and for this reason is unsatisfactory.

The writer's hypothesis is that these logarithmic relations really represent portions of a rectangular hyperbola. The evidence in support of this theory is as follows. This relation is found in the case of many drugs which react with active proteins in a manner which can be measured quantitatively, e.g. carbon monoxide on haemoglobin, and many enzyme poisons.

In the case of some enzyme poisons it can be shown that the relation between concentration and action follows a rectangular hyperbola both when the poisons act on purified enzymes and when they inhibit the enzymatic activity of cells (e.g. cyanides).

In the case of many potent drugs (e.g. acetylcholine and adrenaline) it can be shown that the relation between concentration and action, when studied over the whole range of possible action, follows a rectangular hyperbola and the extremes of action show a clear deviation from the linear relation between log. concentration and effect. The mode of action of these drugs is unknown but the writer considers that the resemblance between the concentration-action curves of these hormones and of enzyme poisons justifies the hypothesis that the hormones form a reversible chemical combination with a limited number of receptors in the cell.

The chief aim of this article is to discover the probable nature of the reaction between drugs and cells and in relation to this problem the hypotheses outlined above are of dominant importance.

---

[1] STORM VAN LEEUWEN, W., and J. W. LE HEUX: Pflügers Arch. **177**, 250 (1919).

The validity of these hypotheses can best be tested by a careful consideration of the evidence existing in the case of drugs that have been studied most fully. Acetylcholine and adrenaline also deserve special consideration, not only because they have been studied exhaustively, but also because a knowledge of their mode of action is of importance in relation to the theory of the humoral transmission of nerve impulses. The narcotics are another group of special interest because our conceptions of the nature of the cell surface are to some extent based on the mode of action of these drugs.

**The Mode of Action of Acetylcholine.** In the case of enzyme poisons a certain amount is known about the relation between the chemical action of the drug and the biological effect produced. For example, if the fermentation of yeast is arrested by a heavy metal it is fairly certain that the inhibition is due to a combination of the metal with the active group of the enzyme. In the case of a hormone such as acetylcholine we only know that, when the drug is brought into contact with certain tissues, a characteristic response follows, but there is no evidence to show what kind of chemical process produces this effect, and we do not even know whether it is due to a chemical reaction between the drug and the cell.

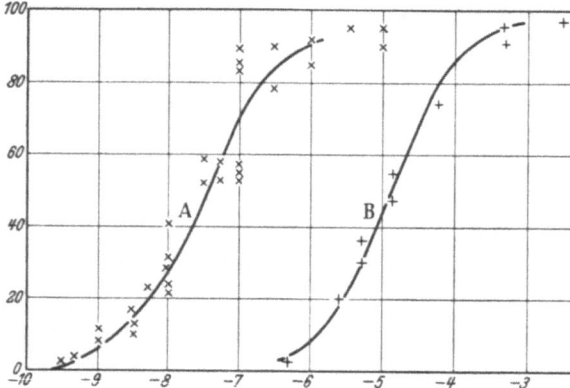

Fig. 16. Concentration-action relations of acetylcholine. Abscissa:— log. molar conc. Ordinate: — per cent. action. *A* Inhibition of isometric response of isolated frog's ventricle. (CLARK, 1927[1].) *B* Contracture of *Rectus abdominis* of frog. (CLARK, 1926[2].)

The first outstanding feature of acetylcholine action is that the relation between concentration and action extends over a wide range of concentrations. The actions of acetylcholine on the frog's heart or rectus abdominis are effects which are exceptionally easy to measure, because the actions are fairly rapidly produced and are fully reversible. Consequently a series of observations can be made on a single tissue and errors due to individual variation in tissues can be eliminated.

Measurements of this type are shown in fig. 16 and the results show with some certainty that an inhibition of 20 p.c. is produced by about one twentieth the concentration needed to produce 80 p.c. inhibition. The scatter of the observations at these two points shows, however, that they are only accurate within ± 5%. The results for concentrations outside this range are even more difficult to measure with certainty. In the case of the frog's ventricle the measurement of a small amount of inhibition is difficult because the activity of the ventricle is not absolutely constant, whilst the accurate measurement of more than 95 p.c. of inhibition can only be made if the method of recording is very free from instrumental error.

In the case of the rectus abdominis measurements of actions less than 10 p.c. of the maximum can, however, be made with considerable accuracy although in this case the maximum effect cannot be determined accurately and hence measure-

---

[1] CLARK, A. J.: J. of Physiol. **64**, 123 (1927).
[2] CLARK, A. J.: J. of Physiol. **61**, 530 (1926).

ments between 80 and 100 p.c. action are uncertain. The frog's heart and rectus abdominis together, however, provided fairly accurate information over nearly the whole range of possible action.

With regard to the curves shown in fig. 16 it is important to remember the following facts.

(a) The relation from 0—30 p.c. action closely approximates to a simple linear relation between concentration and action.

(b) The relation from 0—70 p.c. action can be interpreted as an expression of WEBER's law $[Ky = \log. (ax + 1)]$.

(c) The relation from 30—60 p.c. action can be interpreted as an expression of FREUNDLICH's adsorption formula $[Kx^n = y]$.

The writer found that in actual practice none of these relations expressed the experimental results as closely as did the application of the mass-action formula $\left(Kx = \dfrac{y}{100 - x}\right)$. Moreover this formula has the advantage that it expresses a recognisable physico-chemical process the occurrence of which is possible. It is obvious, however, from the facts mentioned above that a reasonable probability in favour of any formula can only be obtained if the experimental data cover the whole range of possible biological effects. Furthermore, it is unreasonable to expect great accuracy because the data must be subject to many uncontrollable errors: for example, it is highly improbable that all the receptors in the cells of a frog's ventricle are equally accessible to the drug.

Various other writers have noted the fact that acetylcholine produces a graded action over a wide range of concentrations. BEZNAK's (1934)[1] results show the following relations between dosage and action of acetylcholine.

| Dose in μg. of acetylcholine | 0.001 | 0.01 | 0.1 | 1.0 | 3.3 | 5 | 7 | 5 | 10 |
|---|---|---|---|---|---|---|---|---|---|
| Contracture of eserinised leech muscle | 13 | 24 | 54 | — | — | — | — | — | — |
| Per cent inhibition of frog's heart | — | 20 | 39 | 74 | — | — | — | — | — |
| Contracture of eserinised frog's rectus abdominis | — | — | — | 15 | 33 | 41 | 41 | — | 44 |

The contractures of the leech and rectus abdominis are expressed as the rise of the lever measured in mm. The ratio indicated between the concentrations producing 16 and 84 per cent., of maximum effect are about $^1/_{100}$ in the case of frog's heart, $^1/_{20}$ in the case of the rectus abdominis and about $^1/_{100}$ in the case of the leech muscle. BEZNAK's results, therefore, agree with those of the author in showing a graded response to acetylcholine over a wide range of concentration, by both the frog's heart and by the rectus abdominis and they also show that the heart is considerably more sensitive than the rectus abdominis. His results, however, show slopes of different angles from those obtained by the author.

KAHLSON (1934)[2] found a linear relation between the concentration of acetylcholine and the response of the frog's rectus abdominis. His figures only extend, however, over a 5 fold range of concentration. LANCZOS (1930)[3] found in one case with the frog's heart that 1 in $10^9$ produced a visible effect, 1 in $10^8$ produced 75 per cent. inhibition and 1 in $10^7$ produced arrest. This suggests a narrower range of action than obtained by the author, but the latter used ventricles that were stimulated electrically and whose response was measured isometrically. These conditions favour the obtaining of a graded response over a wide range of concentration.

---

[1] BEZNAK, A. B. L.: J. of Physiol. **82**, 129 (1934).
[2] KAHLSON, G. K.: Arch. f. exper. Path. **175**, 198 (1934).
[3] LANCZOS, A. L.: Pflügers Arch. **225**, 710 (1930).

LAUBENDER and KOLB (1936)[1] studied the action of acetylcholine on the rectus abdominis of the frog. Their figures show that a concentration of $2 \times 10^{-7}$ acetylcholine produces a half maximum response, and the relation they found between concentration and action approximates to the formula advanced by the author.

The effect of injections of acetylcholine on the blood pressure or pulse rate of mammals show relations between dosage and action which bear a striking similarity to the results obtained with isolated tissues. Fig. 17 records results obtained by CLARK and WHITE (1927)[2] and this shows a graded response over a 100 fold range of dosage with a ratio of $1/_{35}$ between the doses producing 16 and 84 p.c. actions. GREMELS and ZINNITZ (1933)[3] measured the amount of acetylcholine per minute injected intravenously into cats, and the plateau fall of the blood

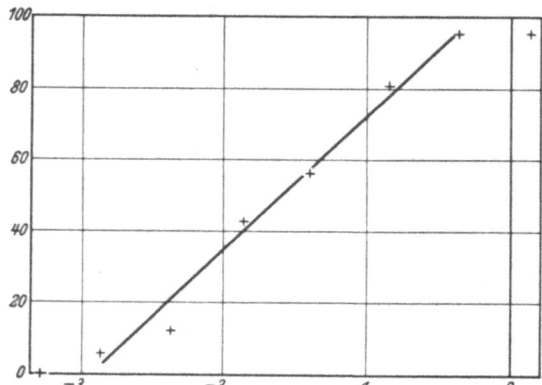

Fig. 17. Action of acetylcholine in reducing heart rate in non-eserinised cat. Abscissa:— log. dose (i. v. i.) in mg./kg. Ordinate:— per cent. reduction in heart rate. (CLARK and WHITE, 1927[2].)

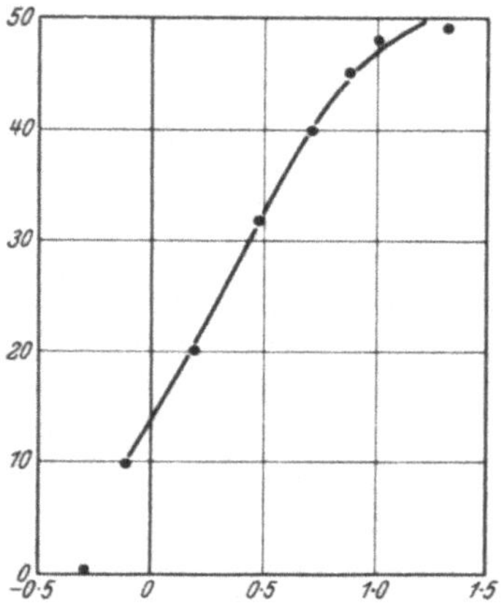

Fig. 18. Action of acetylcholine on blood pressure of eserinised cat. (Continuous intravenous injection.) Abscissa: — log. dosage in $\gamma$ per min. Ordinate: — fall in blood pressure in mm. Hg. (GREMELS and ZINNITZ, 1933[3].)

pressure. Their results are shown in fig. 18. If 55 mm. Hg. be taken as the maximum fall in B. P. then the ratio between dosages producing 16 and 84 p.c. action is $1/_{13}$.

BEZNAK and FARKAS (1937)[4] found that there was an exponential relation between the amount of acetylcholine injected intra-arterially and the amount of saliva secreted by cats both with and without eserine.

The outstanding fact shown by these results is that in all cases acetylcholine shows a graded action over a range of dosage, which in many cases is as much as one hundred fold, and the relation between the logarithm of dosage or concentration and the effect is linear over the greater portion of the range. This curious type of concentration × action relation is seen with systems as different as the leech muscle and the intact cat. It will be seen, however, that the slope of the curve relating log. concentration and action varies widely. Considered as a whole the results support the writer's findings, but are ambiguous as regards the exact relation between concentration and action. Most of these results could be interpreted equally easily either as a hyperbola or as a linear relation between

[1] LAUBENDER, W., and H. KOLB: Arch. f. exper. Path. **182**, 401 (1936).
[2] CLARK, A. J., and A. C. WHITE: J. of Physiol. **63**, 11P (1927).
[3] GREMELS, H., and F. ZINNITZ: Arch. f. exper. Path. **179**, 229 (1933).
[4] BEZNAK, M., and E. FARKAS: Quart. J. exper. Physiol. **26**, 265 (1937).

log. concentration and action. The results suggest, however, the acetylcholine has a similar action on invertebrate and vertebrate tissues and that the action is similar in normal and in eserinised preparations since the concentration-action relations are similar in both cases.

The fact that there certainly is not a simple linear relation between concentration and the amount of action is strong evidence against any simple physical theory of drug action, since, as HILL (1909)[1] pointed out, a simple diffusion process would result in a linear relation between the concentrations at equilibrium inside and outside the cell.

The hypothesis that covers most of the facts observed is that that acetylcholine forms a reversible chemical combination with certain receptors on the heart cell surface. The possibility of this hypothesis can be tested by considering the amounts of drug concerned in the reaction, and the facts known regarding the rate at which the effect is produced.

**Amount of Acetylcholine Acting on Cells.** The potency of acetylcholine has been recognised as a remarkable phenomenon since REID HUNT (1901)[2] showed that a demonstrable action on the blood pressure of a cat (not eserinised) was produced by 0.000,03 $\gamma$ per kilo. CLARK and WHITE (1927)[3] found corresponding figures of 0.004 $\gamma$ per kilo, whilst FELDBERG and VARTIAINEN (1934)[4] found that an eserinised eviscerated cat regularly responded to a dose of 0.002 $\gamma$ acetylcholine. GREMELS (1936)[5] found that a continuous infusion of $1.7 \times 10^{-5} \gamma$ per min. of acetylcholine produced a marked diminution in the oxygen consumption of the isolated heart-lung of the dog. Experiments on isolated tissues have shown that concentrations of 1 in $10^9$ acetylcholine can be demonstrated. The frog's heart shows a very wide individual variation but the author found that a sensitive heart of *R. temporaria* would respond to 1 in $10^9$ acetylcholine, a similar figure was found by FÜHNER (1923)[6] and LANCZOS (1930)[7] found a similar limit with *R. esculenta*. BEZNAK (1934)[8] working with the STRAUB preparation on *R. esculenta* found that in 1000 hearts the majority gave a measurable respone to $10^{-5} \gamma$ in 0.5 c.c., several responded to $10^{-9} \gamma$ in 0.5 c.c. and two extreme cases responded to $10^{-16} \gamma$ in 0.5 c.c. The dose of $10^{-16} \gamma$ corresponds to less than one molecule and, therefore, this result seems doubtful.

ARMSTRONG (1935)[9] made micro-injection experiments with Fundulus embryos (volume 4 cu.mm.) and obtained a positive effect on the heart with a dose of $2.3 \times 10^{-5} \gamma$ acetylcholine. The author made experiments with small drops of fluid added to moist ventricular strips from the frog and found that a dose of 0.02 $\gamma$ per g. tissue produced 50 p.c. inhibition. BEZNAK's figure for the minimum effective dose for the majority of hearts ($10^{-5} \gamma$ per heart) is equivalent to the production of 50 p.c. inhibition by a dose between 0.001 and 0.01 $\gamma$ per g.

SKRAMLIK (1921)[10] states that the average size of the frog's ventricular cells is $131 \times 9$ micra and this gives a surface per cell of 1900 sq.micra and a cell volume of 2,600 cu.micra. The number of cells per g. is, therefore, $3.3 \times 10^8$ and the total cell surface per g. is 6000 sq.cm.

[1] HILL, A. V.: J. of Physiol. **39**, 361 (1909).
[2] HUNT, REID: Amer. J. Physiol. **5**, VII (1901).
[3] CLARK, A. J., and A. C. WHITE: J. of Physiol. **63**, 11P (1927).
[4] FELDBERG, W., and A. VARTIAINEN: J. of Physiol. **83**, 103 (1934).
[5] GREMELS, H.: Arch. f. exper. Path. **182**, 1 (1936).
[6] FÜHNER, H.: Abderhaldens Biochem. Arbeitsmeth. IV. **7**, 421 (1923).
[7] LANCZOS, A. L.: Pflügers Arch. **225**, 710 (1930).
[8] BEZNAK, A. B. L.: J. of Physiol. **82**, 129 (1934).
[9] ARMSTRONG, P. B.: J. of Physiol. **84**, 20 (1935).
[10] SKRAMLIK, E. VON: Z. exper. Med. **14**, 246 (1921).

One gram molecule of acetylcholine (164 g.) contains $6 \times 10^{23}$ molecules and hence the dose of 0.02 $\gamma$ per g. found by the author, contains about $10^{14}$ molecules, which corresponds to $3 \times 10^5$ molecules per cell. BEZNAK's average figure of 0.001 $\gamma$ per g. corresponds to about 15,000 molecules per cell. The author's results show that if each molecule of acetylcholine covers 100 sq. A, then the number of molecules acting on one heart cell could only cover $3 \times 10^7$ sq. A or 0.3 sq. micron and this is only $1/_{6,000}$ of the cell surface, whilst with BEZNAK's results the proportion becomes $1/_{200,000}$. These results show conclusively that acetylcholine cannot possibly cover the whole surface of the heart cells and if the drug exerts a surface action it must act on receptors which only cover a minute fraction of the total cell surface.

**Individual Variation.** The problem of individual variation will be dealt with later, but it may be noted that all workers with extensive experimental experience agree regarding the astonishing individual variation shown by frog's hearts and other tissues in their response to acetylcholine. FÜHNER (1923)[1] found the usual minimum effective concentration was 1 in $10^8$ with a range from 1 in $2 \times 10^9$ to 1 in $10^6$. CLARK (1933, fig. 34)[2] found the mean effective concentration was about 1 in $10^8$ with a range from about 1 in $2 \times 10^9$ to 1 in $2 \times 10^6$. BEZNAK (1934)[3] reported in the case of 1000 hearts that the majority responded to concentrations between the limits of 1 in $5 \times 10^{10}$ and 1 in $5 \times 10^3$.

BEZNAK and FARKAS (1937)[4] noted an individual variation extending over a 33 fold range of dosages in the salivary response of the eserinised cat to intra-arterial injections of acetylcholine.

Table 12 shows the range of variation found with different systems. It is evident that individual variation of a comparable range as regards response to acetylcholine has been found with all systems that have been tested extensively. It occurs equally with normal and with eserinised preparations and, therefore, is not dependent on the action of choline esterase. A remarkably extensive individual variation in response must, therefore, be regarded as one of the outstanding general features of the action of acetylcholine. The possible significance of this remarkable effect will be discussed later.

Table 12. Range of individual variation in various responses to acetyl choline.

| Response | Approximate range of variation as regards dose needed to produce selected response (log. of conc. or dosage) |
|---|---|
| Inhibition of frog's isolated heart (CLARK, 1933[2], fig. 34).. | −9 to −6 (molar) |
| Inhibition of frog's isolated heart (CLARK and RAVENTOS, 1937[5]) | −8.5 to −5.5 (molar) |
| Contracture frog's Rectus abdominis (CLARK and RAVENTOS, 1937[5]) (a) without eserine . . . . . . . . . . . . . . | −6.5 to −4.5 (molar) |
| (b) with eserine . . . . . . . . . . . . | −6.5 to −5.0 (molar) |
| Contracture rat's gut (CLARK and RAVENTOS, 1937[5]) . . . | −7.5 to −6.0 (molar) |
| Contracture leech muscle (BEZNAK and FARKAS, 1937[4]) . . | −7 to −2 ($\gamma$) |
| Depression of blood pressure in eserinised cat (BEZNAK and FARKAS, 1937[4]) . . . . . . . . . . . . . . . . . . | −3 to −1 ($\gamma$) |
| Salivary response of eserinised cat (BEZNAK and FARKAS, 1937[4]) . . . . . . . . . . . . . . . . . . . . . . | −2.5 to −1 ($\gamma$) |

**Site of Action of Acetylcholine.** The experiments by COOK (1926)[6] on the antagonism of acetylcholine by methylene blue, described in chapter 3 (p. 24),

[1] FÜHNER, H.: Abderhaldens Biochem. Arbeitsmeth. IV. 7, 421 (1923).
[2] CLARK, A. J.: The Mode of Action of Drugs on Cells. London: Arnold and Co. 1933.
[3] BEZNAK, A. B. L.: J. of Physiol. 82, 129 (1934).
[4] BEZNAK, M., and E. FARKAS: Quart. J. exper. Physiol. 26, 265 (1937).
[5] CLARK, A. J. and RAVENTOS, J.: Quart. J. exper. Physiol. 26, 375 (1937).
[6] COOK, R. P.: J. of Physiol. 62, 160 (1926).

prove that methylene blue acts on the surface of the frog's heart cells and that this dye when it has penetrated the interior of the cell ceases to produce an antagonistic action. Since methylene blue acts as a specific antagonist to acetylcholine the simplest explanation of these facts is to suppose that methylene blue and acetylcholine both act on the heart-cell surface. The only alternative hypothesis is the potential theory of drug action which will be discussed later.

Another fact is that acetylcholine acts rapidly. Experiments with jets of solution played upon frog ventricle strips show that acetylcholine can produce half action in less than 5 seconds (CLARK, 1927[1]). The interval between preganglionic vagal stimulation and the appearence of vagal inhibition in the cat is about 0.15 sec. (BROWN and ECCLES, 1934[2]) and the delay of the postganglionic nerve endings is about 0.12 sec. BROWN (1934)[3] concluded that the time of transmission from preganglionic fibres to ganglion cells was not more than $20\sigma$, and the shortness of this time has caused a controversy as to whether humoral transmission occurs in ganglion cells.

The fact that acetylcholine acts as a mediator between vagal nerve endings and heart cells is, however, generally accepted. Hence the time required for the drug to produce an effect on mammalian tissue may be taken as less than 0.1 sec., and the shortness of this time suggests a surface action.

A final fact of importance is that all cells upon which acetylcholine produces an action, themselves contain considerable stores of this substance. For example, the frog's heart content of acetylcholine has been estimated by a number of authors (WITANOWSKY, 1925[4]; JENDRASSIK, 1923[5]; ENGELHART, 1930[6]; VARTIAINEN, 1934[7]; BEZNAK, 1934[8]; CHANG and GADDUM, 1933[9]). All agree that the acetylcholine content of the heart is very much greater than the minimum effective heart dose. For example, BEZNAK found that about 10 $\gamma$ of acetylcholine per g. could be extracted from the frog's heart. Press juice from eserinised frog's hearts on the other hand only showed 0.2 $\gamma$ acetylcholine per g. heart, and BEZNAK concluded that the frog's heart contained little, if any, acetylcholine in a free diffusible form. The amount present in a combined form on the other hand was hundreds of times the quantity required to produce inhibition of a heart. FELDBERG and VARTIAINEN (1934)[10] calculated that the acetylcholine store in the superior cervical ganglion was equivalent to the amount released by 2,000 stimuli. These results show that relatively large quantities of acetylcholine can be stored in the cell in such a way that they produce no effect and yet can be released rapidly on stimulation. This suggests the possibility that acetylcholine resembles potassium in that its pharmacological action when within the cell is quite different from its action when applied to the outside of the cell.

This hypothesis will be discussed later but the simplest theory to account for the facts mentioned above is to assume that acetylcholine acts on receptors on the heart surface and that these receptors are not accessible to acetylcholine contained within the cells.

[1] CLARK, A. J.: J. of Physiol. **64**, 123 (1927).
[2] BROWN, G. L., and J. C. ECCLES: J. of Physiol. **82**, 211, 242 (1934).
[3] BROWN, G. L.: J. of Physiol. **81**, 228 (1934).
[4] WITANOWSKY, W. R.: Pflügers Arch. **208**, 694 (1925).
[5] JENDRASSIK, L.: Biochem. Z. **144**, 520 (1923).
[6] ENGELHART, E. J.: Pflügers Arch. **225**, 721.
[7] VARTIAINEN, A.: J. of Physiol. **82**, 282 (1934).
[8] BEZNAK, A. B. L.: J. of Physiol. **82**, 129 (1934).
[9] CHANG, H. C., and J. H. GADDUM: J. of Physiol. **79**, 255 (1933).
[10] FELDBERG, W., and A. VARTIAINEN: J. of Physiol. **83**, 103 (1934).

**Influence of Temperature on Acetylcholine Response.** LAUBENDER and
KOLB (1936)[1] studied the influence of temperature on the response of the Rectus
abdominis to acetylcholine. They obtained the following results.

| Temperature | 5° C | 10° C | 15° C | 20° C |
|---|---|---|---|---|
| Conc. Ac. ch. $\times 10^6$ producing contracture of equal amount | 10 | 25 | 40 | 100 |

The author (1926[2]) measured the effect of varying the temperatures from
11° C to 29° C upon the response of the frog's heart and rectus abdominis to
acetylcholine and found no certain effect. The results regarding the influence
of temperature are, therefore, too uncertain to merit discussion. A fall of temperature will presumably decrease the activity of esterase and this effect might
account for an increase in acetylcholine action on a non-eserinised tissue.

**Specificity of Acetylcholine Action.** Acetylcholine produces a wide variety
of actions, which cannot be classified in any manner that is completely satisfactory. Two groups, however, are fairly distinct, namely, the muscarine-like
and the nicotine-like effects.

The muscarine-like effects are produced by very low concentrations or by
very small doses and are antagonised by low concentrations of atropine.

The nicotine-like effects are produced by much larger concentrations and are
not antagonised by atropine. The actions on the rectus abdominis and on the
leech are intermediate between these groups and hence the classification is
unsatisfactory. The whole subject will be discussed in detail in a later chapter,
but for the purposes of the present discussion the nicotine-like actions may be
ignored, and attention confined to the muscarine-like or parasympathomimetic
effects.

One striking characteristic of acetylcholine is that nearly all alterations in
its chemical constitution reduce enormously the intensity of its pharmacological
action.

Acetylcholine, acetyl-$\beta$-methyl choline and carbamino-choline all have
parasympathomimetic actions of similar intensity, but no other compounds have
actions of comparable intensity. For example, propionyl choline has only $1/20$ the
action of acetylcholine on the cat's blood pressure (HUNT, 1934[3]). General reviews
of this subject have been given by ALLES (1934)[4] and by GADDUM (1936)[5].

It is important to note that changes in the chemical constitution may cause
a decrease in the muscarine-like action of acetylcholine and an increase in its
nicotine-like action. This fact indicates that the combination of acetylcholine
with tissue receptors must be dependent on many factors, and that the relative
importance of these factors must differ in the case of different tissues and even
in the case of different actions on a single tissue. The hypothesis outlined regarding the reaction of acetylcholine with tissues assumes a reaction of a simplicity
comparable to the dissociation of an acid, but it is obvious that the process must
be far more complex. Since the characteristic concentration-action curve of
acetylcholine is one of the few facts that link the action of this drug with any
known physico-chemical process, it seems justifiable to build hypotheses
regarding the drug action upon this definite relation, but is must not be forgotten
that such attempts are only likely to explain a portion of an extremely complex
effect.

[1] LAUBENDER, W., and H. KOLB: Arch. f. exper. Path. **182**, 401 (1936).
[2] CLARK, A. J.: J. of Physiol. **61**, 530 (1926).
[3] HUNT, REID: J. Pharmacol. Baltimore **51**, 237 (1934).
[4] ALLES, G. A.: Physiologic. Rev. **14**, 276 (1934).
[5] GADDUM, J. H.: Gefäßerweiternde Stoffe der Gewebe. Leipzig: Thieme 1936.

**Possible Nature of Acetylcholine Receptors.** The action of acetylcholine is antagonised in a specific manner by methylene blue and by atropine. In the case of atropine this drug is washed out slowly and the author found that it could not be displaced from the heart by introduction of a massive dose of acetylcholine. One cannot, therefore, assume a simple competition for a single receptor between atropine and acetylcholine, such as occurs in the case of oxygen and carbon monoxide in the presence of haemoglobin.

The study of enzyme poisons has, however, shown the possibility of the occurrence of accessory groups, the occupation of which diminishes the activity of a prosthetic group even though this activity is not abolished. Acetylcholine is a strong base and hence the simplest hypothesis regarding its action is to assume that it reacts with carboxyl groups.

In the case of enzyme poisons which react with carboxyl groups (e.g. basic dyes, QUASTEL and YATES, 1936[1]) the concentration required to produce a constant effect $[C_c]$ decreased when the $p_H$ was increased ($[C_c]/[H]$ = constant).

In the case of acetylcholine, however, when the $p_H$ is increased, the concentration of drug needed to produce a given action on the frog's heart is increased rather than decreased (CLARK, 1927[2]; BEZNAK, 1934[3]). This effect of change of $p_H$, therefore, does not throw any light on the mode of action of acetylcholine.

There are many interesting forms of antagonisms of acetylcholine. For example, the action of acetylcholine on the rectus abdominis is antagonised not only by atropine but also by nicotine, curare and novocaine (RIESSER, 1922[4]; SIMONSON, 1922[5]) and even by massive doses of acetylcholine (BEZNAK, 1934[3]).

These complex antagonisms will be discussed later, but at this point it may be stated that the study of these antagonisms does not provide any clear picture of the mode of action of acetylcholine. This is not surprising because the study of drug antagonism involves two unknowns, namely, the mode of action of the drug and the mode of action of the antagonist. Although the action of acetylcholine is intensely specific yet a combination of muscarine-like and nicotine-like actions can be produced by a wide variety of compounds having the general structure of $(Me_3N) \cdot R$. These compounds, however, act in concentrations ranging from $10^{-4}$ to $10^{-5}$ normal, which is more than 1000 times the concentration of acetylcholine that produces corresponding effects.

KÜLZ (1923)[6] showed that quaternary ammonium salts of the series $Me_3NMe$ to $Me_3NAm$ produced a depressant or muscarine-like action on the isolated frog's heart and a contracture of the rectus abdominis and that these actions were antagonised by salts of the series $ET_3NMe$ to $ET_3NOct$. RAVENTOS (1937)[7] has shown that salts of the series $Me_3NMe$ to $Me_3NAm$ produce an additive effect with acetylcholine on the frog's heart, but that $Me_3NOct$ antagonises the action both of acetylcholine and of the lower members of the series.

These results can be partly explained if it be assumed that a number of quaternary ammonium salts can compete with acetylcholine for occupation of the specific receptors in the frog's heart, that some of these ($Me_3NMe$ to $Me_3NAm$) produce a depressant effect and, therefore, are synergists with acetylcholine, whilst many others such as $Me_3NOct$. and $ET_3NMe$ to $Et_3NOct$

[1] QUASTEL, J. H., and E. D. YATES: Enzymologia **1**, 60 (1936).
[2] CLARK, A. J.: J. of Physiol. **64**, 123 (1927).
[3] BEZNAK, A. B. L.: J. of Physiol. **82**, 129 (1934).
[4] RIESSER, O.: Arch. f. exper. Path. **92**, 254 (1922).
[5] SIMONSON, E.: Arch. f. exper. Path. **96**, 284 (1922).
[6] KÜLZ, F.: Arch. f. exper. Path. **98**, 339 (1923).
[7] RAVENTOS, J.: J. of Physiol. **88**, 5P (1936/37) — Quart. J. exper. Physiol. **26**, 361 (1937).

cannot produce this effect and, therefore, antagonise acetylcholine by blocking the specific receptors. This hypothesis assumes that the action of acetylcholine depends on at least two separable factors, firstly, fixation of the drug by certain receptors and, secondly, the power to produce its action after fixation.

**Acetylcholine Esterase.** The concentration-action formula adopted by the author assumes that equilibrium occurs when the rate of association is balanced by the rate of dissociation. The question arises as to whether this hypothesis is in accordance with the known fact that many tissues contain a large quantity of esterase which rapidly destroys acetylcholine. This esterase acts upon acetylcholine in solution, but it is uncertain whether it acts upon acetylcholine when this is fixed by the cells.

The fact that esterase activity is inhibited by physostigmine makes it possible to estimate its influence. The action of acetylcholine on leech muscle is increased more than one thousand fold by eserine (FÜHNER, 1918[1]); the action of acetylcholine on the frog's heart is prolonged by eserine (LOEWI and NAVRATIL, 1926[2]), but this does not cause any marked increase in the intensity of the action produced. In the case of the Rectus abdominis of the frog eserine increases the action of acetylcholine about five fold (CHANG and GADDUM, 1933[3]). The concentration-action curves of acetylcholine acting on these various tissues are similar, a fact which indicates that the form of these curves is not dependent on the activity of the choline esterase. The striking differences shown by the different tissues as regards the influence of eserine is probably related to differences in the rate of action of acetylcholine. This drug can produce its full action on the frog's heart in a few seconds, and the esterase present cannot destroy much of the drug in this time. The actions on the leech and on the Rectus abdominis are much slower and possibly the esterase destroys the drug before it has time to diffuse to its site of action.

**Concentration-action Relations of Adrenaline.** Adrenaline has been studied almost as extensively as acetylcholine. STORM VAN LEEUWEN and LE HEUX (1919)[4] and MURRAY LYON (1923)[5] on the cat's blood pressure and LAUNOY (1923)[6] on the rabbit's blood pressure all obtained figures which showed a linear relation between the logarithm of the concentration of adrenaline and the effect. A similar relation was found by ANREP and DALY (1925)[7] who measured the acceleration produced by adrenaline on the dog's heart-lung preparation, and by CAMERON and MACKERSIE (1926)[8] who measured the response of isolated arterial strips to adrenaline. SHACKELL (1923)[9] found a sigmoid relation between adrenaline concentration and the contraction of arterial rings, and attributed this to individual variation but this result is unlike that obtained by all other recent workers. The results obtained by HUNT (1901)[10] and by MOLINELLI (1926)[11] on the dog's blood pressure show a relation approximating to a hyperbola, and the figures approximate to the curve expressed by the formula $K x^2 = \dfrac{y}{100 - y}$ (CLARK,

[1] FÜHNER, H.: Arch. f. exper. Path. **82**, 51 (1918).
[2] LOEWI, O., and E. NAVRATIL: Pflügers Arch. **214**, 689 (1926).
[3] CHANG, H. C., and J. H. GADDUM: J. of Physiol. **79**, 255 (1933).
[4] STORM VAN LEEUWEN, W., and J. W. LE HEUX: Pflügers Arch. **177**, 250 (1919).
[5] MURRAY LYON, D.: J. Pharmacol. Baltimore **21**, 229 (1923).
[6] LAUNOY, L.: C. r. Soc. Biol. Paris **88**, 848 (1923).
[7] ANREP, G. V., and I. DE B. DALY: Proc. roy. Soc. B. **97**, 450 (1925).
[8] CAMERON, A. T., and W. G. MACKERSIE: J. Pharmacol. Baltimore **28**, 9 (1926).
[9] SHACKELL, L. F.: J. Pharmacol. Baltimore **24**, 53 (1923).
[10] HUNT, REID: Amer. J. Physiol. **5**, VII (1901).
[11] MOLINELLI, E. A.: Tésis, Buenos Aires **1926**.

1933[1], fig. 36). WILKIE (1928)[2] working with isolated strips found a relation between concentration and response which closely followed the formula $Kx = \dfrac{y}{100 - y}$. GADDUM (1926)[3] found a similar sigmoid relation between log. concentration adrenaline and amount of contraction of the isolated rabbit's uterus. GADDUM attributed this to individual variation in the tissue cells, but this explanation implies a range of individual variation of 600 fold between the most sensitive and the least sensitive cells. The difficult problem of the probable influence of individual variation upon concentration-action relations will be discussed later.

ROSENBLUETH (1932)[4] made a systematic study of the relation between adrenaline dosage and its action on various tissues in the cat, namely the contraction of the denervated nictitating membrane, the rise in blood pressure, the alteration in frequency of the denervated heart and the relaxation of the uterus.

In all cases he found that the relation between dosage and action was a rectangular hyperbola. He found that his results could not be fitted by FREUND-LICH's adsorption formula nor did they show a linear relation throughout their course between log. dosage and action. He interpreted the relation by the formula $y = \dfrac{X}{K^1 - Kx}$; this formula was derived from one given by HILL (1909)[5] to express the rate of drug action, but it can be readily transformed to the author's formula $Kx = \dfrac{y}{100 - y}$.

Fig. 19 shows some of ROSENBLUETH's results plotted with the dosage on a logarithmic scale.

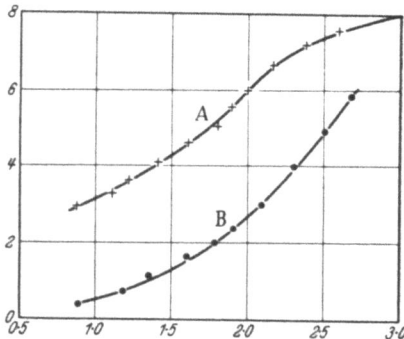

Fig. 19. Concentration-action relations of adrenaline. Abscissa: — log. dose in $\gamma$. Ordinate: — effect in arbitrary units. A Contraction of cat's nictitating membrane. B Rise of blood pressure in dog. (ROSENBLUETH, 1932[6].)

BACQ and FRÉDERICQ (1935)[7] also made studies of the relation between dosage of adrenaline and the response of the nictitating membrane of the cat. Their results (fig. 28) mostly show a linear relation between log. dose and effect, but are not inconsistent with the hypothesis that the relation is a rectangular hyperbola.

A variety of recent work, therefore, supports WILKIE's conclusion that the relation between the concentration and action in the case of adrenaline is a rectangular hyperbola which can be explained as the expression of a chemical reaction between the drug and surface receptors.

**Dosage of Adrenaline.** The minimum effective dosage of adrenaline is of a magnitude comparable to that of acetylcholine. DALE and RICHARDS (1918)[8] obtained a response on the denervated limb vessels in a cat with $5 \times 10^{-6}\ \gamma$ adrenaline per kilo. LIM and CHEN (1925)[9] obtained inhibition of intestinal

[1] CLARK, A. J.: The Mode of Action of Drugs on Cells. London: Arnold and Co. 1933.
[2] WILKIE, D.: J. Pharmacol. Baltimore **34**, 1 (1928).
[3] GADDUM, J. H.: J. of Physiol. **61**, 141 (1926).
[4] ROSENBLUETH, A.: Amer. J. Physiol. **109**, 209 (1932).
[5] HILL, A. V.: J. of Physiol. **39**, 361 (1909).
[6] ROSENBLUETH, A.: Amer. J. Physiol. **101**, 149 (1932).
[7] BACQ, Z. M., and H. FRÉDERICQ: Arch. int. Physiol. **40**, 297 (1935).
[8] DALE, H. H., and A. N. RICHARDS: J. of Physiol. **52**, 110 (1918).
[9] LIM, R. K. S., and T. Y. CHEN: Trans. 6th Congr. Far East Assoc. Trop. Med. **1925**, 1023.

movements of the cat with $7 \times 10^{-4}\,\gamma$ per kilo. The minimum concentration acting on isolated tissues is also very low since the rabbit's intestine is frequently inhibited by a concentration of 1 in $10^9$. The author made experiments on isolated tissues in which the action of small and large volumes of solution were compared and found that the frog's stomach was inhibited when the uptake of adrenaline was not more than $0.06\,\gamma$ per gram moist weight and the corresponding figure found for the rat's uterus was $0.01\,\gamma$. Adrenaline, therefore, resembles acetylcholine in that the quantity of drug which produces an action is too small to cover the cells, and is so small that its effects cannot easily be explained otherwise than by the assumption that the drug occupies certain specific receptors.

The work of Cannon indicates that stimulation of the sympathetic post-ganglionic fibres liberates, not adrenaline, but an allied substance sympathin, and that there may be more than one variety of sympathin. Hence quantitative estimations of drug liberation by nerve stimulation cannot readily be made. The evidence shows, however, that large amounts of sympathin must be contained by cells, because prolonged stimulation does not destroy the sympathin stores. For example, DYE (1935)[1] found that 15 stimuli per sec. for 2 hours (100,000 stimuli) did not exhaust the response of the splanchnic nerves and ORIAS (1932)[2] obtained similar results with the cervical sympathetic. The evidence regarding the mode of action of adrenaline is, therefore, generally similar to that obtained with acetylcholine both as regards the concentration-action relation and as regards the amount of drug needed to produce an effect.

**Concentration-action Relations Found with Various Hormones.** Complete concentration-action curves can only be obtained in favourable cases and with most hormones it is only possible to measure actions of medium intensity. In such cases it is not possible to distinguish between rectangular hyperbolae and linear relations between log. dosage and response.

It is, however, possible to determine whether the response varies as the dosage or as the logarithm of the dosage and in all cases where quantitative measurements are possible the results approximate to the latter relation. This type of relation has been found in the case of insulin, thyroxin, vasopressin and sex hormones.

**Insulin.** The following authors found a linear relation between log. dosage insulin and the amount of fall of blood sugar, MARKS (1926)[3]; MACLEOD and ORR (1924)[4]; GREVENSTUK and LAQUEUR (1925)[5].

GREVENSTUK and LAQUEUR (1925)[5] expressed the opinion that the parabola obtained in these cases had little theoretical significance because there was obviously an upper limit to the possible fall in blood sugar and hence an asymptotic curve was nearly certain to be obtained. EADIE and MACLEOD (1924)[6], however, obtained a similar relationship when they measured the action of insulin in inhibiting the rise of blood sugar produced by a fixed dose of adrenaline and in this case the effect could not have been approaching an upper limit. ALLAN (1924)[7] measured the relation between insulin dosage and the amount of glucose metabolised by a depancreatised dog. MACLEOD (1924)[8] made similar estimations

---

[1] DYE, J. A.: Amer. J. Physiol. **113**, 265 (1935).
[2] ORIAS, O.: Amer. J. Physiol. **102**, 87 (1932).
[3] MARKS, H. P.: League of Nations Publ. Health, C. H. **398**, 24 (1926).
[4] MACLEOD, J. J. R., and M. D. ORR: J. Labor. a. clin. Med. **9**, 591 (1924).
[5] GREVENSTUK, A., and E. LAQUEUR: Erg. Physiol. **23**, 1 (1925).
[6] EADIE, G. S., and J. J. R. MACLEOD: Amer. J. Physiol. **69**, 177 (1924).
[7] ALLAN, F. N.: Amer. J. Physiol. **67**, 275 (1924).
[8] MACLEOD, J. J. R.: Physiologic. Rev. **4**, 21 (1924).

with a diabetic patient. ALLAN found a linear relation between log. dosage (g) and glucose (V), which followed the formula $g = K(V)^{0.15}$.

**Thyroxin.** Since a single dose of thyroxin produces an action for 2 or 3 weeks, it is not practicable to obtain quantitative measurements of the response to a single dose, but the relation between a constant daily dosage of thyroxin and the change in the basal metabolism can be measured. Such measurements have been made on animals by CAMERON and CARMICHAEL (1926)[1], MØRCH (1929)[2], GADDUM and HETHERINGTON (1931)[3]. Similar measurements have been made on myxoedematous patients by BOOTHBY and SANDIFORD (1924)[4]. All these workers found an approximately linear relation between log. dosage and increase in metabolism. The extreme variations in metabolism which can be produced by absence or excess of thyroxin are about $-40$ p.c. to $+50$ p.c. of normal, and hence the subject is not a favourable one for quantitative measurements. KUNDE (1927)[5] indeed concluded that quantitative relations between dosage of thyroxin and effect on dog's metabolism could not be established. This probably is an unduly pessimistic view, but it indicates the difficulty of obtaining accurate quantitative measurements of metabolism, and it is obvious that mathematical analysis of such uncertain data is unprofitable.

**Posterior Pituitary Principles.** These provide another example of active principles that act in very high dilutions. KROGH (1926)[6] found that 1 part of active principle in $10^{12}$ produced melanophore dilatation, and ABEL (1924)[7] found that the minimum effective concentration on the guinea pig's uterus was 1 in $5 \times 10^{10}$. ABEL (1930)[8] also found that $0.05 \gamma$ per kilo produced a rise of cat's blood pressure. The activity of these principles, which have not yet been isolated in a pure state, is comparable to that of acetylcholine.

The dosage-action curve of vasopressin for the rise of blood pressure of the pithed cat was determined by HOGBEN, SCHLAPP and MACDONALD (1924)[9] and their results show that the concentration producing 84 p.c. action is at least 10 times that which produces 16 p.c. action (cf. CLARK, 1933[10], fig. 47).

The concentration-action relations of vasopressin, therefore, resemble those found with other hormones. Most quantitative measures of the action of oxytocin have been made on the guinea pig's uterus and show a sharp all-or-none response. The peculiarities of this tissue will be discussed later, but as far as the writer is aware there is no clear example of oxytocin producing a graded action over a wide range of dosage.

**Sex Hormones.** The action of sex hormones is usually measured by the occurrence of some response that is measured as an all-or-none effect, e.g. induction of oestrus in a castrated mouse. A certain number of graded effects have, however, been measured. Fig. 20 shows relations found between the dosage of oestrone and progesterone and the weight of uteri. This is not a type of response suited for accurate quantitative measurement, but, the results indicate that there is a graded response over at least a ten fold range of dosage.

[1] CAMERON, A. T., and J. CARMICHAEL: Trans. roy. Soc. Canada **8**, 201 (1926).
[2] MØRCH, J. R.: J. of Physiol. **67**, 221 (1929).
[3] GADDUM, J. H., and M. HETHERINGTON: Quart. J. Pharmacy **4**, 183 (1931).
[4] BOOTHBY, W. M., and I. SANDIFORD: J. of biol. Chem. **59**, XL (1924).
[5] KUNDE, M. M.: Amer. J. Physiol. **82**, 195 (1927).
[6] KROGH, A.: J. Pharmacol. Baltimore **29**, 177 (1926).
[7] ABEL J. J.: Johns Hopkins Bull. Hosp. **35**, 305 (1924).
[8] ABEL, J. J.: J. Pharmacol. Baltimore **40**, 139 (1930).
[9] HOGBEN, L. T., W. SCHLAPP and A. D. MACDONALD: Quart. J. exper. Physiol. **14**, 301 (1924).
[10] CLARK, A. J.: The Mode of Action of Drugs and Cells. London: Arnold and Co. 1933.

The action of testicular hormone on the growth of the capon's comb has been studied by many authors (BLYTH et. al., 1931[1], FREUD, 1931[2], FREUD et. al.

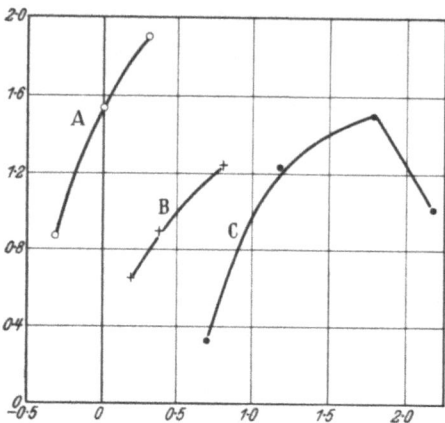

1932[3], GREENWOOD et. al., 1935[4], GALLAGHER et. al., 1935[5]) and all agree that the rate is not a simple linear relation between dosage and comb area, but that there is an approximately linear relation between log. dosage and the increase in the comb area.

These results are in accordance with the fact that oestrone produces a series of effects on mammals and that the dosage needed to produce effects such as mating is enormously greater than the dosage needed to produce the vaginal oestrous changes.

Fig. 20. Relation between dosage of sex hormones and uterine weight. Abscissa:— log. dosage. Ordinate:— weight of uteri. *A* Log. dosage of oestrone in mg. and weight of uteri in g. of immature rabbits. (McPHAIL, 1934[6].) *B* Log dosage of oestrone in γ and weight of uteri as mg. per 100 g. body weight of ovariectomised rats. (BÜLBRING and BURN, 1935[7].) *C* Log. dosage of progestin in LØVEN's units and weight of uteri in g. of immature rabbits. (McPHAIL, 1934[6].)

**Various Alkaloids.** Exponential curves showing an approximately linear relation between log. dosage and response have been described in the case of a number of alkaloids.

**Nicotine.** This alkaloid produces a number of graded effects suitable for quantitative measurement. HILL (1909/10)[8] measured the relation between the concentration of nicotine and the response of the frog's rectus abdominis, and showed that the concentration-response relation could be related by a formula which expressed a simple reversible reaction between the drug and a limited number of cell receptors. This formula can be transposed to the one given below.

CLARK (1933[9], fig. 38) made observations over a wide range of concentrations on the same system and found that the results approximated to the formula

$$Kx = \frac{y}{100 - y}.$$

LAUBENDER and KOLB (1936)[10] also found that this type of formula fitted the concentration-action curve for the contracture of the frog's rectus abdominis produced by varying concentrations of nicotine. They also showed that an increase of temperature from 15° C to 25° C reduced the sensitivity of the muscle and the ratio between the equiactive concentrations at the two temperatures was about 2.2. They concluded, therefore, that the combination between nicotine and the cells receptors was an exothermic process.

The writer hesitates to accept this conclusion as proved by the results because a change in temperature alters the muscle in so many respects that there is no

[1] BLYTH, J. S. S., E. S. DODDS and E. J. GALLIMORE: J. of Physiol. **73**, 136 (1931).
[2] FREUD, J.: Pflügers Arch. **228**, 119 (1931).
[3] FREUD, J., P. DE FREMENY and E. LAQUEUR: Pflügers Arch. **229**, 763 (1932).
[4] GREENWOOD, A. W., J. S. S. BLYTH and R. K. CALLOW: Biochemic. J. **29**, 1480 (1935).
[5] GALLAGHER, T. F., and F. C. KOCH: J. Pharmacol. Baltimore **55**, 97 (1935).
[6] McPHAIL, M. K.: J. of Physiol. **83**, 145 (1934).
[7] BÜLBRING, E., and J. H. BURN: J. of Physiol. **85**, 320 (1935).
[8] HILL, A. V.: J. of Physiol. **39**, 361 (1909).
[9] CLARK, A. J.: The Mode of Action of Drugs on Cells. London: Arnold and Co. 1933.
[10] LAUBENDER, W., and H. KOLB: Arch. f. exper. Path. **182**, 401 (1936).

guarantee that at different temperatures the fixation of equal quantities of drug will produce an equal effect.

STORM VAN LEEUWEN (1923)[1] found a linear relation between dosage of nicotine and the rise of cat's blood pressure, but since this effect is an indirect one caused chiefly by adrenaline release it is obviously unsuited for determination of quantitative relations; moreover, large doses of nicotine cause a subsequent paralysis and hence the drug is not very suitable for quantitative measurements.

**Physostigmine.** This alkaloid is of particular interest because its chief action is to produce a known chemical effect, namely, the inhibition of the choline esterase.

AMMON (1935)[2] gives figures for the inhibition of esterase by physostigmine which show a roughly linear relation between concentration and effect such that $C_{84}$ is 100 times greater than $C_{16}$. The concentration-action relation of physostigmine, therefore, is of a type that can be interpreted as a reversible reaction between the alkaloid and the active group of the esterase.

**Other Alkaloids.** STORM VAN LEEUWEN (1923[3], Chap. IX) was one of the first to attempt a sytematic survey of the quantitative relations between concentration and action of drugs and he made quantitative studies on many systems such as the reflex activity, the blood pressure and isolated tissues. He describes the following drugs as showing an exponential relation between dosage and effect. Morphine on reflex activity of decapitated rabbit (fig. 121); Pilocarpine on isolated cat's gut (fig. 125); Choline on isolated cat's gut (fig. 128); Adrenaline and pituitrin on cat's blood pressure (fig. 129). This author also studied the adsorption of alkaloids by charcoal and serum and showed that the concentration-adsorption curves closely resemble the concentration-action curves. This is to be expected because, as has been pointed out, LANGMUIR's equations for adsorption express equally well certain forms of mass action.

In general it may be said that an approximately linear relation between log. dose and effect is the commonest relation found with potent drugs. Only in certain favourable cases it is possible to get sufficiently extensive evidence to show whether the relation approximates to a hyperbola.

# Chapter 9
# Concentration-action Relations II.
## (3) Linear Relations; Action of Narcotics.

The action of narcotics on ferments, cells and living tissues usually shows an approximately linear relation between concentration and action, a relation which is relatively rare in the case of other drugs. The explanation of these curves is, therefore, associated with the problem of the mode of action of narcotics on cells. Unfortunately any explanation involves assumptions regarding the nature of the cell membrane, which is a controversial matter and since hypotheses regarding the nature of the cell membrane are to a large extent based on the action of narcotics, the subject is a difficult one to discuss.

The concentration-action relations of the action of narcotics on inorganic catalysts, on purified enzymes and on living cells show striking resemblances and, therefore, any theory of narcotic action ought to account for all these phenomena.

---

[1] STORM VAN LEEUWEN, W.: Abderhaldens Biochem. Arbeitsmeth. IV, **7**, 1021 (1923).

[2] AMMON, R. A.: Erg. Enzymforsch. **4**, 102 (1935).

[3] STORM VAN LEEUWEN, W.: Grondbegins. d. alg. Pharmacol. Den Haag: Wolters 1923.

The simplest explanation of the linear relation between concentration of
narcotic and the action on living cells is to suppose that the action is due to
differential solubility. This, however, will not explain why similar effects are
produced on purified enzymes. Hence it seems preferable to accept the adsorption
theory of narcotic action and to assume that the narcotics act by covering
enzymes or cell surfaces. The prolonged controversy between the differential
solubility and the adsorption theory of narcotic action has been summarised by
WINTERSTEIN (1926)[1].

The action of narcotics on enzymes and on certain simple cells has already been
discussed and it has been shown that the simplest method of interpreting the
results is to assume that the narcotics produce their action by adsorption on
surfaces. The effect of such adsorption in the case for instance of alcohols would
be to interpose a layer of $CH_3-CH_2$-groups between the active surface and the
watery solution. Such a barrier can reasonably be expected to depress all forms
of exchange of molecules between the surface and the solution. According to
this theory the biological effect should be proportional to the action of the
narcotic in lowering the surface tension. Investigation shows that as long as
members of any homologous series are compared with each other, a most remarkable parallel is found between biological activity and surface action (cf. fig. 14).
Unfortunately, however, this parallel disappears when members of different
homologous series are compared. This fact is illustrated by the following examples.

| | Molar concentrations | |
|---|---|---|
| | (I) Producing 50 p. c. inhibition of frog heart strip | (II) Reducing air/water surface tension to 63 Dyn/cm. |
| Propyl alcohol . . | 0.17 | 0.14 |
| Ethyl urethane . | 0.13 | 0.26 |
| Amyl alcohol . . | 0.02 | 0,018 |
| Chloral hydrate . | 0.006 | 0.4 |

These figures show that the
simple theory outlined does
not explain the facts, but actually the theory is too simple
to explain the facts observed
with the simplest inorganic
systems: for example RIDEAL
and WRIGHT (1926)[2] showed
that amyl alcohol completely
inhibited the auto-oxidation of charcoal when the amount adsorbed was only
sufficient to cover 0.38 p.c. of the surface.

A fact such as this indicates clearly that any hypothesis regarding the action
of narcotics on such a complex system as the living cell can only be a first approximation. The fact that so many parallels are found between the action of
narcotics on simple inorganic systems and on living cells is, however, very
remarkable and in our present state of knowledge it is unreasonable to hope for
complete theories which will account for all the facts observed.

As regards the site of action of narcotics on cells the most important fact
is that micro-injection experiments have proved that narcotics injected into
amoebae (HILLER, 1927[3]; MARSLAND, 1934[4]) do not produce narcosis and this
can only be explained by the assumption that narcosis is due to some action
produced on the external surface of the cell. The quantity of narcotic fixed by
the cells is far greater than in the case of drugs such as acetylcholine and adrenaline
The author found (1930[5]) that in the case of the higher alcohols (heptyl-dodecyl)
about 0.5 mg. alcohol p.g. frog's ventricle was fixed when 50 p.c. inhibition of
contraction was produced. This is 25,000 times the amount of acetylcholine

[1] WINTERSTEIN, H.: Die Narkose. 2. Aufl. Berlin: Julius Springer 1926.
[2] RIDEAL, E. K., and W. M. WRIGHT: J. chem. Soc. (Lond.) 127, 3182 (1926).
[3] HILLER, S.: Proc. Soc. exper. Biol. a. Med. 24, 427, 938 (1927).
[4] MARSLAND, D.: J. Cell. Comp. Physiol. 4, 9 (1934).
[5] CLARK, A. J.: Arch. int. Pharmacodyn. 38, 101 (1930).

required to produce the same effect. The concentration-action curves obtained with aliphatic narcotics are usually linear, but occasionally other types are observed. Fig. 12 shows typical curves obtained by MEYERHOF (1914)[1] on an inorganic catalyst and on an enzyme. The curve obtained with the inorganic catalyst is clearly an adsorption curve, whilst the other curve is nearly but not quite linear. The latter is exactly similar in shape to concentration-action curves obtained on a wide variety of living tissues. e.g. Urethane on reflexes of decapitated cat (STORM VAN LEEUWEN, 1923[2], fig. 18). Alcohols and urethanes on frog's heart, fig. 15. (CLARK, 1930[3].)

The concentration-action curve of narcotics usually is stated to be linear, but the writer believes that in most cases where the relation has been determined with particular care a shallow curve of the type shown in Fig. 21 has been obtained.

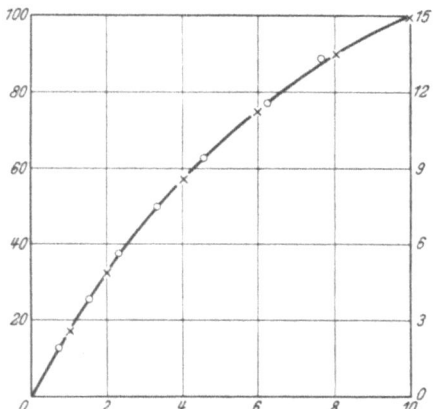

Fig. 21. Concentration-action relations of ethyl ure-thane. Abscissa:— concentration or dosage in arbitrary units. Circles:— Relation between dosage in decapitated cat and per cent. reduction in reflex response (left ordinate). (STORM VAN LEEUWEN, 1923[3].) Crosses:— Relation between concentration and reduction of air/water surface tension (right ordinate, dyne/cm.).

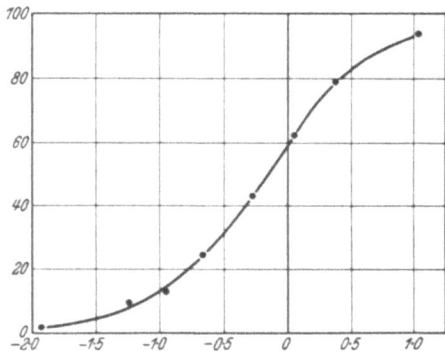

Fig. 22. Relation between log. conc. of ethyl urethane (abscissa) and reduction in air/water surface tension, expressed as per cent. of maximum reduction (73 − 36 = 37 dyne/cm.).

The simplest explanation for this relation is to suppose that it is the lower half of an adsorption curve. Fig. 22 shows the full relation between reduction of surface tension and the log. concentration. It follows the formula $Kx = \dfrac{y}{100 - y}$.

Fig. 21 shows the relation found by STORM VAN LEEUWEN between dosage of ethyl urethane and the amount of inhibition of reflexes in the decapitated cat. The circles show these results and the crosses show points transferred from the curve in fig. 22. The identity of the relations is remarkable. The author found a similar agreement in the case of the depression of the frog's heart.

The comparison of the action of members of homologous series and the study of concentration-action curves in narcotics both show very remarkable parallels between the biological actions of narcotics and their adsorption on air/water surfaces.

MEYER (1937)[4] pointed out that in any aliphatic homologous series many physico-chemical properties changed together when the length of the carbon chain was changed. He argued that few conclusions could be drawn from the comparison of the actions of different members of a single homologous series,

[1] MEYERHOF, O.: Pflügers Arch. **157**, 251 (1914).
[2] STORM VAN LEEUWEN, W.: Grondbegins. d. alg. Pharmacol. Den Haag: Wolters 1923.
[3] CLARK, A. J.: Arch. int. Pharmacodyn. **38**, 101 (1930).
[4] MEYER, K. H.: Trans. Farad. Soc. **1937**.

and that any explanation of narcotic action must correlate the effects produced by members of different homologous series. He found that this test showed a much closer relation between biological activity and oil/water differential solubility than between biological activity and surface activity.

The following examples from his results illustrate this fact.

|  | Narcotic conc. for tadpoles mol/litre | Corresponding equilibrium concentration (mol/litre) in | | |
|---|---|---|---|---|
|  |  | Olive oil | Oleic alcohol | Surface activity |
| Butyl alcohol . . . . . . | 0.03 | 0.02 | 0.02 | +++ |
| Ethyl ether . . . . . . . | 0.024 | 0.05 | 0.05 | ++ |
| Luminal . . . . . . . . | 0.008 | — | 0.048 | + |
| Chloroform . . . . . . . | 0.000,08 | 0.03 | 0.026 | 0 |

The only criticism against this conclusion is that the ratios of biological activity vary widely according to the test used. For example the following data show estimations of the equi-depressant concentrations of the drugs listed above when measured on the isolated frog heart.

|  | Equi-active concentrations (mol/litre) | | |
|---|---|---|---|
|  | Arrest of heart (FÜHNER 1921 [1]) | 50 p. c. depression (CLARK, 1930 [2] and unpublished) | Minimum effective conc. (MEZEY and STAUB, 1936 [3]) |
| Butyl alcohol . . . . . | 0.11 | 0.05 | 0.0043 |
| Ethyl ether . . . . . . | 0.29 | 0.08 | 0.05 |
| Na luminal . . . . . . | — | 0.0004 | 0.0026 |
| Chloroform . . . . . . | 0.007 | 0.002 | 0.0005 |

If the narcotic concentration of chloroform be taken as 1, then the ratios shown below are obtained for the equi-active concentrations.

The results obtained by different authors with the frog's heart vary in a disappointing manner, but they agree in showing a complete divergence from the results obtained with the tadpoles. Obviously if the lipoid/water differential solubility is in agreement with the tadpole experiments it cannot be in agreement with any of the frog heart experiments.

|  | Tadpole expts. | Frog heart expts. | | |
|---|---|---|---|---|
| Butyl alcohol . . | 400 | 16 | 25 | 9 |
| Ethyl ether . . . | 300 | 40 | 40 | 100 |
| Na luminal . . . | 100 | — | 0.2 | 5 |
| Chloroform . . . | 1 | 1 | 1 | 1 |

The drugs mentioned above were a random selection of common narcotics which possessed divergent chemical structures.

The result of this examination suggests that more work must be done to establish the ratios of biological activities before it is possible to correlate these with physico-chemical properties. A general survey of the evidence suggests to the writer that as long as attention is confined to members of a single homologous series, a most gratifying uniformity of results is obtained whether the activities are measured on diverse biological tissues or by physico-chemical means. Unfortunately this uniformity ceases when members of different homologous series are compared, since, not only do the biological and physico-chemical activities diverge, but also divergent results are obtained with different biological systems.

[1] FÜHNER, H.: Biochem. Z. **120**, 143 (1921).
[2] CLARK, A. J.: Arch. int. Pharmacodyn. **38**, 101 (1930).
[3] MEZEY, K., and H. STAUB: Arch. f. exper. Path. **180**, 12 (1936).

## (4) All-or-None Responses.

The concentration-action relations, which follow a sigmoid curve and are termed all-or-none effects, present a difficult problem because these curves can be produced by a large number of different causes. These reactions can be divided into two main groups:—

(a) Cases where the chemical reaction between the drug and the cell is believed to be of a graded character, but the concentration-action relation is distorted by some peculiarity in the cell response.

(b) Cases in which the chemical reaction appears to approximate to the all-or-none type.

This classification is an uncertain one, and the distinction between the two groups depends chiefly on the fact that with some drugs a graded action is found with some tissues and an all-or-none effect with others whilst there are a few drugs that appear to give an all-or-none response with all tissues.

In a large number of cases, however, sigmoid curves when obtained can with some certainty be attributed to the distortion of a graded action. The following causes may produce distortion.

(1) Instrumental errors. — (2) Distortion by the cell of some chemical relation. — (3) The choosing of an obligatory all-or-none response.

(1) **Instrumental Errors.** This is a simple effect, because almost any cellular response can be converted into an all-or-none effect by defective experimental methods. The simplest example is a strip of frog's ventricle. If the mechanical response is recorded with a delicate isometric lever then a graded response can be obtained, but if a relatively heavy isotonic lever be used, then the response may be converted into an all-or-none effect, because feeble contractions will not be recorded, and any contraction powerful enough to overcome the inertia of the lever is likely to give a nearly maximum movement.

(2) **Distortion by the Cell of some Chemical Relation.** The simplest case is when a drug is known to react with some purified cell constituent in a particular manner but this relation is obscured when the drug acts on the same substance inside a living cell. The uptake of oxygen by haemoglobin is a well known example of this effect. The uptake of oxygen by a solution of haemoglobin in distilled water follows the simple law of mass action, but this simple relation disappears even when the haemoglobin is dissolved in saline and also when the haemoglobin is inside a red blood corpuscle. Roughton (1934)[1] has shown that the latter curves can be explained on the assumption that the reaction $Hb_4 + 4O_2 = Hb_4O_8$ proceeds as a chain process in four stages. There is, however, a curious resemblance between the change produced in the oxygen concentration and uptake curve of purified haemoglobin when the haemoglobin is in a corpuscle and the change in the enzyme poison concentration and enzyme inhibition relation when this is measured on cells instead of on purified enzymes. This change can be expressed by measuring the ratios between the concentrations required to produce 84 p.c. and 16 p.c. action. In the case of a hyperbola following the formula $Kx = \dfrac{y}{100 - y}$ the ratio $C_{84}/C_{16} = 27$ and in the case of an exact all-or-none action the ratio would be 1. Examination of haemoglobin oxygen curves (Barcroft and Camis, 1909[2], and Barcroft and Roberts, 1909[3]) shows that with the haemoglobin in solution in pure water the ratio of 24 is obtained, when the haemoglobin is in

---

[1] Roughton, F. J. W.: Proc. roy. Soc. B. **115**, 451 (1934).

[2] Barcroft, J., and M. Camis: J. of Physiol. **39**, 118 (1909).

[3] Barcroft, J., and Fr. Roberts: J. of Physiol. **39**, 143 (1909).

saline solution the ratio falls to 5.6 and in the case of blood in presence of a normal $CO_2$ tension the ratio becomes 4.

A similar effect is observed in the case of the poisoning of invertase by mercuric chloride. With purified invertase the $C_{84}/C_{16}$ ratio is about 50 (MYRBÄCK, 1926[1]) whereas when the drug acts on yeast cells the $C_{84}/C_{16}$ ratio falls to less than 2 (EULER and WALLES, 1924[2]).

These examples show that even in cases where a drug is known to react with a cell constituent according to the laws of mass action, the living cell may cause the concentration-action relation to be distorted into a sigmoid curve.

The examples that have been chosen are simple ones in which the nature of the fundamental chemical reaction is known. In the case of most drugs this is not known and hence the significance of sigmoid curves is obscure.

It may be pointed out that as a general rule reactions that occur in colloidal systems are complex. It is not a matter of surprise that in many cases the relation between the response of the cell and the fundamental chemical reaction causing the response is obscure. A more remarkable fact is that in some favourable cases there appears to be a simple relation between these events.

**(3) Obligatory All-or-None Effects.** There are many events which can only be recorded as all-or-none events. Clear examples of such responses are the death of a cell, and cell division. For example, ethyl alcohol acting on sea urchin eggs shows different concentration-action relations according to the mode in which its action is recorded (fig. 23). A linear relation is found when the oxygen uptake is measured and a sigmoid relation is found when the incidence of cell division is measured. This is a simple example of the form of a concentration-action relation being determined by the form of response selected for measurement. There are other forms of cellular responses which tend to assume an all-or-none character in which the obligatory nature of this type of response is less obvious. Such responses are those dependent on interference with conduction, on injury to membranes and on exhaustion of reserves.

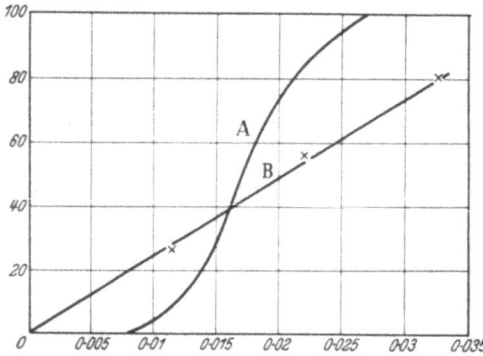

Fig. 23. Relation between molar conc. ethyl urethane (abscissa) and per cent. inhibition of sea urchin eggs (ordinate). *A* Inhibition of cell division. (SCOTT, unpubl. results.) *B* Inhibition of respiration. (MEYERHOF, 1914[3].)

**Interference with conduction.** In the case of a local anaesthetic acting on a nerve trunk, if we accept the hypothesis of decrementless conduction we must admit that as regards the individual nerve fibre the drug produces a sharp all-or-none effect. Either the impulse passes at normal speed or else it is stopped. Similarly, in the case of cardiac tissue, if the response of the ventricle is measured and the response depends on a stimulus passing through the Purkinje tissue, then any depressant of this conduction tissue is likely to produce an all-or-none effect.

**Membrane injury.** The breaking down of the resistance of a semipermeable membrane is an event which is obviously likely to assume an all-or-none character. The haemolysis of red blood corpuscles is a simple example of this kind. It is

[1] MYRBÄCK, K.: Hoppe-Seylers Z. **158**, 161 (1926).

[2] EULER, H. VON, and E. WALLES: Hoppe-Seylers Z. **132**, 167 (1924).

[3] MEYERHOF, O.: Pflügers Arch. **157**, 251 (1914).

now agreed that haemolysis of a corpuscle resembles the bursting of a balloon, there is little leakage until a point is reached at which the membrane bursts.

**Exhaustion of Reserves.** Living tissues usually contain a considerable excess of substances essential for their normal function. If a drug inactivitates an enzyme system, it is quite possible that a considerable reduction in the system may occur without interfering with the cell function, but once a certain limit has been reached any further reduction will produce a sharp depression. The influence of reduced oxygen pressure on cells is a simple example of this fact. Fig. 24 shows the relation between oxygen pressure and the activity of amoebae and similar relations have been recorded with many other systems.

It is obvious that the concentration-action curve does not record how much oxygen is entering the cell, but merely shows the point at which the supply ceases to be adequate for the demand. In the case of oxygen lack, there is the further complication that many tissues can carry on anaerobic activity for a considerable time by means of glycolysis, and this will distort the concentration-action relation still further.

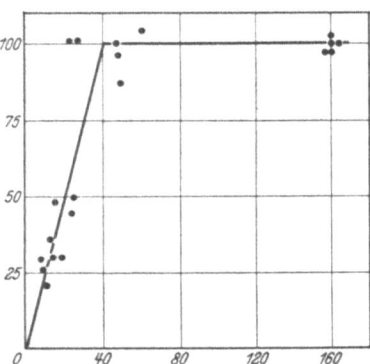

Fig. 24. Relation between oxygen pressure (abscissa, mm. Hg.) and mean velocity of amoebae as per cent normal activity (ordinate). (PANTIN, 1930[1].)

**All-or-None Cellular Responses.** The responses of many types of cells to stimuli have been stated to be of an all-or-none character and it is necessary to consider briefly the suggestion that drugs affect cells in all all-or-none manner and that all concentration-action relations are expressions of individual variations amongst cells.

In the first place this theory cannot be true of all cells because in the case of mobile cells such as amoebae or leucocytes it is possible to observe graded effects of stimulation or inhibition of movement in individual cells. In the second place, there is the important fact that with a single drug-cell system totally different concentration-action relations are obtained when an obligatory all-or-none effect and an effect believed to be a graded action are measured. Thirdly, in the case of the important group of enzyme poisons these drugs in some cases show the same concentration-action relations with pure enzymes and enzymes in cells. The number of enzyme molecules per cell is thousands, if not millions, and there is no justification for the hypothesis that the whole of the population of enzyme molecules in a cell functions as a single unit. It is true that in many cases the concentration-action relations of enzymes in cells are different from the relations found with pure enzymes, and it is possible that the cell membrane interposes a protection against the poison which may be overcome in an all-or-none manner, but this does not justify the extension of such a hypothesis in other cases. Finally it may be noted that the all-or-none principle of stimulation is not firmly established. ROSENBLUETH (1935)[2] has recently discussed this question. The nature of the response of striped muscle fibres to direct stimuli has been a matter of controversy. PRATT and EISENBERGER found a quantal response whilst FISCHL and KAHN (1928)[3], GELFAN (1930)[4] and ASMUSSEN (1932)[5] found

[1] PANTIN, C. F. A.: Proc. roy. Soc. B. **105**, 553 (1930).
[2] ROSENBLUETH, A.: Quart. Rev. Biol. **10**, 334 (1935).
[3] FISCHL, E., and R. H. KAHN: Pflügers Arch. **219**, 33 (1928).
[4] GELFAN, S.: Amer. J. Physiol. **93**, 1 (1930).
[5] ASMUSSEN, E.: Pflügers Arch. **230**, 263 (1932).

a graded response. ROSENBLUETH explains this discrepancy by an explanation based on the results of GELFAN and BISHOP (1933)[1] who observed conducted contractures without action potentials on mechanical stimulation of single striped muscle fibres of the frog. This indicates a dissociation of contraction and the conducted wave of depolarisation. GELFAN and BISHOP (1932)[2] concluded that electrical stimuli produced graded responses on striped muscle fibres when the stimulus skipped the conducted disturbance and acted beyond, presumably on the contractile system itself.

ROSENBLUETH distinguishes between the conducted disturbance in the cell membrane and the response of the contractile mechanism and suggests that whilst conduction is an all-or-none effect yet the contractile response is a graded effect.

This hypothesis appears to cover a large proportion of the observed facts, but involves an old standing controversy regarding the relation between the electrical and mechanical responses of muscle. KATZ (1928)[3] has given full references to this controversy, and references may also be made to the work of BOGUE and MENDEZ (1930)[4] who confirmed Mines' view that the electrical and mechanical responses of the frog's heart could show wide independent variations.

**Concentration-action Curves with Guinea Pig's Uterus.** This tissue is frequently used in pharmacological research, and since it very frequently shows an all-or-none response it is a convenient example of a tissue which tends to respond in an all-or-none fashion.

FROMHERZ (1926)[5] concluded that this tissue always tended to give an all-or-none response, and that when a markedly submaximal response was obtained this was due to a portion of the tissue contracting fully, whilst the remainder remained relaxed. He concluded for instance that a half maximum contraction was due to half the uterus contracting fully.

Oxytocin and histamine cause contraction of the guinea pig uterus in high dilution and most authors agree that the effect is of an all-or-none character. Oxytocin is probably a polypeptide and, therefore, has a considerably more complex structure than most of the hormones hitherto considered, but histamine has a molecular size similar to those of adrenaline and acetylcholine. The peculiar concentration-action relation of these drugs cannot, therefore, be attributed to their molecular size and, since it is difficult to provide a physico-chemical explanation for an all-or-none action, it is necessary to consider whether these responses are due to some peculiarity of the tissue or to the hormones in question producing their effect by some mechanism different from that found with other hormones. CAMERON and MACKERSIE (1926)[6] concluded that there was a linear relation between the concentration of oxytocin and the response of the guinea-pig's uterus. Most workers, however, have found an all-or-none effect (STORM VAN LEEUWEN and LE HEUX, 1919[7]). This can be seen from the results recorded in connection with the biological standardisation of oxytocin since half the dose which produces a maximum response, usually produces a very small response. Results obtained by HSING (1932)[8] are shown in fig. 25. Oxytocin does not

[1] GELFAN, S., and G. H. BISHOP: Amer. J. Physiol. **103**, 237 (1933).
[2] GELFAN, S., and G. H. BISHOP: Amer. J. Physiol. **101**, 678 (1932).
[3] KATZ, L. N.: Physiologic. Rev. **8**, 447 (1928).
[4] BOGUE, J. Y., and R. MENDEZ: J. of Physiol. **69**, 316 (1930).
[5] FROMHERZ, K.: Arch. f. exper. Path. **113**, 113 (1926).
[6] CAMERON, A. T., and W. G. MACKERSIE: J. Pharmacol. Baltimore **28**, 9 (1926).
[7] STORM VAN LEEUWEN, W., and J. W. LE HEUX: Pflügers Arch. **177**, 250 (1919).
[8] HSING, W.: Inaug.-Diss. Frankfurt 1932.

produce many responses suitable for quantitative measurement, but the action of vasopressin on the blood pressure has been shown to be of a graded nature (STORM VAN LEEUWEN, 1923[1]; HOGBEN, SCHLAPP and MACDONALD, 1924[2]). In the case of histamine a number of authors have noted the all-or-none character of the response of the guinea pig's uterus (e.g. LIPSCHITZ and KLAR, 1933[3]; WEBSTER, 1935[4]).

Two questions arise, firstly, whether the guinea pig's uterus always responds in an all-or-none fashion to drugs and, secondly, whether drugs which produce a graded action on other tissues produce an all-or-none action on the guinea pig's uterus.

DEUTICKE (1932)[5] compared the action of adenosin and of histamine on the guinea pig's uterus and his results suggest in both cases an all-or-none effect.

LIPSCHITZ and HSING (1932)[6] found that barium chloride as well as oxytocin showed a sigmoid or all-or-none concentration-action effect on the guinea pig's uterus. WEBSTER (1935)[4] studied the response of the guinea pig's uterus to histamine and to acetylcholine, and her results with the latter drug (fig. 25) show a relation between concentration and response different from that obtained with this drug with most other tissues. In this case the dose of acetyl-

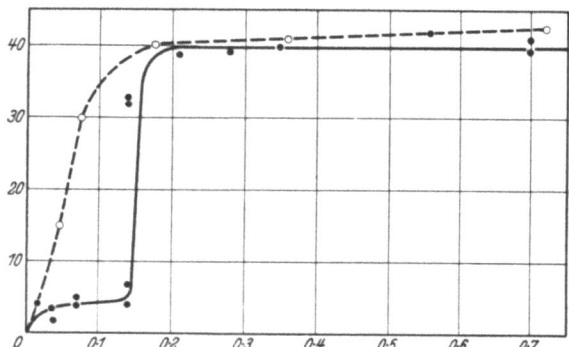

Fig. 25. Relation between conc. of drugs (abscissa) and height of contraction of isolated guinea pig's uterus (ordinate). Circles:— acetyl choline, molar conc. × 10⁸. (WEBSTER, 1935[4].) Dots:— Posterior pituitary extract, Voeghtlin units per litre. (HSING, 1932[7].)

choline producing 84 p.c. response is only about 4 times that needed to produce 16 p.c. response, whereas with most other tissues this ratio is about 25. These results taken together show that the guinea pig's uterus can show a response graded over a certain range of action, but that even in the case of drugs such as acetylcholine, which usually showed a response graded over a wide range of concentration the guinea pig uterus distorts the reaction in the direction of an all-or-none response.

**Drugs Producing All-or-None Effects.** The three substances histamine, potassium chloride and phenol may be taken as examples of agents which usually produce all-or-none responses.

**Histamine.** The activity of this drug on sensitive tissues is of a similar order to that of acetylcholine and adrenaline, since the minimum effective intravenous dose in a cat is $10^{-3}\,\gamma$ per kilo, and the minimum effective concentration for the guinea pig's uterus or ileum is 1 in $10^8$ to 1 in $10^9$. Furthermore the author found that the amount of histamine fixed by the rat's uterus in the case of a minimum effective concentration was about $0.2\,\gamma$ per gramme tissue. The evidence available indicates that histamine tends to produce an all-or-none effect on plain muscle,

[1] STORM VAN LEEUWEN, W.: Abderhaldens Biochem. Arbeitsmeth. IV, 7, 1021 (1923).
[2] HOGBEN, L. T., W. SCHLAPP and A. D. MACDONALD: Quart. J. exper. Physiol. 14, 301 (1924).
[3] LIPSCHITZ, W., and F. KLAR: Arch. f. exper. Path. 174, 223 (1933).
[4] WEBSTER, M. D.: J. Pharmacol. Baltimore 53, 340 (1935).
[5] DEUTICKE, H. J.: Pflügers Arch. 230, 537 (1932).
[6] LIPSCHITZ, W., and W. HSING: Pflügers Arch. 229, 672 (1932).
[7] HSING, W.: Inaug.-Diss. Frankfurt 1932.

even in cases where this is capable of showing a graded response to other drugs. The fact that histamine, like many other drugs, causes an all-or-none action on the guinea pig's uterus has already been mentioned, and tests on other tissues show that histamine frequently tends to produce an all-or-none effect. The gut muscle is, on the other hand, capable of showing a graded response. STORM VAN LEEUWEN (1923)[1] showed that when choline acted on the cat's gut the concentration needed to produce a maximum response was at least 20 times the threshold concentration. BARSOUM and GADDUM (1935)[2] found that adenosin acting on the guinea pig's ileum produced a graded effect over about 100 fold range of concentration, whereas histamine acted over a much narrower range. OLIVECRONA (1921)[3] also found a narrow range of histamine action with the isolated gut of cats and rabbits. The action of histamine in lowering the blood pressure of

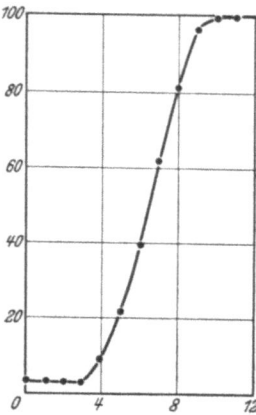

the cat shows a graded response over a certain range of dosage, but BURN (1928)[4] and BEST (1929)[5] found a fairly sharp all-or-none effect, whilst ELLINGER (1929, 1930)[6] found that the response was graded over at least a ten fold range of dosage.

In general it may be said that the evidence regarding the concentration-action relations of histamine is incomplete, but that on the whole it suggests that the drug tends to produce an action over a range of concentration much narrower than is found in the case of drugs such as acetylcholine and adrenaline.

**Potassium Chloride.** Excess of potassium chloride nearly always produces an all-or-none effect. The author (CLARK, 1926[7]) noted this effect in the case of the action of KCl on the mechanical response of the frog's heart and rectus abdominis, but believed that this unusual relation might be due to the action of potassium in interfering with conduction. SOLANDT (1936)[8], however, has shown that potassium chloride excess produces a sharp all-or-none effect on the

Fig. 26. Relation between concentration of potassium chloride (abscissa, millimolar conc.) and resting heat production of isolated frog's sartorius (ordinate, arbitrary units). (SOLANDT, 1936[8].)

resting heat production of the frog's sartorius (fig. 26). Similar results have been recorded by FENN and COBB (1934)[9]. Fig. 26, shows a remarkably steep all-or-none effect, one of the steepest that the writer has encountered, for the ratio between concentrations producing 84 p.c. and 16 p.c. action is 1.8. The simplest explanation of this curve is that potassium chloride produces a sharp all-or-none effect on the cells of the sartorius muscle and that these have a coefficient of variation of 30 p.c. of the median in respect of the potassium concentration needed to produce this effect.

The nature of the effect produced by potassium chloride is, however, more uncertain. The characteristic action on the frog's heart is to produce a gross disturbance of the electrical response, a disturbance far greater than that produced by most other depressant agents. This suggests some interference with the

[1] STORM VAN LEEUWEN, W.: Abderhaldens Biochem. Arbeitsmeth. IV, 7, 1021 (1923).
[2] BARSOUM, G. S., and J. H. GADDUM: J. of Physiol. 85, 1 (1935).
[3] OLIVECRONA, H.: J. Pharmacol. Baltimore 17, 141 (1921).
[4] BURN, J. H.: Methods of Biological Assay. Oxford: Univ. Press 1928.
[5] BEST, C. H.: J. of Physiol. 67, 256 (1929).
[6] ELLINGER, FR.: Arch. f. exper. Path. 136, 129 (1929); 149, 343 (1930).
[7] CLARK, A. J.: J. Pharmacol. Baltimore 29, 311 (1926).
[8] SOLANDT, D. V.: J. of Physiol. 86, 162 (1936).
[9] FENN, W. O., and D. M. COBB: J. gen. Physiol. 17, 629 (1934).

polarisation of the cell membrane (BOGUE and MENDEZ, 1930[1]; DALY and CLARK, 1921[2]). The relation between the action of acetylcholine and potassium ions is at present uncertain. Any theory which seeks to harmonise these two must, however, take account of the fact that acetylcholine is characterised by the wide range of concentrations over which it produces a graded effect whereas potassium ions produce a sharper all-or-none effect than any other drug.

**Action of Phenols.** RONA and his co-workers when studying enzyme poisons found that dinitrophenol was peculiar in that it produced a sharp all-or-none type of poisoning unlike the concentration-action relations found with other enzyme poisons (cf. fig. 1).

The action of phenol as a protein precipitant is of an all-or-none character (cf. fig. 36). The relation between the concentration of phenol and the time required to destroy bacteria or yeast cells (fig. 9) also is of a sharp all-or-none character. These results suggest that the action of phenol depends upon it causing some change in the proteins once it has attained a certain critical concentration in the protein and it seems probable that the action of phenol on cells is of a similar all-or-none character.

There are, other all-or-none relations found with drugs allied to phenol which appear to be the expression of some unusual form of chemical reaction. The all-or-none action of dinitrophenol on invertase has already been discussed, and substituted phenols produce similar effects on cells.

Fig. 11 shows the effect of dichlorphenol on arbacia eggs. The action in inhibiting cell division is an all-or-none effect as is to be expected but the action of the drug in stimulating oxygen uptake also is an all-or-none effect and there is not a priori reason for this.

The similarity of the two curves in fig. 11 may be compared with the gross differences in the curves in fig. 23 which show the action of narcotics in inhibiting cell division and in inhibition of respiration in sea urchin eggs. The phenols, therefore, provide an example of a single class of drug showing a single unusual form of concentration-action with a wide variety of systems.

**Discussion.** Quantitative pharmacological measurements frequently show all-or-none responses over a narrow range of concentrations. In the majority of cases these results are of little theoretical interest, because responses of such a type can be produced in any cell-drug system by errors in recording. Some forms of response (e.g. death, cell division, haemolysis) are of an obligatory all-or-none character and, moreover, some tissues, such as the guinea pig uterus, always tend to show an all-or-none response. The essential character of these all-or-none responses is that there is no graded relation between drug concentration and response, and in consequence, these responses give little information regarding the nature of the reaction between the drug and the cells. On the other hand, for the purposes of biological standardisation it is essential to have a sharp endpoint for comparison between the standard and the unknown preparation, hence all-or-none effects are most suitable in this case.

There is, in addition, definite evidence that certain classes of drugs tend to show an all-or-none effect on systems which with other drugs show graded actions over a considerable range of concentration. The action of phenol and its derivatives may be attributed to the fact that these substances appear to act by altering the state of aggregation of proteins. The action of potassium chloride may be attributed to its producing some change in the permeability of the cell membranes, since this is a type of effect that is likely to be of an all-or-none character. There

---

[1] BOGUE, J. V., and R. MENDEZ: J. of Physiol. **69**, 316 (1930).
[2] DALY, I. DE B., and A. J. CLARK: J. of Physiol. **54**, 367 (1921).

is, however, no obvious explanation for the tendency shown by histamine to produce an all-or-none effect on the tonus of plain muscle. The mode of action of histamine and its relation to anaphylactic shock are subjects of notorious difficulty and our present state of knowledge is insufficient to account for the peculiar mode of action shown by this important drug.

## Chapter 10

## Quantitative Pharmacology and the Theory of Humoral Transmission.

**Introduction.** The physiological importance of acetylcholine and adrenaline has caused these drugs to be the subject of very extensive research and, hence, there is a large amount of quantitative evidence regarding their mode of action. It is of interest to consider what light this evidence throws on the theory of the humoral transmission of the nervous impulse.

It is important in the first place to remember that our direct knowledge is limited to the fact that when tissues are exposed to these drugs certain responses are produced. We have no direct knowledge as to the manner in which the drugs act on the cells.

The following facts have, however, been demonstrated in the last chapter.

Acetylcholine and adrenaline frequently act at dilutions of 1 in $10^9$ and sometimes act in much higher dilutions. The maximum amount of drug which can be fixed by a single cell when certain effects are produced is not more than 100,000 molecules. The action of these drugs is intensely specific since small changes in molecular configuration always change greatly the intensity of the action and may even abolish activity.

The action of the drugs also can be antagonised by a wide variety of other chemicals some of which act in dilutions comparable to the active dilution of acetylcholine.

Finally the concentration-action curves of acetylcholine and adrenaline as determined on a wide variety of tissues resemble closely the curve expressing the uptake of a chemical by an active protein (e.g. CO and haemoglobin).

The only hypothesis based on known physico-chemical processes which provides an explanation for a considerable proportion of these facts is the conception of specific receptors with which the drugs form a reversible combination. This explains the concentration-action curve very simply but the complex details of drug synergisms and antagonisms can only be explained on the theory that the receptors are complex and that the drug action depends first on its being fixed by some particular group and secondly on the molecule as a whole, after fixation, fitting some pattern of the surface mosaic.

In view of the fact that it has been necessary to assume the existence of accessory groups in the active portions of enzyme molecules this hypothesis does not seem unreasonably complex.

There are many facts which cannot readily be explained by the hypothesis outlined above, and certain features of drug tolerance can more readily be explained by the potential theory of drug action, which will be discussed later. It may be here mentioned, however, that there are two serious objections to the potential theory; firstly, it assumes a process which is unknown in physical chemistry and, secondly, it provides no explanation for the quantitative data as a whole.

For these reasons the receptor hypothesis is preferred, and will be adopted as a provisional hypothesis in considering whether the quantitative data regarding the action of acetylcholine and adrenaline are in accordance with the humoral theory of the transmission of nervous impulses.

The chief points upon which the pharmacological and physiological data can be compared are effective dosage, rate of action and concentration-action relations, and the phenomena of synergism and antagonism.

**Quantitative Data.** All the pharmacological evidence agrees in showing that the effective dosage of acetylcholine and of adrenaline is very small, whether this be measured on isolated tissues or on intact animals. BEZNAK's (1934)[1] figures show that in the eserinised frog's heart a measurable response is frequently obtained when the number of molecules of acetylcholine is only a few thousand per cell and the author found that a few hundred thousand molecules per cell produced a 50 p.c. inhibition of the non-eserinised frog's heart. FELDBERG and VARTIAINEN (1934)[2] calculated that the amount of acetylcholine released in the superior cervical sympathetic ganglion of the cat by preganglionic stimulation was 3 million molecules per stimulus per cell.

The pharmacological evidence, therefore, is in quite good agreement with the physiological. In the case of adrenaline the nature of the substance liberated by the post-ganglionic fibres is a matter of dispute and, therefore, the adrenergic fibres are a less favourable subject for discussion than the cholinergic fibres. The pharmacological and physiological facts agree in indicating that vagal inhibition of a tissue such as the frog's heart cell is produced by the appearance around the cell of not more than a few million molecules of acetylcholine. These facts give certain indications regarding the possible site of release of acetylcholine; a problem that was recently discussed by LOEWI (1935)[3] who pointed out that acetylcholine might be released either from the organ or from the nerve ending. The evidence for the existence of relatively large quantities of acetylcholine in the organ (heart cell) has already been discussed. LOEWI agreed that acetylcholine was present in the organ in some labile, non-diffusible combination which was neither active nor liable to attack by esterase.

The evidence also agrees in showing that the potential store of humoral transmitter is large, because very prolonged stimulation is needed to produce signs of exhaustion. These facts alone suggest the organ as the source of humoral transmitter, but LOEWI pointed out that in many cases not every functioning unit received a nerve fibre and he came to the following conclusion:

"According to Stohr, for instance, there is at most only one nerve fibre for every 100 capillaries; but when the nerve is stimulated all the capillaries react. From what point is the transmitter to diffuse, in such cases to the non-innervated parts? In such a case there is, in my opinion, only the nerve ending available as the place of release."

It must, however, be remembered that neuro-humoral transmission is a new subject and probably it will be found to be much more complex than is at present imagined. The action of pituitary secretion and of adrenaline on melanophores is, for example, one of the most primitive examples of humoral transmission. PARKER (1935)[4] has shown that in fish this control is complex, and varies in different species. In the dog-fish the effects can be explained by the production of a melanophore dilator by the pituitary gland and the production of a slowly diffusible melanophore contractor from the nerve endings. In other fish (e.g. Fundulus) the control is, however, entirely through the nerves and Parker

[1] BEZNAK, A. B. L.: J. of Physiol. **82**, 129 (1934).
[2] FELDBERG, W., and A. VARTIAINEN: J. of Physiol. **83**, 103 (1934).
[3] LOEWI, O.: Proc. roy. Soc. B. **118**, 299 (1935).
[4] PARKER, G. H.: Quart. Rev. Biol. **10**, 251 (1935).

postulates two sets of nerves producing oil soluble and slowly diffusible neuro-humoral agents with opposing actions.

Although the mechanisms controlling melanophores are complex and variable, yet in all cases the evidence suggests neuro-humoral agents either carried by the blood or released by nerve endings, and the diffusion of these agents from one area to another can be followed.

ROSENBLUETH and RIOCH (1933)[1] found that if a large fraction (e.g. $^5/_6$) of the nerve supply to an autonomic effector were destroyed, the mechanical response to high frequencies of stimulation (20 per sec.) was equal to that obtained before nerve section, although the response to low frequencies (1 per sec.) was reduced. This result also shows that one nerve fibre can influence a large number of effector elements, an effect that strongly supports the free diffusion of mediator from cell to cell.

Another fact that supports the nervous origin of acetylcholine is that it is possible to abolish the action of acetylcholine on the heart without stopping the post-ganglionic release of the drug. WITANOWSKI (1926)[2] showed this in the case of atropine, ether and hypotonic saline on the frog's heart. FRYER and GELLHORN (1933)[3] showed that heat acted on the nerves since it paralysed the vagus action without abolishing the response of the heart to acetylcholine.

ROSENBLUETH (1935)[4] pictures the course of events as follows. Excitatory state at neuro-effector junction → conducted disturbances in the effector → liberation of mediator → combination of mediator with receptive substance → specific reaction of the effector. This view is much easier to reconcile with the quantitative pharmacological data, and in particular with the quantities of mediator released on prolonged stimulation before exhaustion occurs, for it is very difficult to imagine how these can be produced by post ganglionic nerve endings. On the other hand, this hypothesis is difficult to reconcile with the cell to cell transmission of the mediator, more particularly because the time required for the mediator to produce its effects is so small. Since there is evidence that the mediators act on the external surface of the effector cell it seems clear that if these cells produce the mediator this must be released from the cell surface.

A more fundamental objection to ROSENBLUETH's scheme is that in the heart the wave of electrical excitation does not cause release of the mediators although these are released by sympathetic and vagal stimulation.

The balance of evidence appears, therefore, to be in favour of the hypothesis that the neuro-humoral transmitters are released from nerve endings and act on the cell from the outside. It must, however, be admitted that the facts regarding the amount of stimulation needed to produce exhaustion are extremely difficult to reconcile with this hypothesis.

**Rate of Action.** Pharmacological experiments show that acetylcholine acts rapidly when applied to the frog's heart. The evidence existing shows that it requires not more than a second to produce its action and a considerable proportion of this delay is probably due to diffusion. The delay at the post ganglionic fibres is much less, namely, about 0.12 sec. (BROWN and ECCLES, 1934[5]). The application of a drug to the heart surface by means of a jet is a crude method of administering a drug in comparison with its release close to the cells by means

[1] ROSENBLUETH, A., and D. McK. RIOCH: Amer. J. Physiol. **106**, 365 (1933).
[2] WITANOWSKI, W. R.: J. of Physiol. **62**, 88 (1926).
[3] FRYER, A. L., and E. GELLHORN: Amer. J. Physiol. **103**, 392 (1933).
[4] ROSENBLUETH, A.: Quart. Rev. Biol. **10**, 334 (1935).
[5] BROWN, G. L., and J. C. ECCLES: J. of Physiol. **82**, 211, 242 (1934).

of nerve endings and hence the rates of action observed in these two cases are not discrepant.

According, however, to Brown (1934)[1] the time of delay at the ganglionic synapse is only 20 $\sigma$. Brown, Dale and Feldberg (1936)[2] have explained this difference in time relations between ganglia and heart cells on the ground that the nerve endings are in direct contact with the ganglionic cells whilst the post ganglionic terminations are not in direct contact with the heart cells. This difference is correlated with the fact that in the ganglia where the acetylcholine acts almost instantaneously the destruction by esterase is very rapid, whereas in the case of the heart the destruction is much slower.

The rapidity of action in the ganglia is so great as to be difficult to reconcile with a chemical reaction; it may be possible to reconcile it with a combination of drug with a receptor group on the cell surface, but it seems quite impossible to reconcile this speed of action with any hypothesis that involves the passage of drug through the cell membrane.

Even in the case of the post-ganglionic fibres the rate of action is so great that it supports the hypothesis of a surface action. The time relations in the case of the application of acetylcholine to the heart or of the post-ganglionic action also imply that the combination of acetylcholine with the receptors produces an almost instantaneous biological response.

This narrows down the possible mode of action of acetylcholine, since any alteration in metabolism would only act after a certain period of lag, during which time the store of such substances as phosphagen were depleted. The effect must be on the contractile mechanism, and must immediately render the tissue incapable of responding to a stimulus. The manner in which a comparatively few molecules can produce a change of this magnitude in a contractile tissue is, of course, completely unknown.

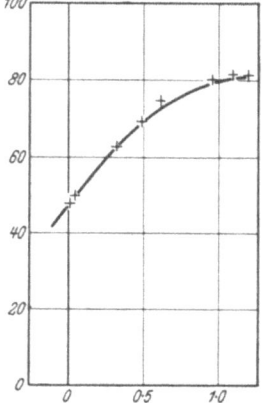

**Concentration-action Relations.** If each stimulus of a post ganglionic fibre causes the release of a fixed amount of acetylcholine, then the total amount released will be directly proportional to the number of stimuli. The effective amount present at the end of stimulation will be equal to the amount released less the amount destroyed by esterase or lost by diffusion. In the case of fairly rapid stimulation the relation between number of stimuli to vagi and amount of inhibition should be similar to the relation between concentration of acetylcholine and amount of inhibition.

Fig. 27. Relation between vagal stimulation (abscissa, log. number of stimuli) and per cent. reduction (ordinate) in amplitude of contraction of tortoise's auricle. (Frédericq, 1935[3].)

Fig. 27 shows the results obtained by Frédericq (1935)[3] and the general shape of the curve resembles the concentration-action curve of acetylcholine. Beznak and Farkas (1937)[4] have compared the effects on the cat's salivary glands of stimulation of the chorda tympani and of intra-arterial injections of acetylcholine. Their results show a remarkable resemblance between the two sets of effects.

[1] Brown, G. L.: J. of Physiol. **81**, 228 (1934).
[2] Brown, G. L., H. H. Dale and W. Feldberg: J. of Physiol. **87**, 394 (1936).
[3] Frédericq, H.: Arch. int. Physiol. **40**, 236 (1935).
[4] Beznak, M., and E. Farkas: Quart. J. exper. Physiol. **26**, 265 (1937).

The dosage-action curve of acetylcholine approximates to a hyperbola and eserine causes the curve to be shifted without altering its slope, with the result that the equi-active doses in the eserinised and non-eserinised animal show a constant proportion; the relation between number of stimuli and effect is similar to that between dosage and effect and is altered in the same manner by eserine. The results are indeed essentially similar to those shown in fig. 28 for the action of sympathetic stimulation and adrenaline on the nictitating membrane of the cat with and without cocaine. BEZNAK and FARKAS also showed that stimulation facilitated the response to a subsequent stimulation and that the same effect could be produced by a series of acetylcholine injections. They made a general study of the relations between frequency and intensity of stimulation and the response produced and showed that a considerable proportion of the relations found could be explained quantitatively on the hypothesis of acetylcholine liberation.

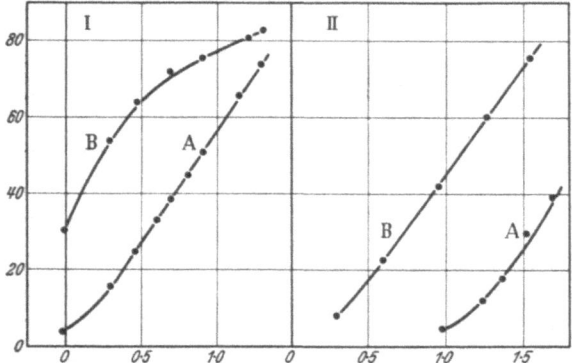

Fig. 28. Relation between contraction of cat's nictitating membrane (ordinate, amplitude of contraction) and (*I*) amount of stimulation of cervical sympathetic, and (*II*) amount in $\gamma$ of adrenaline injected (*A*) normal and (*B*) cocainised. Abscissae:— (*I*) log. number of stimuli. (*II*) log. adrenaline dosage in $\mu$g. (BACQ and FRÉDERICQ, 1935[2].)

In the case of sympathetic stimulation the response of the nictitating membrane of the cat's eye to stimulation of the superior cervical ganglion and to adrenaline injections has proved a suitable material for accurate quantitative measurements. ROSENBLUETH and MORISON (1934)[1] and BACQ and FRÉDERICQ (1935)[2] found that parallel concentration-action curves were obtained with stimuli and with adrenaline injections, and that both were potentiated in a similar manner by cocaine. These effects are shown in fig. 28 where the stimuli and dosage have been plotted as logarithms. It will be seen that three of the curves have a similar slope, and in these cases $C_{84}$ equals 12 times $C_{16}$. This is a steeper slope than that which corresponds to a simple monomolecular action, but in the case of adrenaline, as in the case of acetylcholine, there are many probable sources of error which may distort these relations. There is, however, a clear resemblance between the stimulus-response and the adrenaline-response relation both before and after cocaine.

The examples quoted above show that in the case of autonomic nerves evidence is accumulating which indicates that the relation between frequency or intensity of stimulation and response can in part be interpreted as being dependent on two factors.

(1) The relation between stimulation and amount of acetylcholine or adrenaline liberated.

(2) The relation between the amount of drug liberated and the effect it produces.

The latter relation is probably very complex because any slow effect (e.g. salivary secretion) will depend not only on the concentration of acetylcholine liberated by the stimulation, but also on the duration of its action which will

[1] ROSENBLUETH, A., and R. S. MORISON: Amer. J. Physiol. **109**, 209 (1934).
[2] BACQ, Z. M., and H. FRÉDERICQ: Arch. int. Physiol. **40**, 297 (1935).

be affected both by the rate of wash out by the circulation and the rate of destruction by esterase. The results obtained indicate, however, that the dominant relation between dosage and effect is the mass-action relation.

The literature on the subject of chronaxie is so voluminous and forbidding in its character that one hesitates to risk entanglement by reference to the subject. It is, however, quite clear that many of the effects which have been analysed as purely physical phenomena must, in fact, be dependent on the concentration-action relation.

Unfortunately our methods for following minute chemical changes in tissues are far less sensitive than the methods for following changes of electrical potential, hence the accurate analysis of the chemical changes produced by nerve stimulation is likely to be a very slow and difficult process.

**Specific Antagonisms.** This subject will be considered in detail in a later chapter, but the following points may be mentioned here.

The fact that the motor nerve impulse to voluntary muscles is not antagonised by atropine but is antagonised by curare and cocaine has been regarded as a serious difficulty in accepting the hypothesis that acetylcholine acts as a transmitter in these cases.

A systematic study of the antagonism of either acetylcholine or adrenaline shows at once that this subject is much more complex than is usually assumed. Atropine is regarded as the antagonist of acetylcholine, and hence there is a tendency to ignore as exceptions those cases in which acetylcholine is not thus antagonised. In actual fact these cases are quite numerous and do not follow any easily recognisable law.

The inhibition produced by acetylcholine in the heart of the frog and of *Helix pomatia* is very similar in character; the former is antagonised by atropine but not the latter. On the other hand, muscarine dilates the blood vessels of *Hirudo* and this action is antagonised by atropine (PANTIN, 1935[1]).

Acetylcholine produces contractures that appear to be of a similar character in the rectus abdominis of the frog, in holothurian and in leech muscle; the first two actions are antagonised by atropine but not the last.

The paralysis of motor nerve endings is regarded as the typical curariform effect but curare also antagonises the action of acetylcholine on the rectus abdominis of the frog.

The paralysis of sensory nerve endings is regarded as the typical action of novocaine but this drug also antagonises the action of acetylcholine on frog and leech muscles.

Similarly in the case of the adrenaline-ergotoxine antagonism it may be said that no two actions of adrenaline on the tissues of a single animal, such as the rabbit, are antagonised with the same intensity. The motor response of the uterus to adrenaline is extremely sensitive to ergotoxine, the inhibition of gut tonus is almost unaffected by this drug, whilst a whole range of antagonisms of intermediate intensity can be found.

Drug antagonism, therefore, is a very complex problem, and any attempts to classify drug actions by the manner in which they are antagonised very quickly breaks down if a reasonable variety of drug-cell systems are studied.

This complexity is explicable if it be assumed that the drug receptors in different tissues vary slightly in their pattern and it is difficult to explain these intricate antagonisms by any other general hypothesis of drug action.

---

[1] PANTIN, C. F. A.: Nature (Lond.) **135**, 875 (1935).

Atropine, ergotoxine and nicotine have been such invaluable agents for the analysis of nervous function that it seems ungrateful to belittle their importance. It is, however, very necessary to remember that our knowledge of the mode of action of a single drug on a cell is very imperfect and that the algebraic result of the simultaneous action of two drugs is a much more complex problem. Furthermore, the specificity of these antagonisms always tends to be over-rated because the human mind likes simple generalisations and, hence, awkward exceptions to such rules always tend to be ignored.

**Discussion.** The quantitative evidence which is accumulating regarding the release of transmitters at post-ganglionic fibres agrees in a satisfactory manner with the general theory that the drugs released produce their action by forming a reversible combination with a limited number of receptors on the cell surface. The evidence regarding the amount of transmitter which produces the action and the relation between amount of stimulation and effect produced is in general accordance with the theory outlined. On the other hand, it seems to the author to be very difficult to explain these phenomena on the potential theory of drug action.

The chief unsolved problem is the source of the chemical transmitter. The evidence points to this coming from the nerve endings but it is difficult to understand how these can contain quantities sufficient to resist exhaustion in the manner observed. Furthermore, this hypothesis provides no explanation for the occurrence of large amounts of acetylcholine in the tissues on which the nerve acts.

The antagonism and potentiation of drugs will be dealt with later, but it may be mentioned that in the case of acetylcholine and adrenaline their potentiation by physostigmine and cocaine respectively, and their antagonism by atropine and ergotamine respectively, also harmonise with the general theories outlined. These drugs act in a similar manner on the humoral transmitters whether these are produced by nerve stimulation or injected intravenously. Moreover, the quantitative relations can be explained as a fairly simple example of the mass-action laws, and can be paralleled by examples of antagonistic drugs acting on enzymes. Finally it may be noted that it is evident that the evidence which, at present, is accumulating so rapidly regarding humoral transmission will necessitate a revision of theories regarding the relation between nerve stimulation and the effect produced.

## Chapter 11

## Kinetics of Drug Action.

**Sources of Error in Kinetic Measurements.** It is very easy to make fairly accurate measurements of the rate of action on a cell population of a particular concentration of drug (time-action curve) and from a series of such curves, which cover an adequate range of concentrations, the relation between concentration and the time until a selected action appears (time-concentration curve) can be determined.

The interpretation of these curves presents, however, peculiar difficulties. The fundamental difficulty is the uncertainty of the nature of the processes causing delay.

The kinetics of heterogenous systems are notoriously complex and BAYLISS (1911)[1] pointed out that reactions in such systems involved a chain of processes,

---

[1] BAYLISS, W. M.: Proc. roy. Soc. B. **84**, 81 (1911).

namely, diffusion to the site of adsorption, condensation on surface and finally, a chemical reaction between the adsorbed layer and the adsorbent.

In the case of colloidal solutions he concluded that diffusion and condensation would be more rapid processes than the chemical reaction, and hence the rate of combination would measure chiefly the last process.

Living cells, however, present a more complex problem, because in addition to the factors mentioned, the time spent in diffusing through the cell surface must be taken into account in the case of drugs that act upon the interior of the cell. Moreover, when we measure the response of a cell we do not measure the time at which a chemical change has occurred but the time at which this change has produced a biological response. In some cases this interval may be very short and in other cases it certainly is very large. Hence time measurements mean very little unless the extent of this biological lag is known. The general impression the writer has gathered from the study of the kinetics of drug action is that this is a subject of great difficulty, and that most of the data available are of doubtful significance, because the nature of the process that causes the delay that is measured is wholly unknown. Therefore, it is necessary to consider the errors inherent in this type of measurement before considering the data available.

### (1) Kinetics of Reactions in Heterogeneous Systems.

There are certain important characteristic of reactions in heterogeneous systems which it is necessary to remember when considering the action of drugs on cells. The rate of reactions in such systems usually follows a monomolecular course and NERNST pointed out that this did not prove that reactions in heterogeneous systems were as a class simpler than reactions in homogeneous systems, but merely showed that in the former case the rate of reaction was usually regulated by a diffusion process.

The following are a few examples of various reactions in heterogeneous systems which follow approximately a monomolecular course.

Solution of solids in water and in acids (NOYES and WHITNEY, 1897, 1900[1]; BRUNNER, 1901, 1903, 1906[2]); the evolution of gases from liquids (PENMAN, 1898[3]); uptake of carbon dioxide by caustic soda (CLARK, 1933[4], fig. 44); coagulation of a sol of $Al(OH)_3$ by KCl (GANN, 1916[5]).

Diffusion is a physical process with a low temperature coefficient and, hence, many authors have tried to distinguish between delay due to diffusion and delay imposed by some chemical process, by the study of the temperature coefficient of the rate of action of drugs. In nearly all cases the rate of drug action shows a high temperature coefficient ($Q_{10}$ 2 to 4) whereas a process whose rate is regulated by diffusion ought to show a low temperature coefficient ($Q_{10}$ 1 to 1.5).

| $\mu$ | $Q_{0-10}$ | $Q_{30-40}$ |
|---|---|---|
| 5,000 | 1.37 | 1.28 |
| 10,000 | 1.93 | 1.68 |
| 20,000 | 3.65 | 2.85 |
| 25,000 | 5.00 | 3.75 |

Temperature coefficients are expressed most simply as $Q_{10}$ or can be expressed by the value of $\mu$ in ARRHENIUS' well known formula. Within the biological range of temperature ($5°$ to $35°$ C) the relations shown above hold between the values of $\mu$ and $Q^{10}$ (i.e. the increase produced by a rise of temperature of $10°$ C).

---

[1] NOYES, A. A., and W. R. WHITNEY: Z. physik. Chem. **23**, 689 (1897); **35**, 283 (1900).
[2] BRUNNER, E.: Z. anorg. u. allg. Chem. **28**, 314 (1901); **35**, 23; **37**, 455 (1903) — Z. physik. Chem. **47**, 56 (1906).
[3] PENMAN: Chem. Soc. Trans. **73**, 511 (1898).
[4] CLARK, A. J.: The Mode of Action of Drugs and Cells. London: Arnold and Co. 1933.
[5] GANN, J. A.: Kolloid-Beih. **8**, 64 (1916).

ARRHENIUS (1915)[1] showed that in the case of haemolysis by lysins and by chemical agents and of agglutination of bacilli by agglutinins the value of $\mu$ lay between 20,000 and 40,000. In the case of haemolysis or precipitation of proteins by heat the value of $\mu$ lies between 60,000 and 200,000.

The significance of temperature coefficients of changes in heterogeneous systems is, unfortunately, difficult to interpret. GASSER (1931)[2] reviewed this subject and concluded that "Chemical reaction in heterogeneous systems can have very low temperature coefficient and physical qualities can be cited which have temperature coefficients covering the whole range possible for chemical reactions and extending beyond it".

The temperature coefficient of a reaction in any heterogeneous system provides somewhat uncertain evidence, but in the case of living cells there is the further difficulty that a change of temperature not only alters the activity of the drug but also produces a series of changes in the properties of the cells, e.g. change in viscosity, change in metabolic rate, etc.

In cases where a chemical reaction between the drug and the tissue is measured directly, this source of error may not be serious, but in cases where the drug action is estimated by means of a biological response the temperature coefficient may either express a change in the rate of the chemical reaction or a change in the rate at which the chemical reaction evokes a biological response.

In more general terms it may be stated that the temperature coefficient of any chain process only estimates the alteration in the rate of the slowest process in the chain and provides no information about the changes produced in the remainder of the chain process. For these reasons the writer believes that the measurement of the temperature coefficient of the actions of drugs on cells provides uncertain information as to whether these are of a chemical or physical nature.

## (2) Kinetics of Cell Reactions.

The time between the introduction of a drug and the appearance of a biological response in a cell population may be occupied by any or all of the following chain of events.

(1) Diffusion of drug to cell surface. — (2) Diffusion of drug into cell. — (3) Chemical reactions in the cell. — (4) Interval between chemical change and biological response.

The rate at which any chain process occurs is determined by the rate of the slowest process in the chain of events. The relative speeds of the different processes mentioned above will differ with different drugs and with different cell populations. Hence, kinetic measurements in different cell-drug systems are likely to measure processes wholly different in nature.

The study of the kinetics of drug action is, therefore, of a qualitative rather than a quantitative nature. It is perfectly easy to obtain attractive curves relating time and action, and the ease with which these curves can be fitted by simple formulae is very striking. The difficulties begin when an attempt is made to analyse the factors that must be concerned with the delay.

The writer proposes to discuss first the factors which are known to cause delay in the action of drugs and then to discuss the significance of the curves actually found.

**Delays in Drug Action Due to Diffusion to Cell Surface.** Diffusion may affect either the time taken for a drug to reach cell surfaces or the time taken

---

[1] ARRHENIUS, S.: Quantitative Laws in Biological Chemistry. London: Bell and Sons 1915.
[2] GASSER, H. S.: Physiologic. Rev. **10**, 35 (1930).

for the drug to penetrate the cell. Drugs acting on cell surfaces are only affected by the former type of delay and this is of chief importance in the case of relatively thick tissues such as isolated organs. The system in which delay due to diffusion will be minimal is a suspension of isolated cells acted upon by a drug which reacts with the cell surface. Even in this case, however, there will be some delay due to diffusion owing to the presence of a NOYES-WHITNEY layer of undisturbed fluid around the surface of the cells, which persists even when the suspension is stirred violently. The thickness of this layer has been found to be about 50 micra (BRUNNER, 1906[1]; DAVIS and CRANDALL, 1930[2]) in the case of particles subjected to stirring more violent than could be applied to living cells.

In the case of large tissues such as muscles the delay represented by the time taken by the drug to diffuse up to the cell surfaces may be very much greater and unless special precautions be taken the rate of action of the drug will in such cases express chiefly this time of diffusion. The frog's heart is a relatively favourable tissue as regards diffusion, because of its sponge-like character. The writer made measurements of the relation between concentration of various drugs such as acetylcholine and narcotics, and the time until half action, and at first obtained results of 10 to 30 sec. BERNHEIM and GORFAIN (1934)[3] and WEBSTER (1935)[4] found times of a similar duration in the case of acetylcholine and histamine acting on the isolated gut and uterus of the guinea pig. In the case of the frog's heart, however, further investigation showed that the results were expressions of experimental error since the time of half action could be reduced to less than 2 sec. by applying the drug solution to the tissue in the form of a vigorous jet instead of simply mixing the solution in which the tissue was bathed. Even the latter results probably do not represent the actual time taken for chemical combination between such a drug as acetylcholine and the receptors on which it acts, because BROWN and ECCLES (1934)[5] found that the latent period between the moment of stimulation at a vagal nerve ending and the appearance of a biological response lay between 0.08 and 0.14 sec. In this case, therefore, the time taken by the actual chemical reaction must be very small in comparison with errors due to diffusion. The frog's heart is a far more favourable tissue for time studies than such objects as isolated plain or skeletal muscle and, hence, the time relations of drug actions on such tissues provide very little information. For example, ING and WRIGHT (1932)[6] found that 2 millimolar octyltrimethyl ammonium iodide produced 50 p.c. reduction in response of the frog's gastrocnemius in 13 min. when the muscle was suspended in drug solution and in 0.25 min. when the drug solution was perfused.

The rate of action of local anaesthetics on nerve trunks is another example of delay due to diffusion. A drug such as cocaine produces paralysis in a few seconds when applied to nerve endings by intra-dermal injection, but it may take many minutes to produce the same effect on a nerve trunk. The difference in the latter case must be due to delay in penetrating the medullary sheath.

The writer is of the opinion that it is scarcely worth while discussing time-action relations obtained with relatively thick tissues unless it can be shown that delays of a similar magnitude occur when gross errors due to diffusion have been excluded.

[1] BRUNNER, E.: Z. physik. Chem. **47**, 56 (1906).
[2] DAVIS, H. S., and G. S. CRANDALL: J. amer. chem. Soc. **52**, 3757 (1930).
[3] BERNHEIM, F., and A. GORFAIN: Pharmacol. Baltimore **52**, 338 (1934).
[4] WEBSTER, M. D.: J. Pharmacol. Baltimore **53**, 340 (1935).
[5] BROWN, G. L., and J. C. ECCLES: J. of Physiol. **82**, 211, 242 (1934).
[6] ING, H. R., and W. M. WRIGHT: Proc. roy. Soc. B. **109**, 337 (1932).

**Penetration of Cells.** The physical chemists have introduced the convenient term "sorption" to cover the adsorption of a chemical on a surface and its subsequent diffusion into and reaction with the material on which it has been adsorbed. In most cases the initial adsorption is much more rapid than the subsequent changes.

It is probable that in many cases the uptake of drugs by cells is a sorption process, and in some cases the two stages of initial fixation and subsequent penetration can be easily distinguished. The action of heavy metals is a favourable example because their action at the initial adsorption stage can be arrested by sulphuretted hydrogen.

When enzymes are poisoned by heavy metals an immediate inhibition is produced due to combination of the metal with an active group; this effect can be reversed by $H_2S$, but this initial action is followed by a slower irreversible effect due to the denaturation of the protein carrier by the metal. A somewhat similar effect has been demonstrated in the case of heavy metals and other disinfectants acting on bacteria. The evidence in the case of heavy metals has already been discussed (p. 47) and this shows clearly that there is first a rapid process of adsorption at which stage the action can be stopped by sulphuretted hydrogen, and secondly a process of penetration, the rate of which varies according to the thickness of the cell wall, and which finally results in the death of the cell. In the case of anthrax spores the process of penetration may take several days, whereas in the case of thin walled cells it may only take half an hour. Similarly, in the case of phenol acting on proteins or on bacteria, COOPER (1912)[1] concluded that there was a rapid initial fixation which was followed by a slower process of protein denaturation.

These facts show that there is unlikely to be any close connection between the rate of fixation of a drug by cells and the rate at which it produces its biological effect. This is unfortunate because it limits the value of quantitative analysis in the study of the kinetics of drug action. Most measurements of drug action measure the time of the response of the cell population and these measurements are subject to errors due to the lag in biological response, which is perhaps the most important of all the errors that beset kinetic measurements.

Direct measurements of the rate of entry of drugs into cells can, however, be made in the case of oxygen uptake of red blood corpuscles and the entrance of dyes into large cells such as *Valonia* and *Nitella*. These results are of special interest because they are of a different order of accuracy to the usual kinetic measurements of drug action.

The studies of HARTRIDGE and ROUGHTON (1927)[2] of the rate of uptake of oxygen by haemoglobin in solution and by red blood corpuscles show clearly the amount of delay imposed by a cell membrane in a system specially favourable for rapid diffusion. These workers found that, whereas the half saturation of a haemoglobin solution with oxygen took about 0.004 sec., half saturation of a suspension of red blood corpuscles took about 0.07 sec. They showed that this lag was not due to deficient mixing, but was due to some event which occurred within the corpuscles. The red corpuscles are small cells whose special function is to permit the rapid uptake and output of oxygen, and hence, one may reasonably assume that errors due to diffusion are less in this system than in almost any other biological system.

It is obvious that in this case the measurement of the rate of uptake of oxygen by red blood corpuscles gave no indication of the rate at which oxygen

---

[1] COOPER, E. A.: Biochemic. J. **6**, 362 (1912).
[2] HARTRIDGE, H., and F. J. W. ROUGHTON: J. of Physiol. **62**, 232 (1927).

could combine with haemoglobin, and the example illustrates the general law that in most cases the rate of action of a drug on a cell is regulated by diffusion processes.

**Entrance of Dyes into Cells.** The entrance of non-toxic dyes into cells provides direct evidence regarding both the rate at which chemical substances penetrate the cell membrane and the influence of concentration on this rate. In this case the amount of drug entering the cell is measured directly and hence the number of unknown variables is greatly reduced. Extensive experiments with dyes and other substances have been carried out on the large celled algae *Nitella* and *Valonia*. OSTERHOUT (1933)[1] has summarised this evidence as follows. The entrance of dyes into *Nitella* follows a course resembling a monomolecular reaction (BROOKS, 1926[2] and IRWIN, 1925/26[3]) and this also applies to the exit of dyes from cells (IRWIN, 1925/26)[3] and to the entrance of bromine into *Nitella* (HOAGLAND, HIBBARD and DAVIS, 1926/27[4]). In the case of *Valonia* curves following the course of a bimolecular reaction have been found for the entrance of carbon dioxide (JACQUES and OSTERHOUT, 1929/30[5]) and for the entrance of dyes (BROOKS, 1926[6]). BROOKS and OSTERHOUT pointed out that this approximation to a bimolecular curve might be due to individual variation in the cells. OSTER-

HOUT stated "For if the time curve were really of the first order and in some cells penetration were completed more rapidly than in others a general average would indicate a process appearing to proceed more rapidly at first and then slowing down, as compared with a process of the first order". He also pointed out that "When a process of the second order has its velocity constant calculated by using the equation for a process of the first order it is seen that the velocity constant falls off as the process proceeds". OSTERHOUT here touched on one of the great difficulties of quantitative pharmacology, i.e. that where data are distorted by some source of error such as individual variation, the results often approximate to some other recognised physico-chemical process.

The simplest data are those relating to dyes whose entrance follows the course of a monomolecular reaction, such, for instance, as those of IRWIN (1925)[3] who measured the rate of entrance of the dye cresyl blue into the central vacuole

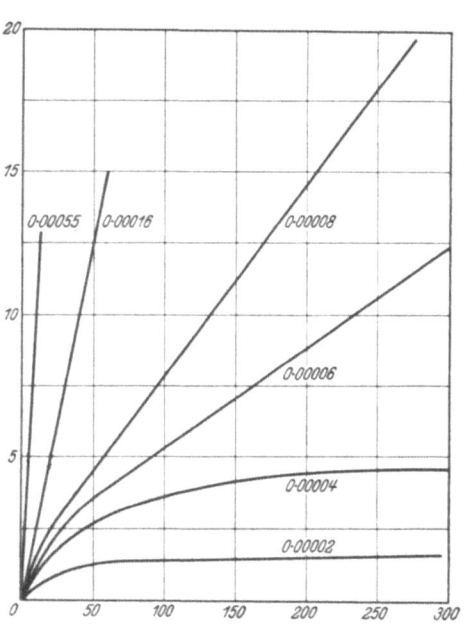

Fig. 29. Rate of entrance of cresyl blue into central vacuole of *Nitella*. Abscissa:— time in minutes. Ordinate:— molar conc. × 10,000 in vacuole. The curves show the rate of entrance at various external molar concentrations. (IRWIN, 1925/26[3].)

of *Nitella*. In this case it is certain that the figures express the passage of a drug through a cell membrane and a layer of protoplasm. The observations

[1] OSTERHOUT, W. J. V.: Erg. Physiol. **35**, 967 (1933).
[2] BROOKS M. M.: Protoplasma **1**, 305 (1926).
[3] IRWIN, M.: J. gen. Physiol. **8**, 147 (1925/26).
[4] HOAGLAND, D. R., P. L. HIBBARD and A. R. DAVIS: J. gen. Physiol. **10**, 121 (1926/27).
[5] JACQUES, A. G., and W. J. V. OSTERHOUT: J. gen. Physiol. **13**, 695 (1929/30).
[6] BROOKS, M. M.: Amer. J. Physiol. **76**, 360 (1926).

covered a range of concentration from 0.00001 molar to 0.002 molar and each point on each curve was the average of about 100 experiments. When the external concentration was kept constant the rate of entrance of the dye resembled that occurring in a monomolecular reaction and was expressed by the formula,

$$Kt = \log \frac{a}{a-x}$$

$a =$ uptake of dye at equilibrium and $x =$ uptake at time $t$. A selection of IRWIN's time-penetration curves are shown in fig. 29.

The study of the entrance of dyes into cells shows, in this case that it is a fairly slow diffusion process and that the rate of entrance follows the mono-molecular formula.

**Delay in Biological Response.** The rate of drug action is usually estimated by the rate of appearance of some biological response and in many cases it is obvious that the rate of appearance of the response does not measure the rate of combination of the drug with the tissue.

The action of monoiodoacetic acid on the frog's heart is a simple example of this fact. The times at which this drug in a concentration of 1 in 20,000 produces death of the heart are roughly as follows. Heart deprived of oxygen 10—20 min. Heart supplied with oxygen 2—3 hours. Heart supplied with oxygen and sodium lactate >3 hours.

In this case the chief action of the drug is to abolish glycolysis and the time before this effect produces death depends chiefly on the alternative source of energy available. Even the first figure given above does not measure the rate of action of the drug in abolishing glycolysis, because if the heart be first poisoned with I. A. A. in presence of oxygen, and then deprived of oxygen, about 5 minutes asphyxia is required to arrest the heart. The I. A. A., therefore, reduces glycolysis to a low level in about 5 min. less than the time until arrest as measured under anaerobic conditions.

This is an obvious example of a case where the rate of appearance of the biological response (mechanical arrest) to a fundamental chemical effect (arrest of glycolysis) is dependent on a large number of conditions and unless these conditions are controlled carefully the rate of arrest will give no information regarding the rate of chemical action. In the case of I. A. A. the chemical effect (arrest of glycolysis) can be measured directly, and it is of interest to note that the results indicate a very wide variation in the case of different tissues. FIELD and FIELD (1931)[1] measured the rate of inhibition by I. A. A. of glycolysis produced by *Streptobacterium casei* and found a latent period of 10 min. after which the reaction followed a bi-molecular course. In the case of yeast LUNDS-GAARD (1930)[2] found that glycolysis was stopped by I. A. A. after 2 hours. In the case of intact skeletal muscle, LUNDSGAARD (1930)[3] and GHAFFAR (1935)[4] found arrest of glycolysis after 30—60 min. and LOHMANN (1931)[5] found a similar rate in the case of muscle pulp. All these results indicate a very slow chemical reaction but CLARK, EGGLETON and EGGLETON (1932)[6] found that the anaerobic frog's heart was arrested in about 10 min. by exposure to N/10,000 I. A. A. and about half this period must have been occupied by depletion of the oxygen and phosphagen present in the tissues.

[1] FIELD, J., and S. M. FIELD: Proc. Soc. exper. Biol. a. Med. **29**, 733 (1931).
[2] LUNDSGAARD, E.: Biochem. Z. **220**, 1 (1930).
[3] LUNDSGAARD, E.: Biochem. Z. **217**, 162 (1930).
[4] GHAFFAR, A.: Quart. J. exper. Physiol. **25**, 61 (1935).
[5] LOHMANN, K.: Biochem. Z. **230**, 444 (1931).
[6] CLARK, A. J., M. G. EGGLETON and P. EGGLETON: J. of Physiol. **75**, 332 (1932).

It is possible that the anaerobic glycolytic activity of the frog's heart is dependent on enzyme molecules at the cell surface and that these are very rapidly inhibited by enzyme poisons, and that there are also intra-cellular enzymes which are less easily attacked but which are unable to maintain anaerobic cardiac activity.

This explanation is unproven but the facts mentioned show clearly that the rate at which I. A. A. inhibits glycolysis is determined by complex factors at present unknown, and hence it cannot be regarded as the expression of the rate of a simple chemical reaction between the drug and an enzyme.

The I. A. A. poisoning of muscle is an extreme example of the manner in which the interval between a chemical reaction and a biological response may vary, but the conditions under which it is safe to assume that the biological response actually measures the occurrence of a reaction between the drug and a cell constituent are relatively rare. The inhibition of enzymatic activity provides certain examples in which a chemical action produces an immediate biological effect. In certain other cases such as acetylcholine and adrenaline, the evidence existing suggests that the combination of these drugs with cell receptors produces an instantaneous change in the activity of the cell.

In a large number of cases, however, it is certain that an extensive delay is imposed by the tissue, because many tissues show a considerable delay between the application of a physical stimulus (e.g. mechanical or electrical) and their biological response. It is interesting to note that definite relations can be measured in such cases between intensity of stimulus and time before response. PORODKO (1926)[1] found that in the case of plants responding to mechanical stimuli the relation between intensity of stimulus ($x$) and the time before response was $t \cdot x^m = K$. This is the same relation as is often found between drug concentration and time before response.

In certain cases it is fairly obvious that the tissue is so sluggish that its response is very unlikely to give an accurate time measurement of any chemical reaction. For example in the case of the rectus abdominis of the frog the writer found that an instantaneous change of state such as an alteration in the load produced a sluggish response which took several minutes to be completed. The response of such a tissue to a stimulant drug is, therefore, unlikely to give any certain information regarding the rate of reaction of the drug with a cellular constituent but must measure chiefly the biological lag in the response.

HILL (1909)[2] found, however, that the course of the nicotine contracture of the rectus abdominis could be fitted accurately by the formula $y = K(1 - e^{\lambda t})$ ($y$ = height of response, $t$ = time and $K$ and $\lambda$ are constants), whilst the relaxation on washing out was fitted by the formula $y = Ke^{-\lambda t}$. This again provides an example of the manner in which kinetic measurements fit formulae which express chemical reactions although it is fairly certain that the times measured do not measure directly the rate of occurrence of the reaction.

The complex nature of the latent period for the action of a drug on a simple system is illustrated very clearly by BOEHM's description (1920)[3] of experiments previously made by him (1910)[4] in which the frog's gastrocnemius was immersed in solution of curarine (0.1 to 0.01 p.c.). His description is as follows:—

„Nach einer größeren Versuchsreihe führte der Aufenthalt im Giftbade während 1 bis 30 Sekunden die Vollwirkung nach 60—80 Minuten herbei; hat die Einwirkung eine Minute

[1] PORODKO, T. M.: Ber. dtsch. Bot. Ges. **44**, 71 (1926).
[2] HILL, A. V.: J. of Physiol. **39**, 361 (1909).
[3] BOEHM, R.: Heffters Handb. exper. Pharmakol. **2**, 187 (1920).
[4] BOEHM, R.: Arch. f. exper. Path. **63**, 219 (1910).

lang gedauert, so vergiftet sich der Muskel ebenso schnell, wie wenn er dauernd bis zum Eintritt der maximalen Wirkung in der Giftlösung verblieben wäre (ca. 27 Minuten).

Es wurde weiterhin konstatiert, daß ein Froschmuskel im Curarin-Bade das Vielfache der zur maximalen Wirkung ausreichenden Giftmenge festhält. Hängt man neben einem so vergifteten Muskel in Ringerscher Flüssigkeit frische unvergiftete Gastrocnemien auf, so reicht das durch Osmose langsam von den vergifteten Muskeln wieder abgegebene Curarin aus, um mehrere frische Muskeln maximal zu vergiften, ohne daß die Lähmung des ersten Muskels in dieser Zeit zurückgeht."

In this case the diffusion of the drug out of the muscle proves that its entry into the muscle was not necessarily an irreversible process, but it would appear that an effective dose of the drug was fixed at or near its site of action within a minute, and that this fixation was followed by some slow complex process which took from 30 to 60 minutes.

These experiments provide a clear example of the fact that the interval between the commencement of the exposure to the drug and the appearance of a biological effect may be occupied by two distinct processes, namely, penetration of the drug to the site of action and the subsequent action.

### (3) Maximum Rate of Drug Action.

There are a large number of factors which are bound to impose a delay between the application of a drug to cells and the appearance of a biological response.

It is of interest to consider the maximum rate at which drugs can produce biological responses in cells when the conditions are most favourable for accurate measurement. The uptake of oxygen by red blood corpuscles in 0.07 sec. (HARTRIDGE and ROUGHTON, 1926[1]) has already been mentioned and in this case the actual chemical combination only occupied 0.004 sec. Studies of enzyme activity have proved that each active group combines with many molecules of substrate per sec. These rates vary greatly, one of the highest figures is that for the splitting of $H_2O_2$ by oxidase (100,000 mol. per active group per sec.) whilst in the case of pepsin the figure is much lower but is calculated to be more than 10 $-CO-NH-$ groups per sec. (LANGENBECK, 1933[2]).

The rate of inhibition of enzyme activity by poisons usually is too rapid to measure, but it would appear probable that once the poison comes into contact with the active group the chemical reaction only takes a fraction of a second. The maximum rate of action of acetylcholine on tissues is a problem of consider-able physiological importance and it is interesting to note that when gross errors due to diffusion are present the rate appears to be of the order of 30 seconds but that this can be reduced to about 1 second by elimination of errors, whilst the rate of vagal response indicates that the true rate of reaction between the drug and the receptors is not more than 0.1 sec. If the theory that acetylcholine is the mediator between nerve ending and cell in ganglia is correct, then the drug must react in less than 0.01 sec. and there must be no measurable lag between chemical action and physiological response. The evidence regarding enzyme activity suggests that this is not an impossible assumption.

Examples such as this indicate the difficulty of kinetic studies of drug action. If acetylcholine can combine with a receptor and induce a biological response in a time of the order of 0.01 sec. then it is clear that, if several seconds elapse between the introduction of the drug and the appearance of the response, the measurements of such times will give no information about the nature of the chemical reaction. The general trend of evidence suggests that the reaction

---

[1] HARTRIDGE, H. and F. J. W. ROUGHTON: J. of Physiol. **62**, 232 (1927).
[2] LANGENBECK, W.: Erg. Physiol. **35**, 470 (1933).

between the drug and the cell constituent with which it combines is usually a rapid process and indeed more rapid than the majority of the numerous and varied processes constituting the chain of events that intervenes between the administration of a drug and the appearance of its biological effect.

## Chapter 12

### The Rate of Action of Drugs on Cells.

The rate of response of a tissue to the action of a drug can be studied in two way:

(1) Measurement of some graded action. The following are simple examples of this type of response: the contracture of plain or of skeletal muscle; the inhibition of the mechanical response of cardiac muscle; the relaxation of plain muscle.

(2) Measurement of the rate of incidence of some all-or-none effect. The following are important measurements of this type: death of micro-organisms; haemolysis of red blood corpuscles; paralysis or death or small organisms.

These two types of time-action curves present separate problems and therefore will be considered separately.

### (1) Curves Relating Time and Graded Action.

HILL (1909)[1] was one of the first to attempt to analyse the reaction between drugs and cells by means of action curves. He studied the action of nicotine in producing contracture of the frog's rectus abdominis, and he showed that the course of contraction was expressed by the formula $y = K(1 - e^{-at})$ and that the course of relaxation on wash-out was expressed by the formula $y = Ke^{-\lambda t}$. In these formulæ $y =$ amount of contraction, $t =$ time and $K$ and $\lambda$ are constants. HILL considered the problem whether the drug action was of a chemical or physical nature and concluded that it was of the former type, firstly because the curves could be fitted by the above formulae which express chemical processes and secondly because the temperature coefficients of these processes were high $Q_{10} = 3 - 4$.

ROSENBLUETH (1932)[2] showed that these formulae expressed the course of the contraction of the nictitating membrane of the cat's eye and of the rise of cat's blood pressure produced by adrenaline, and concluded that from HILL's formulae it was possible to derive relations between concentration and effect produced at equilibrium, which gave the relation $y = \dfrac{x}{K' - Kx}$.

Unfortunately there is no evidence that the times measured in these cases have any direct relation with any chemical process. It already has been pointed out that the curve of isotonic response of the rectus abdominis to an instantaneous physical change, such as change in load, is a slow change in length which resembles in shape and time relations the changes produced by the action of a drug; this fact is shown in fig. 30. Furthermore there is a striking difference between the forms of the isometric and isotonic responses to drugs of a muscle such as the Rectus abdominis. Figs. 30, 31 and 32 show measurements obtained by the writer of the isotonic and isometric responses of this muscle to nicotine, caffeine and potassium chloride respectively. The isotonic time-action curves are similar in the three cases and are of an exponential form which approximates to HILL's

---

[1] HILL, A. V.: J. of Physiol. **39**, 361 (1909).
[2] ROSENBLUETH, A.: Amer. J. Physiol. **101**, 149 (1932).

formula. The isometric time-action curves are however completely different in the three cases. Nicotine shows an exponential curve, caffeine a sigmoid curve with a long latent period and potassium chloride a sharp twitch. The writer concludes from these facts that it is almost impossible to draw any conclusions regarding the rate at which a chemical process is occurring from the course of the isotonic response of the Rectus abdominis and that probably the curves express chiefly the interval between some chemical change and the resulting change in shape of the muscle. Probably the same is also true of most if not all of the responses given by plain muscles.

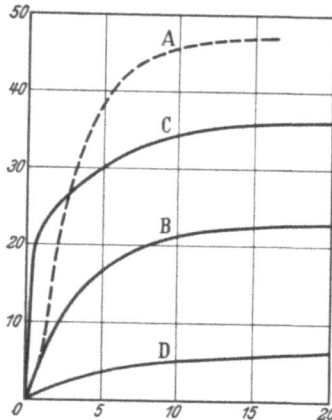

Fig. 30. Responses of frog's *Rectus abdominis*. Abscissa: — time in minutes. *A* Isometric response to nicotine 1 in 500,000. Added tension in g. × 10. *B* Isotonic response to nicotine 1 in 1,000,000. Lever movement in mm. *C* Isotonic lengthening in response to addition of one g. to load. *D* Isotonic shortening in response to removal of 2 g. from load. (CLARK, unpubl. results.)

The rate of response of isolated muscles to drugs also is subject to errors due to diffusion. The experiments of ING and WRIGHT (1932)[1] on the rate of paralysis of the frog's gastrocnemius by quaternary ammonium salts have already been quoted (p. 99), and show that the rate of action on the muscle immersed in solution is an expression of the rate of diffusion, because nearly the whole of the delay can be abolished by perfusion of the muscle.

In some cases the error due to biological lag and diffusion can be estimated approximately by establishing a concentration-action curve and estimating the minimum time of action when the

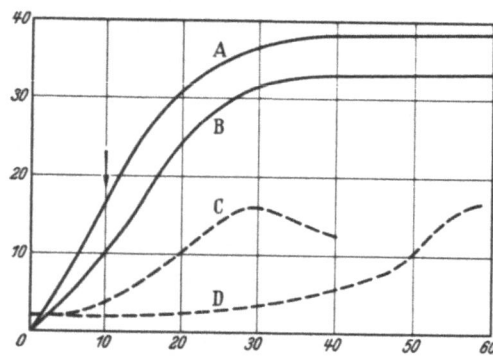

Fig. 31. Responses of frog's *Rectus abdominis* to caffeine (0.08 per cent.). Abscissa: — time in minutes. *A* and *B* Isotonic responses. In case of *A* solution removed at arrow. *C* and *D* Isometric responses. Tension in g. (CLARK, unpubl. results.)

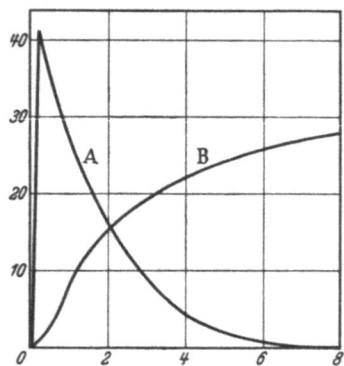

Fig. 32. Response of frog's *Rectus abdominis* to potassium chloride (0.2 per cent.). Abscissa: — time in minutes. *A* Isometric response, added tension in g. × 10. *B* Isotonic response. (CLARK, unpubl. results.)

concentration approaches the maximum. If this time is very small in comparison to the times measured with ordinary concentrations then these errors may be of secondary importance.

The time-graded action curves produced by drugs on muscles have very attractive shapes which invite mathematical analysis. It appears to the writer however that it is useless to try to build up a theory of drug action from such curves, because the nature of the time measured is unknown. The only practic-

---

[1] ING, H. R., and W. M. WRIGHT: Proc. roy. Soc. B. **109**, 337 (1932).

able method of approach is first to work out the possible or probable causes of delay, and until this knowledge has been obtained the time-action curves provide little information. One of the chief methods of investigating the nature of "time" is the study of time-concentration relations and this will be considered later (cf. p. 123).

The rate of inhibition of cellular enzymes appears to be a more promising method for determining the rate of action of drugs. The inhibition of enzymes cannot however be measured rapidly in most cases and hence slow acting poisons are the most suitable for study.

The example of iodo-acetic acid has already been mentioned (p. 102); in this case the rate of action on bacteria follows the course of a bimolecular reaction, but the significance of this fact is greatly reduced by the fact that the rate of action of I. A. A. varies very greatly when a variety of tissues are studied and these variations cannot be attributed to errors due to diffusion.

The rate of action of ergotamine in producing inhibition of the response of tissues to adrenaline has been measured by various workers. BRAUN (1925)[1] and GADDUM (1926)[2] both found that the rate of action of ergotamine on the rabbit's uterus was very slow, and concluded that the amount of effect was directly proportional to the duration of exposure, but MENDEZ (1928)[3] showed that equilibrium probably was attained after one or two hours. In the case of the isolated intestine of the rabbit on the other hand ergotamine produces its full action in a few minutes (ISSEKUTZ and LEINZINGER, 1928[4]; ROTHLIN, 1929[5]; NANDA, 1931[6]). The tissues under consideration namely the uterus and the gut are of similar thickness and hence these gross differences in the rate of action of ergotamine cannot be attributed to delays due to diffusion. The effect of ergotamine (inhibition of adrenaline response) is the same in all cases and hence it seems probable that the fundamental chemical action is similar.

The fact that similar reactions occur at completely different rates in different tissues shows that these rates of action depend on factors that at present are unknown. It appears to the author that until something is known about the nature of these factors there is little profit in attempting to apply mathematical methods of analysis to the results.

**The Shapes of Time-action Curves.** In some cases gross differences in the shape of the time-action responses of a tissue to a drug can be observed. For example WEBSTER (1935)[7] noted that the response of the guinea pig's uterus to moderate concentrations of acetylcholine and of histamine differed in an obvious manner. The acetylcholine time-action curve was an exponential shape, whereas the histamine response was a steep sigmoid curve. This difference in the shape of the response can be correlated with differences in the concentration-action. Acetylcholine produces a graded response over a fairly wide range of concentration, whereas histamine produces an all-or-none effect.

If it be assumed that these drugs diffuse relatively slowly into the uterus then it is to be expected that when acetylcholine is applied the uterus will commence contracting as soon as a small amount has entered the muscle and that the effect of the drug will not be completed before the diffusion is completed. In the case of histamine on the other hand no effect is to be expected until a

---

[1] BRAUN, I.: Arch. f. exper. Path. **108**, 96 (1925).
[2] GADDUM, J. H.: J. of Physiol. **61**, 141 (1926).
[3] MENDEZ, R.: J. Pharmacol. Baltimore **32**, 451 (1928).
[4] ISSEKUTZ, B. VON, and M. V. LEINZINGER: Arch. f. exper. Path. **128**, 165 (1928).
[5] ROTHLIN, E.: J. Pharmacol. Baltimore **36**, 657 (1929).
[6] NANDA, T. C.: J. Pharmacol. Baltimore **42**, 9 (1931).
[7] WEBSTER, M. D.: J. Pharmacol. Baltimore **53**, 340 (1935).

threshold concentration is attained in the muscle, and this results in there being a long latent period but once this threshold has been attained a maximum effect is produced. Figs. 30, 31 and 32 show that the isometric responses of the Rectus abdominis to nicotine, caffeine and potassium chloride are completely different in character, although these differences are obscured when the responses are recorded isotonically.

These different forms of isometric response can be correlated with differences in the mode of action of the drugs. Nicotine probably forms a reversible chemical combination with some cell constituent. Caffeine produces an irreversible injury to the muscle. Potassium chloride appears to produce some instantaneous change in the physico-chemical condition of the cell membrane. The general shape of the time-action curve may therefore give an indication of the probable nature of the action of the drug on the tissue even though it does not provide an accurate measure of the rate of occurrence of the drug action.

In the case of drugs which produce an all-or-none effect, the response of the tissue is always of a sigmoid character. This is to be expected because it is impossible for the drug to reach all parts of the muscle at the same moment, hence the response to the drug will be distorted by individual variation in respect of the time at which different muscle cells commence to contract.

In some cases the curve of response to weak concentrations of drug is of a sigmoid character, whilst with strong concentrations it approximates to a hyperbola.

GRAY (1932)[1] investigated an extremely simple system, namely the rate of poisoning of single trout eggs by aniline. The rate of poisoning was estimated by the rate of diffusion outwards of the cell contents. Strong concentrations of aniline produced a curve resembling a hyperbola, and this can be attributed to sudden breakdown of the cell membrane and consequent loss of cell contents following the laws of diffusion. Weak concentrations showed however a sigmoid time-action curve. GRAY accounted for this effect by the hypothesis that the weak solution gradually broke down the resistance of the cell and that certain patches of the cell membrane were rendered permeable more quickly than others. Here again it is evident that the study of the rate of action of the drug on the cell, as measured by the diffusion, does not give any information regarding the nature of the chemical reaction between the drug and the cell surface.

### (2) Curves Relating Time and All-or-None Effects.

The interpretation of these curves is a matter of some difficulty because the subject has become entangled in a curious controversy. HENRI in 1905[2] observed that there was a linear relation between the logarithm of the survivors and the time of action when fowl's red blood corpuscles were haemolysed by dog's serum. He concluded that this fact proved that haemolysis was due to a monomolecular reaction between the lysin and the cells (one molecule of lysin reacting with one cell), and this conclusion started a controversy that has continued ever since.

Similar monomolecular curves were found for the destruction of bacteria by disinfectants, heat and drying (CHICK, 1908[3]) and for the precipitation of proteins by heat (CHICK and MARTIN, 1910, 1911 and 1912[4]). Fig. 33 shows examples of the curves obtained by CHICK. ARRHENIUS (1915)[5] gave his powerful support

[1] GRAY, J.: J. of exper. Biol. **9**, 277 (1932).
[2] HENRI, V.: C. r. Soc. Biol. Paris **58**, 37 (1905).
[3] CHICK, H.: J. of Hyg. 8, 92 (1908).
[4] CHICK, H., and C. J. MARTIN: J. of Physiol. **40**, 104 (1910); **43**, 1 (1911); **45**, 61 (1912).
[5] ARRHENIUS, S.: Quantitative Laws in Biological Chemistry. London: Bell and Sons 1915.

to the hypothesis that these curves proved that a monomolecular reaction occurred in these cases. The scope of the controversy was extended by BLAU and ALTENBURGER (1922)[1] who found that the destruction of micro-organisms by radiations gave monomolecular curves and concluded that this proved that death of cells was produced by one, or at most a few quanta of energy.

CHICK (1930)[2], RAHN (1930, 1935)[3] and the writer (CLARK, 1933[4]) have in recent years made collections of the evidence upon which this prolonged controversy has been based. The subject will therefore be dealt with here as briefly as possible but unfortunately it cannot be ignored because the acceptance of the monomolecular theory of drug actions is incompatible with most of the hypotheses regarding the action of drugs advanced in this article. The nature of the difficulties that arise if the monomolecular theory of drug action be accepted are as follows.

BROOKS (1919)[5] pointed out that:

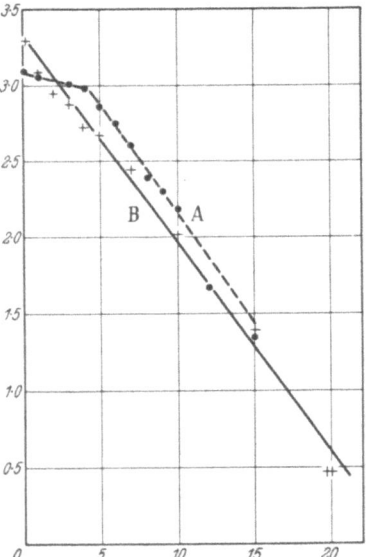

Fig. 33. Rate of destruction of bacteria. Abscissa:— time in minutes. Ordinate:— log. survivors. *A Staphylococcus pyogenes aureus* and 0.6 per cent. phenol at 20° C. *B B. typhosus* and water at 49° C. (CHICK, 1910[6].)

"The acceptance of such an explanation makes it necessary to assume that loss of viability like the breaking up of a single molecule of saccharase during inversion takes place in a single step; in other words, that the disinfectant cannot have any cumulative effect on the viability of single cells."

The chief postulates of this hypothesis may be formulated as follows.

(a) In a population of cells there is no important individual variation as regards response to lethal agents.

(b) Death of a cell is produced by one or at most a few molecules of drug or quanta of radiant energy.

(c) The action of drugs or radiations on cells is non-cumulative and a cell when exposed to such influences is unaffected until the lethal event occurs.

The mere statement of these postulates appears to the writer to constitute a *reductio ad absurdum*. Variation is one of the fundamental characteristics of living organisms and variation in response to drug action actually constitutes one of the most serious and ever present difficulties in quantitative pharmacology. The number of molecules of drug combining with single cells can be measured in certain cases and is usually of the order of millions. Finally it is in many cases possible to demonstrate graded sub-lethal actions produced by lethal agents on individual cells.

The apparent simplicity and exactitude of the monomolecular theory of drug action has however given it a wide popularity. Most of the writers who have

[1] BLAU, M., and K. ALTENBURGER: Z. Physik 12, 315 (1922).
[2] CHICK, H.: Med. Res. Counc. System of Bacteriol. 1, 179 (1930).
[3] RAHN, O.: J. gen. Physiol. 13, 179, 396 (1930); 14, 319 (1931) — Symposia Quant. Biol. 2, 76 (1935).
[4] CLARK, A. J.: The Mode of Action of Drugs on Cells, p. 163—168. London: Arnold and Co. 1933.
[5] BROOKS, S. C.: J. gen. Physiol. 1, 61 (1919).
[6] CHICK, H.: J. of Hyg. 10, 237 (1910).

adopted the theory have made no attempt to consider its implications. ARRHENIUS (1915)[1] however produced a reasoned argument in its defence. He recognised the existence of individual variation in cell populations but argued that the linear relation obtained (e.g. fig. 33) proved that this variation did not produce any significant effect. He concluded as follows:

> "The different lifetime of the different bacteria does not therefore depend in a sensible degree on their different ability to resist the destructive action of the poison. Instead of this a certain fraction of the bacilli still living dies in one second, independent of the time during which they have been in contact with the poison."

He suggested that at any particular moment only a few molecules of protein were vulnerable to attack by drugs and that this made a monomolecular reaction between drugs and cells a possibility. It is obvious that a physico-chemical theory regarding the mode of action of drugs, which has received the support of ARRHENIUS must be considered carefully, particularly since its acceptance would modify or rather annihilate most other hypotheses advanced in connection with this subject.

The controversy has spread over such a large range that it is most convenient to consider separately the various problems raised. The frequency with which monomolecular curves have been obtained with biological material is very surprising, but the writer believes that this is due to the fact that they express a skew distribution of variation, and does not mean that biological material customarily reacts with chemicals in a manner so simple as to be very uncommon even in the simplest inorganic systems.

The kinetics of protein precipitation will therefore be first considered and then the problem of the influence of individual variation on the time-action curves.

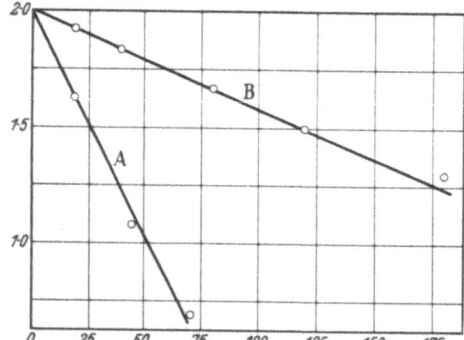

Fig. 34. Rate of precipitation of haemoglobin. Abscissa:— time in minutes. Ordinate:— log. of per cent. unprecipitated. *A* 3 per cent. solution at 62.6° C. 8—10 min. allowed for heating solution. (CHICK and MARTIN, 1911[2].) *B* 1 per cent. solution at 60.5° C. and $p_H$ 7.21. (LEWIS, 1926[5].)

**Kinetics of Protein Precipitation.**
The precipitation of a protein from a watery solution by exposure to a suitable temperature follows a remarkable course, since a linear relation is found to exist between the time of exposure and the logarithm of the amount left in solution. That is to say a fixed proportion of the protein in solution is precipitated in each unit of time. This relation which is shown in fig. 34, has been demonstrated in the case of egg albumen (CHICK and MARTIN, 1911[2]; LEWIS, 1926[3]) and in the case of haemoglobin (CHICK and MARTIN, 1910[4]; LEWIS, 1926[5]; HARTRIDGE, 1912[6]).

CHICK and MARTIN (1911)[2] concluded that denaturation occurred in two stages. Firstly a chemical reaction between the protein and water and secondly an agglutination and separation of the product. They concluded that under suitable

[1] ARRHENIUS, S.: Quantitative Laws in Biological Chemistry. London: Bell and Sons 1915.
[2] CHICK, H., and C. J. MARTIN: J. of Physiol. **43**, 1 (1911).
[3] LEWIS, P. S.: Biochemic. J. **20**, 978 (1926).
[4] CHICK, H., and C. J. MARTIN: J. of Physiol. **40**, 404 (1910).
[5] LEWIS, P. S.: Biochemic. J. **20**, 965 (1926).
[6] HARTRIDGE, H.: J. of Physiol. **44**, 34 (1912).

conditions the rate of the second process greatly exceeded that of the first process and hence the measurement of the rate of formation of the precipitate measured the rate of the first reaction.

LEWIS concluded that the mechanism of denaturation was a localised hydrolysis of relatively labile links situated at various points on a large heavily hydrated molecular unit. FISCHER (1936)[1] studied the heat precipitation of serum globulin and found that it followed an exponential curve, but that the process could be greatly accelerated if a "starter" of partly coagulated globulin were added. He concluded that there was no evidence that hydrolysis of the proteins occurred. He found that addition of formaldehyde delayed or inhibited the denaturation and concluded that the denaturation was due to the appearance of amino groups on the surface of the protein molecules, which resulted in their aggregation.

The nature of protein coagulation is therefore uncertain. The modern conception of a protein molecule in solution is however that it is spherical (SVEDBERG, 1930[2]; ASTBURY et al., 1935[3]) with a molecular weight which is a multiple of 34,000. It is therefore improbable that the aggregation of units of this size should be produced by the alteration of a single side chain. It seems more probable that aggregation depends on the occurrence of a number of events, and that the course of precipitation expresses the individual variation in the protein molecules.

**Precipitation of Protein by Phenol.** The precipitation of egg white by phenol follows a course somewhat similar to heat aggregation. The following figures were obtained by COOPER and HAINES (1928)[4].

Action of 1 p.c. phenol on solution of egg white at 30° C.

| Time in min. . . . . . . . . . . . . . | 0 | 20 | 35 | 50 | 90 | 150 | 240 | 300 |
|---|---|---|---|---|---|---|---|---|
| Egg white remaining in sol. (mg. p. 100 c.c.) | 714 | 653 | 614 | 600 | 576 | 560 | 536 | 532 |

The figures suggest that about 530 mg. of the egg white would never be coagulated and if this quantity be subtracted then a linear relation can be obtained between time and the log. of the coagulable egg white left in solution (fig. 35). This fact has no apparent theoretical significance but the figures show that the precipitation of protein by a chemical may proceed in a very slow manner and that the course of the reaction may approximate to a die-away curve.

COOPER (1912)[5] measured the process of protein precipitation by varying

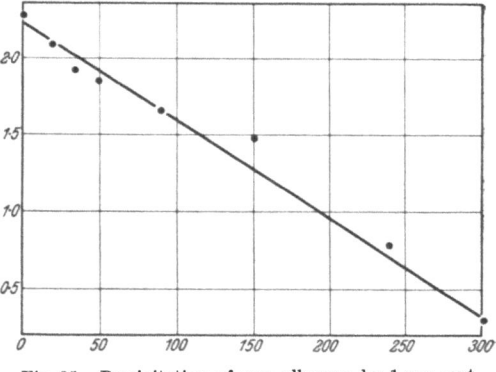

Fig. 35. Precipitation of egg albumen by 1 per cent. phenol. Abscissa:— time in minutes. Ordinate:— log. of quantity unprecipitated less quantity unprecipitated at end of experiment. (COOPER and HAINES, 1928[4].)

concentrations of phenol and the results are shown in fig. 36. The uptake of phenol by protein suggests it is regulated by differential solubility, but when a

[1] FISCHER, A.: Nature (Lond.) **137**, 576 (1936).
[2] SVEDBERG, T.: Kolloid-Z. **51**, 10 (1930).
[3] ASTBURY, W., S. DICKENSON and K. BAILEY: Biochemic. J. **29**, 2351 (1935).
[4] COOPER, E. A.: and R. B. HAINES: J. of Hyg. **28**, 162 (1928).
[5] COOPER, E. A.: Biochemic. J. **6**, 362 (1912).

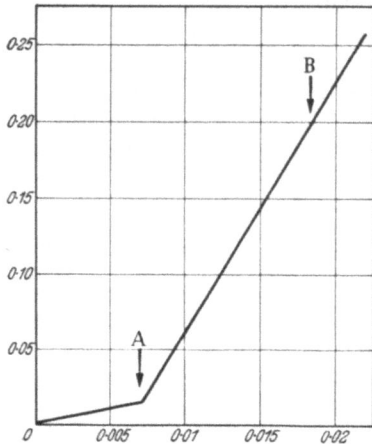

Fig. 36. Combination of phenol with egg albumen. Abscissa:— phenol left in solution (g. per c.c.). Ordinate:— phenol fixed by albumen (g. per g.). *A* Precipitation commencing. *B* Precipitation complete. (COOPER, 1912[1].)

concentration of 0.8 p.c. is attained precipitation commences and the differential solubility increases abruptly Protein precipitation commences when the concentration of phenol in the protein is 1—5 p.c. and is completed when the concentration is 20 p.c. An equimolecular mixture of phenol (94) in egg albumen (34,000) would contain only 0.28 p.c. phenol, which is much less than the concentration at which precipitation commences.

The precipitation of proteins by heat and by phenol does not therefore provide any definite evidence in favour of the monomolecular theory. The time curves expressing the course of precipitation are curious but the writer considers that the most probable explanation for these curves is individual variation in the changes undergone by the large protein molecules.

### (3) Time Action Curves as Expressions of Variation.

GEPPERT (1889)[2] attributed the shape of the time-action curves obtained in haemolysis to the individual variation in the population studied, and MIONI

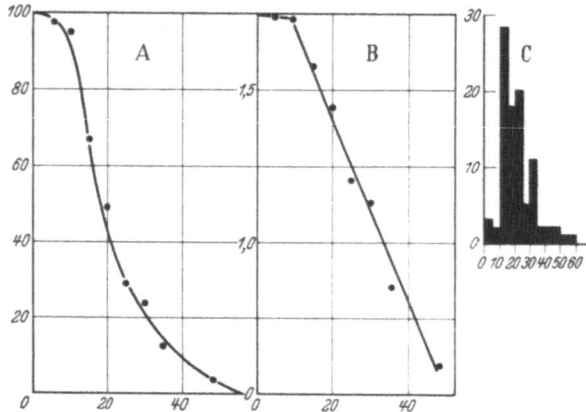

Fig. 37. Rate of destruction of *Colpidium* by 0.2 m. molar. mercuric chloride. Abscissae:— time of exposure in minutes. Ordinates:— (*A*) Per cent. survivors. (*B*) Log. per cent. survivors. (*C*) Per cent. dying at 5 minute intervals. (PETERS, 1920[4].)

(1905)[3] pointed out that HENRI's assumption that the time-action curve of haemolysis represented the course of a monomolecular reaction was invalid because it neglected the fact that there was an extensive individual variation in the resistance of red blood corpuscles. Since that date a number of writers have pointed out that logarithmic curves of the types shown in fig. 34 can be explained if a skew variation in the sensitivity of the cells be assumed. The results obtained by PETERS (1920)[4] may be taken as an example. He measured the death rate of colpidium exposed to mercuric chloride (about 0.2 milli molar). The results are shown in fig. 37. Inspection of curve *A* shows that it is a typical curve of skew variation, and the analysis of the deaths per equal interval of time shown in *C* confirms this fact.

[1] COOPER, E. A.: Biochemic. J. **6**, 362 (1912).
[2] GEPPERT, J.: Berl. klin. Wschr. **26**, 789, 819 (1889).
[3] MIONI, G.: C. r. Soc. Biol. Paris **58**, 192 (1905).
[4] PETERS, R. A.: J. of Physiol. **54**, 260 (1920).

If however the time is plotted against the logarithm of the survivors the linear relation shown in $B$ is obtained and this can be interpreted as expressing a monomolecular reaction commencing after a lag of 10 min. This lag which occurs frequently in disinfection curves (cf. fig. 34) can be explained on the assumption that death is due not to a single event but to a few events. This fact was pointed out by YULE (1910)[1] and the explanation has been elaborated by RAHN (1930, 1931)[2]. The point is not of great importance since the fundamental objection to the "monomolecular theory" is that it does not accord with the known biochemical and biological facts and this objection holds equally against the assumption that the action of drugs on cells is produced by a few molecules.

The interpretation of these curves as expressions of individual variation involves no obvious absurdities, but it is necessary to remember that any form of curve can be explained as expressing individual variation, provided that we are allowed to assume any distribution that we please for the variation. Hence explanations based on individual variation are scarcely more satisfactory than the monomolecular theory unless some explanation can be provided for the unusual manner in which the variation is distributed.

The problem therefore is to find a rational explanation for a skew distribution of variation which will produce an approximately linear relation between the logarithm of the survivors and the time.

GALTON (1879)[3] and MACALISTER (1879)[4] pointed out that skew distributions of variation would occur when non-linear relations occurred between cause and effect. KAPTEYN (1916)[5] also dealt with this subject. REINER (1933)[6] expressed the principle in relation of time action curves as follows:

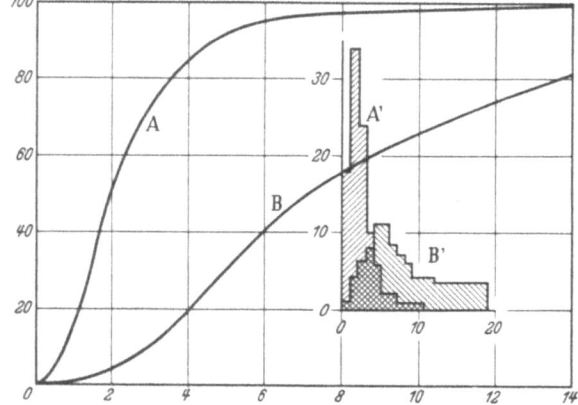

"Asymmetry is to be expected whenever the time which registers the event is a non-linear function of the parameter on which the occurrence of the event depends, even though the variation of the same follows the probability rule."

REINER (1936)[7] has provided a mathematical treatment to relate survival time with toxicity and resistance. Fig. 38 illustrates the obvious fact that the distribution of variation in a population differs according to the character measured. In this case particles of the emulsion show an extreme skew variation when classified according to their diameter ($A$ and $A_1$). On the other hand if

Fig. 38. Distribution of droplets in an emulsion of liquid paraffin. Abscissa: — diameter of particles in micra. Ordinate: — per cent distribution of population. ($A$) According to number of particles. ($B$) According to volume of particles. (SIBREE, 1930[8].)

---

[1] YULE, J. UDNY: J. Statist. Soc. **73**, 26 (1910).
[2] RAHN, O.: J. gen. Physiol. **13**, 179, 396 (1930); **14**, 315 (1931).
[3] GALTON, F.: Proc. roy. Soc. **29**, 365 (1879).
[4] MACALISTER, D.: Proc. roy. Soc. **29**, 367 (1879).
[5] KAPTEYN, J. C.: Rec. Trav. bot. néerl. **13** (2), 105 (1916).
[6] REINER, L.: Proc. Soc. exper. Biol. a. Med. **30**, 574 (1933).
[7] REINER, L.: J. gen. Physiol. **19**, 419 (1936).
[8] SIBREE, J. O.: Trans. Farad. Soc. **26**, 26 (1930).

the volume of paraffin present in particles of different size be measured a slightly skewed sigmoid curve is obtained ($B$ and $B_1$).

This example is instructive because it illustrates the fact that the normal curve of error is an expression of the distribution of variation that may be expected under particular conditions, and unless these conditions obtain there is no reason why the variation should be distributed, in this, rather than any other, form.

The size of particles is apparently regulated chiefly by some process in which there is a non-linear relation between cause and effect and hence the distribution of particles as regards size is of a skew character (curve $A$). The fact that the distribution calculated according to volume (curve $B$) is less skewed does not imply in this case that it is a more correct method of calculating the variation.

This point is of importance because the majority of distributions of individual variation in response to drugs are skewed and there is a tendency to regard these as abnormalities. The normal curve of error represents the simplest distribution of variation and it will be assumed in the calculations made below, but there is no evidence for the assumption of this particular form of distribution.

**Calculation of Time-action Curves.** IRWIN's (1925/26)[1] experiments (fig. 29) provide direct evidence regarding the rate at which a substance (cresyl blue) penetrates a cell (Nitella). These data provide a basis for the calculation based on the following assumptions.

(1) The drug is assumed to enter a cell at the rate shown by IRWIN's experiments and to produce death when a certain concentration $x$ is attained in the cell.

(2) The individual cells are assumed to vary as regards the lethal concentration $x$ and this variation in susceptibility is assumed to follow the normal curve of error. These assumptions permit the calculation of the rate at which the individual cells will die when exposed to the drug (time-action curve).

IRWIN found that the rate of entrance of cresyl blue into *Nitella* followed the mono-molecular formula $\left(Kt = \log \dfrac{a}{a - x}\right)$. The action of a drug in a cell may be assumed to vary as the amount of drug that has diffused into the cell ($x$ in the above formula). Fig. 39, curve $A$, shows the relation between uptake of drug ($x$) and time ($t$). Curve $B$ shows the distribution of incidence of response in relation to concentration in a population of cells which shows a symmetrical variation in respect of the amount of drug needed to produce the selected biological effect. It is assumed that the median concentration is 0.000,25 molar and that the standard deviation is 33 p.c. of the median.

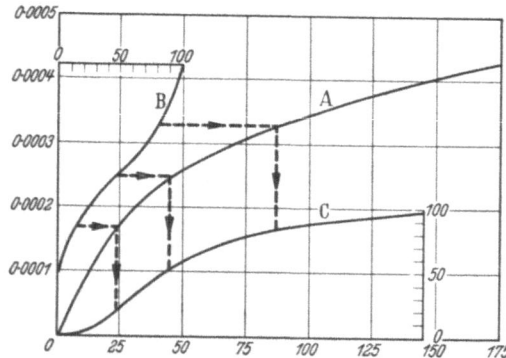

Fig. 39. Conversion of symmetrical to skewed variation. Curve $A$. Diffusion of cresyl blue into Nitella when external concentration is 0.000,4 molar. Abscissa:— time in minutes. Ordinate:— molar conc. of cresyl blue in sap. (IRWIN, 1925/26[1].) Curve $B$. Distribution of variation of response of organisms to be expected if mean effective conc. is 0.000,25 molar and $\sigma = 30$ per cent. of mean. Curve $C$. Distribution of variation of response in respect of time calculated from curves $A$ and $B$.

Curve $C$ shows the manner in which the symmetrical variation shown in curve $B$ will be distorted if the variation of the response be measured in relation to the time of its occurrence.

[1] IRWIN, M.: J. gen. Physiol. **8**, 147 (1925/26).

Fig. 40 shows curve $C$ fig. 39 plotted as a time-action curve i.e. log. survivors × time.

The result shows the commonest type of time-action curve, found with disinfectants for there is an initial lag period of 25 min., after which there is a fairly exact linear relation between log. survivors and time for the next 100 min.

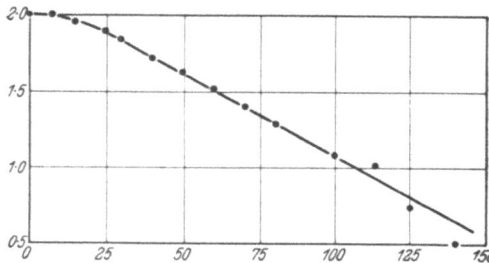

This calculation shows that it is quite simple to account for the logarithmic time-action curves as being expressions of individual variation distorted by an exponential relation between amount of diffusion and time. The general principle is as follows. Suppose three processes or events

Fig. 40.   Curve $C$ in fig. 39 plotted as log. survivors × time.

$A$, $B$ and $C$ are related so that variations in $A$ cause variations in $B$ which cause the appearance of effect $C$. If then the incidence of $C$ shows a symmetrical variation as regards changes in $B$, then the only condition under which variations in $C$ will be distributed symmetrically in relation to changes in $A$, will be when there is a simple linear relation between $A$ and $B$.

This is an important general principle in quantitative pharmacology, because most processes studied are chain processes and figures usually express relations between the extremes of the chain. On the other hand simple linear relations are rare in pharmacology whilst exponential relations are common. Hence skew variations are very frequently found.

**Time Relations of Toxic Action of Copper on Algae.** The toxic action of copper was studied in detail by COOK (1925/26)[1] and the results provide an interesting example of the manner in which a complex process may show relatively simple time relations.

Microchemical experiments on *Valonia* showed that copper chloride penetrated into the cell sap in 5 min. and this relatively rapid rate of penetration was confirmed by experiments on *Nitella* for when the exposure of this organism to copper was stopped after 2 min. it was found that some of the cells subsequently showed signs of injury.

Measurements of the action of copper in reducing carbon dioxide production of *Aspergillus* showed however a latent period of some 15 min. after which the toxic action was produced. If the exposure to copper chloride was terminated after three minutes, the usual latent period was observed and then the toxic action commenced.

These results show that the copper entered the cells rapidly, and produced there some relatively slow chemical process, the end effect of which was to inhibit carbon dioxide production. The course of inhibition followed a monomolecular curve after the initial latent period had been completed.

The time measured in this case therefore expresses the time occupied by two processes, firstly the diffusion of drug into the cell, which, although rapid, occupies a significant proportion of the total time, and secondly the time occupied by the subsequent chemical action which ultimately results in inhibition of the carbon dioxide consumption. The time relation observed is a latent period followed by an inhibition which follows the monomolecular course.

---

[1] COOK, S. F.: J. gen. Physiol. **9**, 575, 631, 735 (1925/26).

The experiments mentioned show that the duration of the latent period is longer than the time needed for diffusion and the simplest explanation of the facts is to suppose that after the copper has diffused into the cell it is converted into some activated form which reacts with some enzyme essential for the production of carbon dioxide. The evidence regarding the poisoning of enzymes by heavy metals shows that this type of reaction is frequently of a monomolecular character.

The time-action curve of copper can therefore be interpreted as expressing three processes, namely: (a) Diffusion of copper chloride into cell; (b) some unknown process activating the copper chloride, and (c) a monomolecular reaction between the activated metal and an enzyme.

The entrance of cresyl blue into *Nitella* and the poisoning of *Aspergillus* by copper both follow the monomolecular formula $\left(Kt = \log \dfrac{a}{a-x}\right)$, but it must be noted that the formula expresses completely different processes in the two cases. In the case of the entrance of cresyl blue $a =$ uptake of dye at equilibrium and $x =$ the uptake at time $t$, whilst in the case of copper poisoning $a =$ normal amount of active enzyme as measured by carbon dioxide production and $x =$ amount of enzyme poisoned at time $t$.

It is interesting to note that these measurements of the rate of action do not provide any direct information regarding the rate of entrance of the drug. They can be interpreted as expressing a monomolecular reaction between the drug and an enzyme, but it is necessary to assume that a large portion of the time is occupied by processes of an unknown nature which cause activation of the copper. This fact somewhat reduces the theoretical importance of the mathematical interpretation of the time-action curve. The formula also provides no information regarding the relation between drug concentration and rate of action, and the value of $K$ in the formula $Kt = \log\left(\dfrac{x}{a-x}\right)$ changes when the concentration of copper chloride is changed.

Cook studied the relation between $K$ and concentration ($c$) and found that the time-concentration curve showed a linear relation between $\log K$ and $\log c$. Log $K$ varied as $^1/_3 \log c$ and this relation was found to hold over a thousandfold range of concentration.

If the time for 50 p.c. inhibition at varying concentrations be considered then the following arguments apply. With all concentrations $\dfrac{a}{a-x} = \dfrac{100}{100-50} = 2$, and hence $Kt =$ constant.

The relation between $K$ and concentration ($c$) is expressed by the formula $K = K_1 c^{\frac{1}{3}}$. Hence $K_1 c^{\frac{1}{3}} t =$ constant, or $c^{\frac{1}{3}} t =$ constant.

The occurrence of a latent period complicates the direct measurement of the time-concentration curve, but Cook (1925/26)[1] found that the duration of the latent period resembled the velocity of reaction in that it varied inversely as (concentration)$^{\frac{1}{3}}$.

This resemblance in the time relations of the latent period and rate of action when the concentration is varied is curious because the time-action curves indicated that the processes occupying the latent period were different from those occupying the subsequent time.

The simplest explanation appears to be to assume an initial adsorption process of such nature that the surface concentration of the adsorbed drug varies as the cube root of the external concentration. If the rate of activation of the copper

---

[1] Cook, S. F.: J. gen. Physiol. **9**, 575, 631 (1925/26).

were proportional to its surface concentration and the rate of action of copper on the enzyme were proportional to the amount activated then the uniform relation between concentration and rate of action would be explained.

This example has been considered at some length because the evidence is more complete than in most cases. The general result is to show that although the time-action curves at first sight suggest a simple chemical process, yet further investigation indicates the occurrence of a complex chain process involving adsorption and diffusion as well as chemical changes of an unknown nature which ultimately result in enzyme poisoning.

The effects of copper considered above were of a graded character but Cook (1925/26)[1] made further observations relating the concentration of copper chloride and the production of a uniform amount of injury on individual cells of *Nitella*. Large populations of these cells were exposed to copper chloride solutions and the proportion of the population showing a certain amount of injury at different times was measured. In this case the time ($t$) required to produce equal action (50 p.c. death) was expressed by the formula $C^n t$ = constant ($n = \frac{1}{3}$). This result agrees with the observations on the inhibition of carbon dioxide production of *Aspergillus*. This agreement is to be expected because in both cases the times measured were those until the appearance of an equal biological effect although the nature of the effect selected was different in the two sets of experiments. The course of destruction of the populations actually followed skew sigmoid curves. These curves when plotted as log. survivors against time show an initial lag period and then a linear relation (fig. 41). According to the monomolecular theory which has already been described, this fact indicates that each cell of *Nitella* is killed by a few molecules of

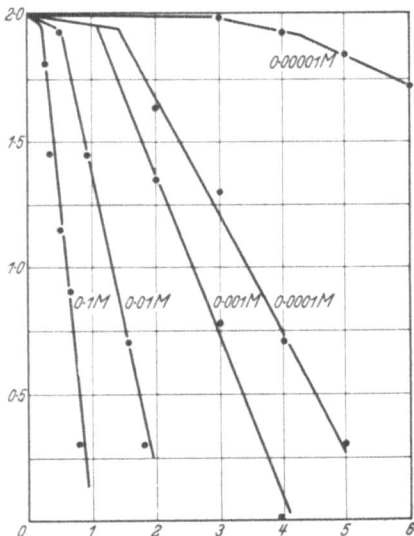

Fig. 41. Time-action curves of copper chloride (0.000,01 to 0.1 molar) on Nitella. Abscissa:— time in hours until loss of turgidity. Ordinate:— log of per cent. of survivors. (Cook, 1925/26[2].)

copper. The *Nitella* cells are 2 to 5 cm. long and 1 mm. in diameter and this hypothesis appears too absurd to permit discussion. The evidence however for the monomolecular theory is just as good in this case as in the case of bacteria, and it is merely the difference in size which makes the explanation seem more ridiculous in the case of *Nitella*.

In this case the rate of inhibition of a graded response ($CO_2$ production of aspergillus) is known to follow a monomolecular curve, whilst the incidence of an all-or-none effect (injury to *Nitella*) has been shown to give logarithmic time-action curves. Fig. 39 show the manner in which an exponential relation between graded effect produced and time of action can distort a symmetrical individual variation and produce a logarithmic time-action curve, and this seems an adequate explanation for the results obtained in the case of copper poisoning. Copper poisoning of algae is therefore a case in which there is fairly complete evidence regarding the processes which eventually result in the appearance of a logarithmic time-action curve.

[1] Cook, S. F.: J. gen. Physiol. **9**, 735 (1925/26).

[2] Cook, S. F.: J. gen. Physiol. **9**, 575, 631, 735 (1925/26).

## (4) Implications of Monomolecular Theory.

The theory that a cell is killed by the action of one or a few molecules of drug and that the action is an all-or-none effect equally likely to occur at any period during the exposure conflicts with the whole of the quantitative evidence regarding the action of drugs. The hypothesis can be tested as regards two obvious points, namely the evidence regarding the amount of drug fixed by cells, and the evidence regarding the processes that occur when drugs act on cells. These subjects have been dealt with previously but in view of the importance of this subject some of this evidence may be recapitulated.

**Quantitative Measurements of Drug Uptake.** The monomolecular theory of drug action implies that one or a few molecules of drug kill one cell and that nothing which happens before the lethal event occurs affects the likelihood of the occurrence of this event. The probability of these hypotheses can be estimated by a consideration of the quantitative data regarding the uptake of drugs by cells.

Measurements of the amount of drug taken up by the cells show that even in the case of small cells such as bacteria the number of molecules fixed per cell at the time of death is very large. Comparative measurements of the rate of fixation of drug and the rate of appearance of biological effects show that the fixation of the drug usually occurs much more rapidly than does the appearance of the biological effect.

These facts are illustrated by the following examples. Fig. 9 shows the uptake of drug from varying concentrations of phenol by yeast cells. The results indicate that the uptake of phenol depends on differential solubility, but that the differential solubility increases abruptly when the concentration of phenol in the water reaches about 0.8 p.c. The reason for this change is indicated in fig. 36 since protein precipitation commences at this point, and COOPER (1912)[1] has shown that whereas the differential solubility between water and soluble protein and water is about $^3/_1$, the differential solubility between precipitated protein and water is about $^{10}/_1$.

Fig. 36 shows clearly that as the concentration of phenol in the watery phase is increased the concentration in the protein rises until at a certain critical point precipitation occurs, and fig. 9 shows a similar course of events. The chief difference is that in the latter case the differential solubility of phenol between cells and water is much lower, namely about $^1/_2$. Fig. 9 shows that when the cellular concentration of phenol reaches 0.26 p.c. lethal effects commence and that all the organisms are killed at a concentration of 0.36 p.c.

These figures permit the calculation of the number of molecules of phenol fixed per cell.

If the volume of a yeast cell be taken as 200 cu.micra then a concentration of 0.3 p.c. phenol corresponds to $3 \times 10^9$ molecules per cell. Similar calculations can be made regarding the reaction between phenol and bacteria.

REICHEL (1909)[2] found that the distribution coefficient between B. pyocyaneus and a watery solution of phenol lay between $^6/_1$ and $^{20}/_1$. If the volume of a bacterium be taken as 4 cu.micra and the phenol concentration in the bacterium as 10 p.c. then there will be about $10^{10}$ molecules of phenol per bacterium.

Similar results are obtained from measurements of the action of mercuric chloride on yeast. RAHN and BARNES (1933)[3] found that the death rate of yeast cells exposed to 0.025 p.c. mercuric chloride followed an exact logarithmic curve.

[1] COOPER, E. A.: Biochemic. J. **6**, 362 (1912).
[2] REICHEL, H.: Biochem. Z. **22**, 149 (1909).
[3] RAHN, O., and M. N. BARNES: J. gen. Physiol. **16**, 579 (1933).

HERZOG and BETZEL (1911)[1] measured the uptake of mercuric chloride by yeast, and found with an outside concentration of 0.015 p.c. an uptake of 0.08 p.c. This corresponds to about $10^8$ molecules per cell.

These examples suffice to show that the number of molecules of lethal agent fixed per cell is very large, and the theory that out of this huge population only one molecule produces any effect is extremely improbable. Calculations of this type can be repeated indefinitely. The number of molecules fixed per cell in the case of lethal agents usually works out between $10^8$ and $10^{10}$. Even in the case of potent drugs acting at dilutions of 1 part in $10^9$ or more the number of molecules per cell required to produce a demonstrable action is seldom less than 10,000.

**Drug Actions as Chain Processes.** The monomolecular theory also implies that the action of drugs is due to one or to a few events and that until these events occur the cell is in no way effected.

There is however a fair amount of evidence that in these cases a chain of reactions occurs. The first step is the fixation of the drug and this is followed by a series of chemical changes which ultimately result in the event that is measured.

Chain processes of this type are frequent in reactions in heterogeneous systems. For example GARNER (1926)[2] found that at $1000°$ C. the adsorption of oxygen by charcoal was practically instantaneous but that the heat liberated by this process was liberated over periods varying from 1 to 2 minutes. Hence even in this very simple system the rate of adsorption could not be measured by the rate of heat production.

In the case of the precipitation of proteins by phenol COOPER (1912)[3] found that the uptake of phenol by protein proceeded very rapidly and was completed in about 12 min. whilst the actual precipitation took a much longer time. Similarly in the case of phenol acting on bacteria there is evidence that the fixation of the drug is the first of a chain of processes which culminate in death.

KÜSTER and ROTHAUB (1913)[4] measured the rate of uptake of phenol by anthrax bacilli and the time of death. They found that the fixation of the phenol was completed within 24 hours but that death did not occur until 3 or 4 days. Hence the rate of death of the bacteria gave no indication of the rate of uptake of the drug.

COOPER and WOODHOUSE (1923)[5] concluded that the absorption of phenol by bacteria was only the initial stage in the process of disinfection and that the germicidal action which followed was not a chemical reaction but a physicochemical process, namely the de-emulsification of the colloidal suspension. Similarly in the case of haemolysis with weak acids. CHRISTOPHERS (1929)[6] showed that these substances might be fixed by the corpuscles in less than 5 minutes whilst haemolysis might not occur until an hour later.

Similar evidence exists to show that when mercuric chloride acts on cells it is first fixed on the cell surface and then slowly diffuses into the cell The rate of diffusion is relatively rapid in the case of thin-walled cells and very slow in the case of spores COOK's experiments on the action of copper chloride on algae showed that the action was certainly divided into three stages namely

[1] HERZOG, R. A., and R. BETZEL: Hoppe-Seylers Z. **74**, 221 (1911).
[2] GARNER, W. E.: Trans. Farad. Soc. **22**, 433, 461 (1926).
[3] COOPER, E. A.: Biochemic. J. **6**, 362 (1912).
[4] KÜSTER, E., and ROTHAUB: Z. Hyg. **73**, 205 (1913).
[5] COOPER, E. A., and D. L. WOODHOUSE: Biochemic. J. **17**, 600 (1923).
[6] CHRISTOPHERS, S. R.: Indian J. med. Res. **17**, 544 (1929).

entrance of drug into cell, intermediate and unknown chemical changes and finally the poisoning of the cell.

The quantitative data just considered appear to the writer to constitute a disproof of the monomolecular theory as definite as is ever likely to be obtained in a subject as uncertain as quantitative pharmacology.

The number of molecules of common poisons known to be present in each cell when death occurs ranges from $10^4$ to $10^8$ and usually is nearer the latter number. The hypothesis that only one molecule of this huge population produces a lethal action is extraordinarily improbable, indeed the only analogous case is the fertilisation of an ovum by the entry of one out of a huge population of spermatozoa. The evidence that drugs are rapidly fixed by the cell, and then slowly exert a lethal action is also directly adverse to the monomolecular theory which states that the chance of death for any cell is the same after a few molecules of drug have penetrated as after the penetration of relatively large quantities of drug. The individual variation theory supposes that death occurs after the production of a certain amount of chemical injury and that the cells vary, probably as regards several factors such as thickness of cell wall and the amount of drug which must enter the cell in order to produce death.

Pharmacological evidence is so uncertain that it is seldom possible to produce an absolute proof or disproof of any hypothesis, but judged from the standpoint of probability the monomolecular hypothesis appears to verge on the impossible.

### (5) Mortality Curves.

The monomolecular theory of destruction of organisms has exercised a strange fascination on a variety of workers. BROWNLEE (1919)[1] concluded that the formulae for estimating rates of mortality advanced by GOMPERTZ in 1825 and modified by MAKEHAM could be regarded as expressing a monomolecular reaction. He considered that these formulae suggested that:

"The substances or capacities on which life depends decay according to the law of the unimolecular reaction, that is that the amounts present at the end of equal intervals of time can be represented by the terms of a geometrical progression."

PEARL (1928)[2] pointed out that if the logarithm of survivors in a population were plotted against the time three types of curve might be obtained.

(a) Nearly rectangular. This will occur in the case of a uniform population whose survival depends on individual resistance rather than on the chance occurrence of fatal events. Human mortality curves for ages above 10 years approximate to this type.

(b) Linear relation. This indicates a constant death rate   Pearl obtained figures approximating to this type with vestigial drosophila.

(c) Concave relation. This indicates a decreasing death rate   This type of curve is obtained with human infants.

SZABO (1931)[3] found that curves of this last type also expressed the duration of life of oak trees.

GOWEN (1931, 1934)[4] has published mortality curves of mice of various strains exposed to three lethal agents, ricin poisoning, infection with mouse typhoid and infection with pseudo-rabies. When plotted as log. survivors × time, the ricin curves were nearly linear, the mouse typhoid curves convex and the

[1] BROWNLEE, J.: J. roy. Statist. Soc. **82**, 34 (1919).
[2] PEARL, R.: The Rate of Living. New York 1928.
[3] SZABO, I.: Quart. Rev. Biol. **6**, 462 (1931).
[4] GOWEN, J. W.: J. gen. Physiol. **14**, 463 (1931) — Symposium quantit. Biol. **2**, 128 (1934).

pseudo-rabies curves were concave. This author also found with drosophila populations under optimum conditions that normal flies showed the usual convex mortality curve but that an abnormal intersex variety provided a mortality curve which showed a latent period of about a day and then was nearly exactly linear for 70 days.

Curves of all these types may be obtained with micro-organisms, not only when exposed to disinfectants, but also when exposed to a wide variety of unfavourable conditions. For instance CHESNEY (1916)[1] gives figures for the dying out of pneumococci from old cultures which show a constant death rate (linear relation between log. survivors and time). HENDERSON SMITH (1921)[2] measured the rate of death of *Botrytis* spores exposed to phenol He found that old resistant spores showed sigmoid death curves, whereas young susceptible spores showed logarithmic curves. These observations provide direct proof that the shape of the death curves is an expression of the variation of the resistance of the population on which the drug acts. Populations of mice, drosophila, algae and micro-organisms therefore show essentially similar mortality curves.

In all cases some of the curves show a constant death rate (monomolecular curves). If these curves in the case of bacteria poisoned with phenol are interpreted as proof of the occurrence of a monomolecular reaction between bacteria and the drug, then they prove equally the occurrence of a monomolecular reaction between mice and ricin. It appears to the writer that the improbability in the two cases is not greatly dissimilar.

### (6) Action of Radiations.

The destruction of micro-organisms by radiations (radium, X-rays or ultraviolet light) provides curves similar to those provided by disinfectants.

BLAU and ALTENBURGER (1922)[3] suggested that the occurrence of logarithmic curves proved that the death produced by radiations was due to the absorption of one or a few quanta per cell. This theory has been developed by CROWTHER (1926)[4], P. CURIE (1929)[5], HOLWEEK and LACASSAGNE (1930)[6], WYCKOFF (1930)[7], PUGSLEY, ODDIE and EDDY (1935)[8]

PACKARD (1931)[9] has summarised the evidence and literature. The essentials of the controversy are exactly similar to the controversy in relation to the action of disinfectants. The curves obtained are sometimes sigmoid and sometimes logarithmic. The quantum theory implies that radiations produce death in an all-or-none fashion and do not produce graded actions There is however a mass of evidence which shows that radiations can produce graded, sub-lethal effects on cells. The quantum theory also implies that there is no extensive individual variation in the resistance of cells. This assumption is contrary to the known laws of biology.

In the case of radiations it is very difficult to estimate directly the number of quanta arrested per cell, but WYCKOFF (1932)[10] made such measurements in

[1] CHESNEY, A. M. C.: J. of exper. Med. **24**, 387 (1916).
[2] HENDERSON SMITH, J.: Ann. appl. Biol. **8**, 27 (1921).
[3] BLAU, M., and K. ALTENBURGER: Z. Physik **12**, 315 (1922).
[4] CROWTHER, J. A.: Proc. roy. Soc. B. **100**, 396 (1926).
[5] CURIE, P.: C. r. Acad. Sci. Paris **188**, 202 (1929).
[6] HOLWEEK, F., and LACASSAGNE A.: C. r. Soc. Biol. Paris **103**, 766 (1930).
[7] WYCKOFF, R. W. G.: J. of exper. Med. **52**, 435, 769 (1930).
[8] PUGSLEY, A. T., T. H. ODDIE and C. E. EDDY: Proc. roy. Soc. B. **118**, 276 (1935).
[9] PACKARD, C.: Quart. Rev. Biol. **6**, 253 (1931).
[10] WYCKOFF, R. W. G.: J. gen. Physiol. **15**, 351 (1932).

the case of ultraviolet light acting on bacteria and found that each bacterium absorbed millions of quanta.

The quantum theory is not so obviously absurd as the monomolecular theory of drug action because there is so much less quantitative evidence in the former case. It does however involve a number of very improbable if not impossible assumptions and only explains a portion of the curves obtained.

A far simpler and more rational explanation is to suppose that the radiations produce chemical changes inside the cells which cause disorganisation of the protoplasm, possible by denaturation of the proteins. The logarithmic curves can be explained in exactly the same manner as can the similar curves obtained with drugs.

### Discussion.

The author's objection to the monomolecular theory of drug action is that it is opposed to the majority of facts established regarding quantitative pharmacology. The general conception of an organism such as a bacterium or a yeast cell is that it is a structure composed of millions of protein molecules and carrying on its activities by means of a large population of enzyme molecules. The number of different kinds of enzymes in a cell is large but the number of enzyme molecules of any one kind in a cell is in most cases very large. The enzymatic activity is correlated in a manner that is at present unknown.

A cell is killed by a drug after it has taken up a large number of drug molecules, and in many cases the lethal action is produced slowly, and there is evidence for the occurrence of a chain of reactions. The usual conception of drug action is that the drug gradually disorganises the cell organisation by such actions as enzyme poisoning or protein denaturation and at a certain stage of disorganisation the cell is killed.

The monomolecular theory of drug action assumes however that the drug produces only a single significant effect on the cell, namely the destruction of some vital centre or as RAHN (1935)[1] terms it, an essential gene  This effect is supposed to be produced by a single or at most a few molecules of drug and to be as likely to occur at the commencement as at the end of the exposure to the drug. The slow processes of uptake and penetration of the drug are supposed not to predispose the cell to the final lethal event.

The writer's objection to this hypothesis is on the grounds of its extreme vitalistic character, since it assumes a type of organisation in the living cell that is unknown to physical chemistry. The writer does not suggest that our present knowledge of cellular biology or of physical chemistry is adequate to explain the behaviour of the cell by the laws of physical chemistry, but he considers that every endeavour should be made to explain cellular behaviour without assuming unknown forms of organisation.

The other outstanding objection to the monomolecular theory is that it denies the existence of individual variation. The individual variation of organisms in response to drugs is however one of the most outstanding features of drug action observed when the relation between dosage and effect is studied. In this case time is allowed for equilibrium to be attained and hence the individual variation observed cannot possibly be explained as an expression of the monomolecular theory.

If we recognise the undoubted fact that all cell populations vary and that skew distributions of variation are bound to occur when the relation between

[1] RAHN, O.: Symposia Quant. Biol. **2**, 70 (1935).

incidence of death and duration of exposure to drug is considered, then there is no difficulty in explaining not only the linear relations between log survivors and time of action, but also the convex and concave relations which are frequently found.

## Chapter 13

## Time-concentration Curves.

### (1) Form of Curves and Possible Significance.

The discussion of the kinetics of drug action in chapter 11 showed that the rate of action of drugs on living tissues often could be expressed by simple formulae, but that closer examination of the processes involved showed that the processes in most cases were of a complex chain character and that the theoretical significance of the formulae was very doubtful.

Time-concentration curves express the relation between concentration and the time needed to produce some selected effect; they are derived from time-action curves and obviously, if the theoretical significance of the latter is unknown, it is impossible to determine the theoretical significance of time-concentration curves. Consequently these latter curves do not provide much help in the analysis of the mode of action of drugs. On the other hand time-concentration curves are of great practical importance because it is necessary in many cases to know the relation between the concentration (or dosage) and the time needed to produce an action. This knowledge is of particular importance in the case of disinfection and disinfestation, and for the calculation of the effects of exposure of human beings to noxious gases. Owing to its practical importance the subject has been studied extensively and there is an abundance of data, but the relations established must in most cases be regarded as empirical.

In view of the character of the evidence the theoretical aspects of the problem will be reviewed briefly and then the importance of the empirical relations found with different classes of drugs will be considered.

The variety of time-concentration curves is particularly large because these curves are exceptionally easy to obtain. It is only necessary to expose a series of cell populations to a series of concentrations or doses of a drug and to measure the time until some selected effect is produced. The effect selected may be either a particular stage in a graded action (e.g. 50 p.c. inhibition of a frog's heart) or an all-or-none effect (e.g. any selected percentage mortality in a population of small organisms).

The study of time-concentration curves can best be commenced by a consideration of the relation between concentration of drug and the time taken for a constant amount to enter the cells. The penetration of *Nitella* by a dye is a particularly simple case because the time measured is simply the time taken by the dye to enter the cell, and no question arises as to how much of the time measured is occupied by the delay between the fundamental chemical action and the biological response. Fig. 42 shows the rate of entrance of cresyl blue into Nitella at varying concentrations (IRWIN, 1925/26[1]). The possible reasons for the shape of these curves were discussed in chapter 11.

Owing to the wide range of times and concentrations covered the curves are shown on logarithmic scales. A time-concentration curve can be obtained by choosing some particular effect (e.g. attainment of $20 \times 10^{-5}$ molar concentration in cell vacuole) and measuring the time taken by varying concen-

---

[1] IRWIN, M.: J. gen. Physiol. 8, 147 (1925/26).

Table 13.  Time-concentration relations of uptake of cresyl blue by *Nitella*.
(IRWIN, 1925/26[1].)

| Molar conc. cresyl blue $\times 10^5$ | 3 | 4 | 6 | 8 | 16 | 25 | 55 | 103 | 207 |
|---|---|---|---|---|---|---|---|---|---|
| Time in min. until $20 \times 10^{-5}$ molar conc. in vacuole | 44.7 | 28.2 | 17.4 | 14.5 | 7.08 | 5.0 | 2.8 | 1.6 | 1.1 |
| c. t. | 135 | 113 | 104 | 116 | 113 | 125 | 152 | 165 | 228 |
| (c —0.7) (t —0.6) | 102 | 92 | 90 | 102 | 100 | 112 | 119 | 102 | 104 |

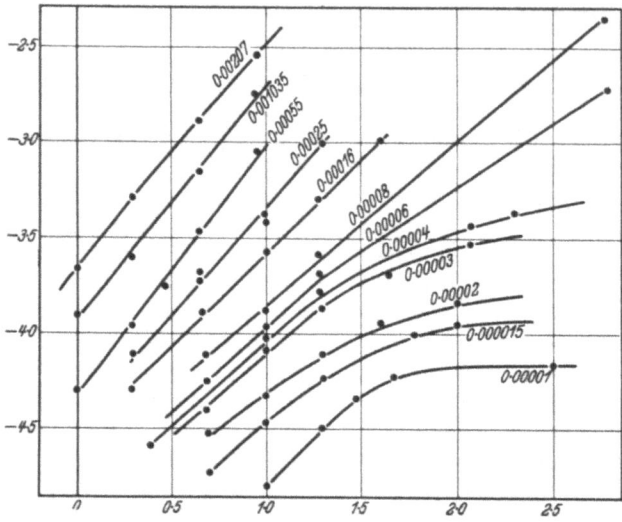

Fig. 42.  Rate of entrance of cresyl blue into Nitella at varying concentrations. Abscissa:— log. time in minutes. Ordinate:— log. molar conc. of dye in central vacuole. The numbers on the curves show the external molar conc. of dye. (IRWIN, 1925/26[1].)

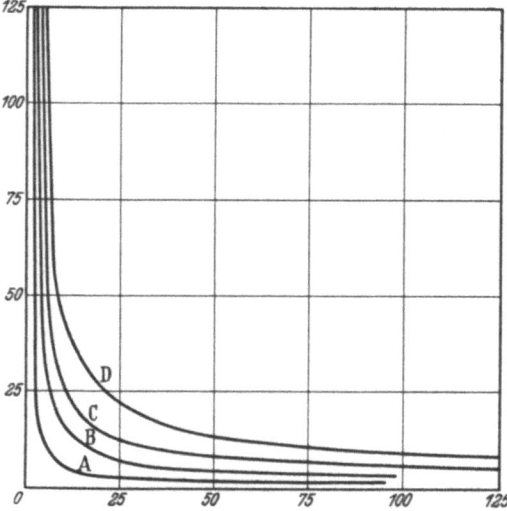

Fig. 43.  Time-concentration curves of entrance of cresyl blue into *Nitella*. Abscissa:— time in minutes. Ordinate:— molar conc. × 100,000. The curves show the times (taken from fig. 42) at which the following internal molar concentrations are attained:— (A) 0.001; (B) 0.000,5; (C) 0.000,2; (D) 0.000,1.

trations to produce this effect. These figures are shown in Table 13, and a series of curves for a range of concentrations are shown in fig. 43.

Inspection of the figures in Table 13 shows that the product c.t. is clearly not constant but rises at the two extremes. The curves in fig. 42 show however that the lowest concentration that will produce an internal concentration of 0.000,2 molar dye is slightly more than 0.000,02 molar. Consequently it seems justifiable to subtract a threshold value from the concentration. It is certain that there must be a minimum time required for penetration of the cell by the dye, however high the concentration and in fact the time-action curves for the highest concentrations, as shown in the original article, provide evidence of a lag period of nearly one minute. If these adjustments are made the relation:—
$$(c - c_m)(t - t_m) = \text{constant, is approximately correct.}$$

This relation holds for any internal concentration that is chosen as an end point, although $c_m$ differs with each end point chosen.

This is a simpler relation between concentration and time till equal action than is found in the case of many drug actions. The penetration of *Nitella* by dye cannot be a simple

[1] IRWIN, M.: J. gen. Physiol. 8, 147 (1925/26).

diffusion process, because the internal concentration is much higher than the external concentration, hence this provides an example of a complex process which has simple time relations.

IRWIN obtained the following figures relating the concentrations of dye outside and inside the cell when equilibrium had been attained.

| Molar conc. outside $\times 10^5$ ($C_1$) . . . . . . | 1 | 2 | 3 | 4 |
|---|---|---|---|---|
| Molar conc. inside $\times 10^5$ ($C_2$) . . . . . . | 7 | 14 | 32 | 48 |

These figures approximate to the relation $(C_1)^{1.5} = C_2$.

Unfortunately they cover only a narrow range because higher concentrations killed the cells before equilibrium was established. It is interesting to note that the internal concentration at equilibrium varies as a low power of the external concentration even though the relation between the two concentrations suggests the occurrence of an adsorption process.

It may be noted that there is no reason why the relation between the external concentration and the internal concentration at equilibrium should be similar to the relation of the external concentration and the reciprocal of the time required for equal uptake of dye, because the latter measure will be a different fraction of the equilibrium concentration at each external concentration investigated.

This example is simpler than any that will be considered subsequently but even in this case a simple relation between concentration and time does not occur. The formula $ct = $ constant is indeed an impossible one in the case of drugs acting on biological material because it implies that an infinitely small concentration of drug will produce the selected action in infinite time, and conversely that a sufficiently high concentration will produce an instantaneous effect. In some cases $ct = $ constant gives an approximate fit, but this merely implies that

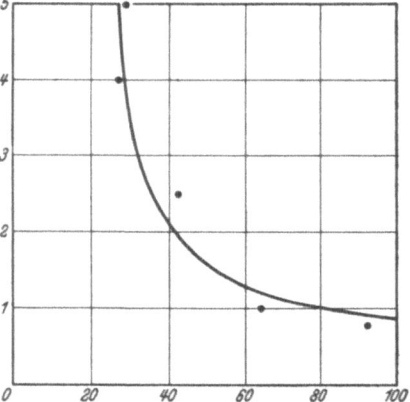

Fig. 44. Time-concentration curve for the production of systolic arrest of the frog's isolated heart by g-strophanthin. Abscissa:— time in minutes. Ordinate: – conc. in parts per 10 million. (HOLSTE, 1912[1].)

$c_m$ and $t_m$ are so small as not to produce a measurable error.

The time-concentration relation of ouabain acting on the heart (figs. 44 and 45) may be taken as a simple example of the relation between concentration and time until the appearance of a biological response. The time measured in this case is considerably more complex than the time measured in the case of cresyl blue penetration since the interval between exposure to drug and response of the heart includes not only the time of drug fixation but also the interval between the drug fixation and the time until appearance of a biological response.

Inspection of fig. 44 shows that in this case the time of action of the highest concentrations of drug would be about 20 min. and it also shows the well known fact that there is a minimum concentration below which the drug will not produce the biological effect. The curve in actual fact follows the formula

$$(c - 0.5)(t - 20) = \text{constant} = 30.$$

[1] HOLSTE, A.: Arch. f. exper. Path. **70**, 433 (1912).

The mode of action of cardiac glucosides on the frog's heart has been studied carefully and in this case there is a certain amount of information regarding the processes that cause the relatively long delay before the action is produced.

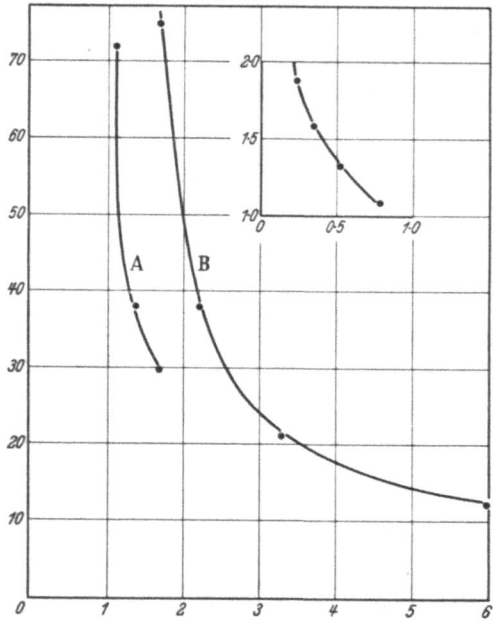

This evidence has been summarised by WEESE (1936)[2] and by LENDLE (1935)[3]. This work has been carried out chiefly on the frog's heart, and there is a general agreement that the action can be divided into three phases, namely (a) membrane phase, (b) fixation phase, and (c) action phase (FISCHER, 1928[4]; CLOETTA, 1929[5]). FISCHER's results with digitoxin are summarised in Table 14. The membrane phase is not included in this table but it is so short (about 10 sec.) that it can be ignored. During this phase the drug is loosely fixed and is immediately removed by washing out.

Fig. 45. Time-concentration relation of action of scillaren (*A*) and of ouabain (*B*) on cat's heart-lung preparation. Abscissa:— conc. in parts per million. Ordinate:— time in minutes until arrest. Inset. Curve *B* plotted as log. $t$ × log. $c$. (ROTHLIN, 1934[1].)

This stage of loose adsorption is followed by a fixation phase during which the drug is firmly fixed and can only be removed by thorough and prolonged washing. If the fluid is changed during this phase a biological effect usually follows after a certain interval.

The amount of drug fixed is proportional to the duration of exposure to the drug, and the figures for the fixation time show that the rate of fixation is directly proportional to the concentration of the drug. During this period of fixation the biological response appears, this proceeds slowly and culminates in systolic arrest. Table 14 shows that the latent period as well as the duration of fixation is inversely proportional to the concentration of the drug.

Table 14. Time-concentration relations of action of digitoxin on the isolated frog's heart. All times in minutes. (FISCHER, 1928[4].)

| Concentration parts per million | (a) Time till systolic arrest | (b) Fixation time | (c) Latent period (time till commencement of biological response) | a—c |
|---|---|---|---|---|
| 166 | 7 | — | — | 7 |
| 83 | 9 | — | — | 9 |
| 40 | 8.5 | — | — | 8.5 |
| 20 | 8—10 | 3—4 | 1 | 8 |
| 10 | 12—13 | 6—8 | 2 | 10 |
| 5 | 24 | 12—16 | 4 | 20 |
| 4 | 84 | — | — | — |

The interval between the commencement and the termination of the biological effect (last column Table 14) shows however an obscure time relation. There

[1] ROTHLIN, E.: Helvet. med. Acta **1**, 460 (1934).
[2] WEESE, H.: Digitalis, p. 127 ff. Leipzig: Georg Thieme 1936.
[3] LENDLE, L.: Heffters Handb. exper. Pharmakol. Ergänzbd. **1**, 1 (1935).
[4] FISCHER, H.: Arch. f. exper. Path. **130**, 111 (1928).
[5] CLOETTA, M.: J. amer. med. Assoc. **93**, 1462 (1929).

appears to be a minimum period of about 8 min. but when the concentration falls below 10 parts per million this period rapidly increases.

It may be mentioned that the distinction between loose adsorption and firm adsorption is a relative one, for if a heart is washed sufficiently thoroughly the action of the drug can be reversed even after systolic arrest has been produced. The ease of reversal varies greatly in the case of different glucosides, but even in the case of the very firmly adsorbed digitoxin, reversal can be produced by sufficiently thorough washing (KINGISEPP, 1936[1]).

The action of digitalis glucosides on the frog's heart is peculiar in two respects, firstly it is a slow action which is favourable for analysis and secondly it has been studied carefully. The results show clearly a complex process comprising initial adsorption followed by slower unknown chemical or physical actions which finally result in a biological response. There appears to be a simple relation between concentration and time until initiation of the biological effects, but the time until systolic arrest, which is the clearest end point is evidently a complex time, with a long minimum period of biological lag.

WEESE (1928)[2] using the cat's heart-lung apparatus found the relation of $ct$ = constant with cardiac glucosides, but more recent experiments by ROTHLIN (1934)[3] with the same method obtained the results shown in fig. 45 which indicate both a threshold concentration and also a minimum time of response. The figures in curve $B$ (fig. 45) are fitted by the formula $(c - 1.2)\ (t - 6)$ = constant = 32. These results show that the relation between the concentration of cardiac glucosides and the time required for an equal biological effect follows a regular course, and the results can be fitted by a simple formula. It is however necessary to subtract threshold values for time and concentration and the expression of the relation by a formula does not add much to our knowledge of the nature of the mode of action of the drugs on the cells.

The nature of digitalis action is unknown; it presumably produces some physico-chemical alteration in the cardiac cell membranes, but it is not known if it combined chemically or acts in some physical manner nor is it known whether it acts on the proteins or on the lipoids. The temperature coefficient of digitalis action has been determined by several workers (SOLLMANN et al., 1914[4]; ISSE-KUTZ, 1924[5]; ZIPF, 1927[6]; FISCHER, 1928[7]). All have found a temperature coefficient ($Q_{10}$) of more than 2 and FISCHER showed that the $Q_{10}$ of both the fixation phase and the action phase was $2 - 3$; these results favour the hypothesis that a chemical reaction occurs between the drug and the tissue.

The analysis of time-concentration relation of the action of ouabain on the heart shows therefore that the action is a complex chain process, proceeding in several stages, but that the general relation between concentration and time until action can be expressed by a simple formula.

The next types of time-concentration relations that may be considered are those expressing the destruction of small organisms. This is a problem of practical importance in relation to disinfection and disinfestation and hence a very large amount of evidence is available. The forms of the curves obtained are of a wide variety and it is necessary to have some method by which they can be described.

[1] KINGISEPP, G.: J. Pharmacol. Baltimore 55, 377 (1936).
[2] WEESE, H.: Arch. f. exper. Path. 135, 228 (1928).
[3] ROTHLIN, E.: Helvet. med. Acta 1, 460 (1934).
[4] SOLLMANN, T., W. H. MENDENHALL and J. L. STINGLE: J. Pharmacol. Baltimore 6, 533 (1914).
[5] ISSEKUTZ, B. VON: Pflügers Arch. 202, 371 (1924).
[6] ZIPF, K.: Arch. f. exper. Path. 124, 259 (1927).
[7] FISCHER, H.: Arch. f. exper. Path. 130, 111 (1928).

Fig. 44 may be taken as a general type of time-concentration curve. The curve in this case consists of a central portion over which the product $C \cdot t$ is approximately constant and two extremities which show $C$ and $t$ approaching infinity when $t$ and $C$ respectively approach certain minimal values. Since $C \cdot t$ is nearly constant over the median portion, there will be a linear relation over this portion if log. $C$ is plotted against log. $t$, whilst the extremes of the curve will run to infinity with minimum values of $C$ and $t$. The advantage of this method of plotting time-concentration relations is that a linear relation will be obtained not only when $C \cdot t =$ constant but also when $C^n t =$ constant, moreover the value of $n$ can be easily measured from the curve.

The chief practical difficulty arises in relation to the extremes of the curve. In many cases the threshold concentration and the threshold time are both small and neglect of these values does not seriously distort the central portion of the curve. Sometimes however these values are large and in such a case no portion of the curve log. $C \times$ log. $t$ will be linear. The inset in fig. 45 shows an

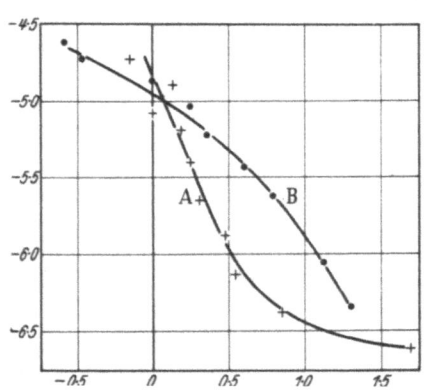

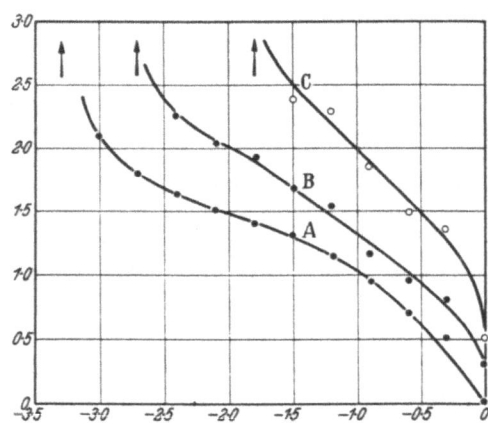

Fig. 46. Time-concentration curve showing destruction of *Spirostomum ambiguum* by alkali. Abscissa: — log. time until death in hours. Ordinate: — log. $C_{OH}$. (A) Tap water and carbonate. (B) Borax buffer. (JENKINS, 1926[1].)

Fig. 47. Time-concentration curve of destruction of *Paramoecia*. Abscissa: — log. conc. Ordinate: — log. time until death in hours. (A) and (B) Quinine on normal and on quinine tolerant forms respectively. (C) Arsenious acid. (NEUSCHLOSS, 1914[1].)

example of this fact. Figs. 46 and 47 show examples of time-concentration relations of the destruction of small organisms plotted as log. $c \times$ log. $t$. Fig. 46, curve $A$ shows a typical form, namely a straight central portion with the time value deviating towards infinity when the concentration falls to a minimum value. Curve $B$ in fig. 46 is however atypical since the extremes of the curve deviate in the opposite direction and indicate that above a certain $p_H$ death is instantaneous and that the organisms do not survive in the medium used beyond a certain period even when the solution is neutral.

The central and approximately linear portions of curves $A$ and $B$ also show different relations, since curve $A$ shows the relation $C^2 t =$ constant and curve $B$ the relation $Ct =$ constant. Since curves $A$ and $B$ both express the action of acid on the same organism it is not possible to provide any theoretical explanation for this difference and these curves provide an example of the exceedingly uncertain evidence provided by time-concentration curves.

Another result is shown in fig. 47 which gives results obtained by NEUSCHLOSS (1914)[2] on paramoecia. The curves show a linear relation between log. time and

[1] JENKINS, P. M.: Brit. J. exp. Biol. 4, 365 (1926).
[2] NEUSCHLOSS, S.: Pflügers Arch. 176, 223 (1914).

log. concentration over the middle of their course. With minimum effective concentrations the curves are deflected, and this could be corrected by subtracting a threshold concentration. With high concentrations the rates of action of the drugs are however accelerated and this can only be explained on the assumption that when the drug concentration rises above a certain figure a change in the poisoning process occurs.

In this case the median portions of these curves are fitted by the following formulae. Quinine on normal paramoecea:— $c^{0.5}t = $ constant; quinine on quinine resistant paramoecea:— $c^{0.72}t = $ constant; arsenious acid $ct = $ constant.

The fact that the value of $n$ is different in the case of normal and of resistant paramoecia suggests that we cannot regard these time concentration relations as a simple expression of a reaction between the drug and the organisms.

Fig. 48 shows the rate of poisoning of *Nitella* by copper chloride; in this case the concentration was varied over a 10,000 fold range but the time only changed about 20 fold and the curve follows the relation $C^{\frac{1}{3}}t = $ constant.

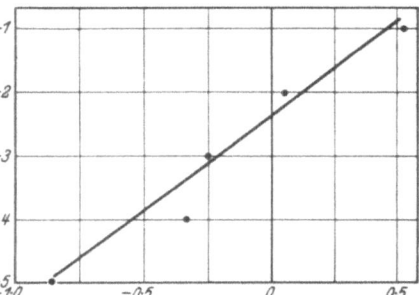

Fig. 48. Time-concentration curve of destruction of *Nitella* by copper chloride. Abscissa:— log. $1/t$ ($t = $ time in hours). Ordinate:— log. molar conc. (COOK, 1925/26[1].)

The examples given show that in the case of drugs acting on small organisms a linear relation over a considerable range of concentrations is obtained when the logarithms of the time and of the concentration are plotted. The writer collected a considerable number of examples in which time-concentration relations for the destruction of small organisms had been measured (CLARK, 1933[2]). He found that in all cases a linear relation was found over a considerable range of concentrations between log. concentrations and log. time. The value of $n$ in the formula $c^n t = $ constant varied from 0.3 to 1.3.

It may be said therefore that it is not difficult to describe time-concentration relations because if log. $C$ be plotted against log. $t$ a linear relation over a considerable range of concentrations is obtained, and the curve can be interpreted by the simple formula $C^n t = $ constant. There is however a considerable difficulty in assigning any definite significance to this formula. The value of $n$ varies greatly in different systems but the variation is not a completely random one. For example heavy metals give values for $n$ of less than 1 with a wide variety of tissues, a number of drugs such as anaesthetics and cardiac glucosides show values of $n$ approximating to unity, whilst phenol regularly shows high values of $n$. The relation between concentration and rate of action depends therefore more upon the drug that is used than upon the biological material on which it acts.

The difficult problem is to relate these variations in $n$ with any probable physico-chemical process. The most likely process to cause delay in the entrance of drugs is diffusion through the cell membrane. The diffusion of substances into cells has been investigated extensively by OSTERHOUT (1933)[3]. He postulates a non-aqueous but liquid surface film in living cells and believes that the rate

[1] COOK, S. F.: J. gen. Physiol. **9**, 735 (1925/26).
[2] CLARK, A. J.: The Mode of Action of Drugs on Cells, Table 10, p. 89. London: Arnold and Co. 1933.
[3] OSTERHOUT, W. J. V.: Erg. Physiol. **35**, 967 (1933).

of entrance of electrolytes and dyes into cells is largely regulated by the rate of passage through this film. OSTERHOUT's general formula for the rate of entrance of electrolytes is

$$\frac{dMi}{dt} = V_M(Mo - Mi)$$

$Mi$ and $Mo$ = internal and external concentrations and $V_M$ = velocity constant.

IRWIN's results upon the entrance of dye into Nitella have been shown to approximate to the formula

$$(c - c_m)(t - t_m) = \text{constant}.$$

In this case $c$ = external concentration and $t$ = time needed to produce a given internal concentration.

These results and conclusions are therefore consistent with the general theory that the rate of entrance of dye into the cell is directly proportional to the concentration gradient between the outside and inside of the cells.

This result is an empirical one for STELLA (1928)[1] showed that the rate of diffusion of a substance into or out of a jelly followed the formula

$$\text{Amount diffusing} = 2c\sqrt{\frac{kt}{\pi}}, \text{ where } c = \text{initial difference in concentration.}$$

This formula has been shown to express the rate of diffusion from agar jelly of lactate, phosphate and creatine (EGGLETON, EGGLETON and HILL, 1928[2]) and of iodides into and out of skeletal muscles (GHAFFAR, 1935[3]). One series of studies on diffusion therefore indicate that the probable relation between concentration and time is $ct = $ constant, whilst the other set of studies shows that $c\sqrt{t} = $ constant or $c^2 t = $ constant. These results show that wide differences in time-concentration relations occur in the case of different living tissues.

Direct chemical measurement shows therefore that the rate of diffusion of non-toxic substances into cells may vary from the relation $ct = $ constant to $c^2 t = $ constant.

Hence any time-concentration relations found with drugs within the ranges $n = 1$ to $n = 2$ are quite probably expressions of rates of diffusion. It may however be noted that the entrance of dye into Nitella measured by IRWIN certainly was not a case of simple diffusion. It is true that the rate of entry was fitted approximately by the formula:—

$$\frac{dx}{dt} = K(a - x),$$

and the time-concentration curve by the formula:—

$$(c - c_n)t = \text{constant},$$

but as is shown in fig. 42 the concentration of the dye in the internal vacuole is about 10 times as great as the external concentration, an effect which could not be produced by simple diffusion.

The fact that time-concentration curves can be fitted by a formula expressing a simple diffusion process therefore does not prove that such a process is occurring and this greatly reduces the theoretical significance of such results.

A considerable proportion of the time-concentration relations found show values of $n$ less than unity. Values between 0.5 and 1.0 are very common and values below 0.5 are not uncommon. Low values of $n$ (i.e. $n = < 1$) are found

---

[1] STELLA, G.: J. of Physiol. **66**, 19 (1928).
[2] EGGLETON, G. P., P. EGGLETON and A. V. HILL: Proc. roy. Soc. B **103**, 620 (1928).
[3] GHAFFAR, A.: Quart. J. exper. Physiol. **25**, 241 (1935).

particularly frequently with heavy metals. Ostwald (1907)[1] suggested that since the fixation of drugs by organisms was an adsorption effect and since adsorption equilibrium was expressed by the formula $K c^{\frac{1}{n}} = \frac{x}{m}$ ($c = $ external concentration; $\frac{x}{m} = $ drug adsorbed per unit weight of adsorbent) therefore the formula $K c^{\frac{1}{n}} = \frac{1}{t}$ ought to express the time relations of fixation. It is an undoubted fact that in cases of substances which are readily adsorbed we frequently find that the rate of action varies as some low power of the concentration and an explanation of Ostwald's formula can be obtained if we regard the process of drug uptake as proceeding in two stages, firstly a fairly rapid process of adsorption on the cell surface and secondly a slower process of inward diffusion from the surface. The rate of inward diffusion will depend on the concentration of adsorbed drug on the surface, and the concentration of adsorbed drug on the surface will vary as some power of the external concentration less than unity. It is of course unlikely that the rate of inward diffusion will be exactly proportional to the surface concentration, but in cases where the surface adsorption varies as $\sqrt{c}$ or $\sqrt[3]{c}$, this relation is likely to dominate all subsequent stages in the chain of processes. An explanation of this form for the time-concentration curves attained by Krönig and Paul (1897)[2] with disinfectants was advanced by Morawitz (1910)[3].

Cook (1926)[4] measured the velocity constant of the inhibition of respiration of *Aspergillus niger* with various concentrations of salts of copper, silver, mercury and hydrochloric acid. In all cases he found the same relation, namely:— velocity varies as $c^{0.4}$. This result with heavy metals is in accordance with the adsorption theory outlined above, and agrees with the time-concentrations relations of the disinfectant action of heavy metals and of their action on *Nitella* (fig. 48). The fact that hydrochloric acid showed the same relation can scarcely be explained in this manner, and differs from results obtained with acids on other tissues, for in most cases these approximate to $ct = $ constant.

The final case is where $n$ is much larger than unity, for instance in the case of phenol killing bacteria, where the time until destruction varies as a high power (at least the cube) of the concentration. Watson (1908)[5] suggested that this proved the occurrence of a polymolecular reaction. Nernst however pointed out that polymolecular reactions depended on the simultaneous collisions of a number of molecules and that such reactions could only attain a measurable velocity under quite exceptional conditions. A consideration of the curves relating concentration of phenol and precipitation of protein shows that the conditions in this case are exceptional. When protein is exposed to phenol the drug distributes itself between protein and water and there is a constant distribution coefficient until a certain critical concentration is attained and then the distribution coefficient rises rapidly and precipitation of the protein commences.

The time-concentration relations of an action such as 50 p.c. precipitation of protein would show $t = \infty$ until the critical concentration of phenol was attained $(c_m)$, after this, however, every increment in concentration would produce a great increase in the rate of action because of the change in the distribution coefficient induced. The action indeed resembles a case of auto-catalysis. High values of $n$ are found when the lethal action of phenol on cells is studied,

[1] Ostwald, Wo.: Pflügers Arch. **120**, 19 (1907).
[2] Krönig, B., and T. Paul: Z. Hyg. **25**, 1 (1897).
[3] Morawitz, H.: Kolloid-Beih. **1**, 317 (1910).
[4] Cook, S. F.: J. gen. Physiol. **9**, 575 (1926).
[5] Watson, H. E.: J. of Hyg. **8**, 536 (1908).

an effect which probably is due to protein denaturation. On the other hand the anaesthetic action of phenol, which is a reversible effect has a totally different time relation. SHACKELL (1922)[1] found that the rate of paralysis of *Limnoria* by phenol approximated to the formula $c^{0.3} t =$ constant, a relation which suggests a surface adsorption.

A study of the formulae expressing time-concentration curves shows therefore that these are not quite so incomprehensible as appears at first sight, since most time-concentration relations can be expressed by the formula $C^n t =$ constant and the values for $n$ fall into three classes namely:—

$$\text{(a) } n = 0.3{-}0.5 \qquad \text{(b) } n = 1{-}2 \qquad \text{(c) } n = {>}3$$

Most of the relations falling into the first class can be explained on the assumption that adsorption occurs, that the concentration of drug on the surface varies as a low power of the concentration in the solution and that the rate of toxic action is dominated by the surface concentration. The relations of the second class can be ascribed to diffusion processes dominating the rate of action of the drug. The relations of the third class can be ascribed to the production of an all-or-none type of effect.

In all cases the formulae applied probably represent an extreme simplification of the processes actually occurring. The rate of uptake of electrolytes and water by proteins and other colloids is a much simpler process than the uptake of drugs by cells, it has been studied intensively and all workers agree that the factors involved are very complex and only partially understood. JORDAN LLOYD (1930)[2] concluded for example that at least three factors regulated the uptake of water by gelatine namely imbibition or restoration of water to a preformed structure, osmotic pressure due to unequal solvent pressures in the solution and in the jelly and swelling of hydration.

A final point must be mentioned, namely that any physico-chemical significance that can attach to time-concentration curves depends on an assumption which is very doubtful, namely that the appearance of an equal biological effect indicates the uptake of an equal quantity of drug by the cell.

SHACKELL (1922)[1] found that this was not true in the case of Limnoria paralysis because animals paralysed by exposure to a high concentration of phenol for a short time took much longer to recover after removal from the drug than did animals paralysed by a long exposure to low concentrations.

Time-concentration curves therefore give relatively little information regarding the physico-chemical basis of drug action. In many cases it is important to know the rate at which poisons exert their effect and in other cases such as local anaesthetics they are the only method by which the activity of a drug can be expressed as a graded effect. In both these cases it is a great convenience to obtain a linear expression of the relation between time until action and concentration. This can usually be obtained over a wide middle range of concentrations by plotting the logarithms of the concentrations and the times. If a linear relation over the whole range of concentration is desired it usually is necessary to subtract threshold values of time and concentration.

The curves thus obtained are convenient for the comparison of the relative rates of actions of drugs but the writer is of opinion that they provide singularly little information regarding the fundamental nature of drug action.

A general study of the literature shows that the known complexity of any process varies not as the complexity of the biological system studied but as

---

[1] SHACKELL, L. F.: J. gen. Physiol. **5**, 783 (1922).
[2] JORDAN LLOYD, D.: Biochemic. J. **24**, 1460 (1930).

the extent and accuracy of the investigations. The kinetics of simple colloidal systems which have been studied at all accurately are known to be extremely complex whereas the kinetics of the action of drugs on mammals often appear quite simple. The simple formulae used to express effects such as the last mentioned are a great convenience, but the results are so variable that it is useless to try to apply more accurate mathematical treatment. It is however important to remember that the formulae applied in no way indicate the probable complexity of the processes which are occurring and that the real reason for their simplicity is the inaccuracy of the data.

The following general points in the use of time relations for biological standardisation may be noted. The measurement of concentrations producing equal actions in an equal time is favourable if the value of $n$ in the formula $c^n t = $ constant is not less than unity because in such cases the differences in time are at least proportional to the differences in concentration. In cases where $n$ is less than unity the method is unfavourable because the changes in time are smaller than the changes in concentration. Finally, if this method of estimating any action is used, it is important to remember that small differences in temperature may cause large differences in the rate of action.

### (2) Time-concentration Curves of Nerve Paralysis.

The paralysis of sensory nerves is a typical all-or-none effect and hence cannot readily be measured as a graded action.

Hundreds of organic compounds with local anaesthetic action have been prepared and it is convenient to have some method for comparing their activity. The usual method is the estimation of the minimum effective concentration (M.E.C.) but this always is an unsatisfactory method, because the nearer a threshold concentration is approached the more inaccurate do the measurements become.

The activity of local anaesthetics can be measured in two ways: (a) relation between concentration and time until paralysis is induced, e.g. paralysis of frog's sciatic nerve, paralysis of nerve endings on frog's skin. (b) Relation between concentration and duration of anaesthesia, e.g. anaesthesia of rabbit's cornea, anaesthesia of human wheal.

Both these methods of measurement can be most conveniently expressed by plotting the logarithm of the concentration and time which gives a linear relation over a considerable range.

The rate of action of cocaine gives figures which follow the formula $C^n t = $ constant with $n$ equal to 0.5 to 1.0. The duration of action of cocaine gives figures which follow the formula $t \cdot \frac{1}{c^n} = $ constant.

The author has estimated the values of $n$, from the experimental data of various authors in the cases of cocaine hydrochloride and of novocaine hydrochloride. The results are shown in Table 15.

Inspection of this table which deals only with two drugs shows that there is a wide variety in the time-concentration results obtained by different observers. The results appear to centre around the relation $c^{0.8} t = $ constant and there appears to be no certain difference between cocaine and novocaine.

Another interesting point is the similarity between the slopes of the curves relating concentration and rate of production of anaesthesia and those of the curves relating concentration and duration of anaesthesia of the cornea or the wheal.

Table 15. Values of constant "$n$" expressing slope of time-concentration curves of local anaesthetics.

| Action | Cocaine hydrochloride | | Novocaine hydrochloride | |
|---|---|---|---|---|
| | $n$ | Author | $n$ | Author |
| I. Rate of action. | | | | |
| (a) Paralysis of frog's sciatic nerve . . . | 0.7 | Sollmann (1917)[1] | 0.65 | Schulz (1925/26)[2] |
| | 0.8 | Gross (1910)[3] | 0.8 | Gross (1911)[4] |
| (b) Anaesthesia of | | | 0.8—1.0 | Meeker (1925/26)[5] |
| frog's skin . . . . | 0.5 | Gramaccioni (1931)[6] | 1.0 | Gramaccioni (1931)[6] |
| II. Duration of action. | | | | |
| (a) Anaesthesia of rabbit's cornea . . | 0.4 | Uhlmann (1930)[7] | 1.0 | Gessner et al. (1932)[8] |
| | 0.7 | Régnier (1923)[9] | | |
| | 0.7 | Schmitz and Loewenhart (1924)[10] | | |
| | 0.75 | Cohen (1925/26)[11] | | |
| | 0.85 | Sinha (1935)[12] | | |
| | 2.0 | Copeland and Notton (1925)[13] | | |
| (b) Anaesthesia of human wheal . . . | 0.43 | Meeker (1925/26)[5] | 0.44 | Sollmann (1918)[14] |
| | 0.44 | Sollmann (1918)[14] | 0.66 | Gessner et al. (1932)[8] |
| | 0.85 | Sinha (1935)[12] | 0.7 | Meeker (1925/26)[5] |

The duration of anaesthesia of the intra-dermal wheal must depend on the rate of which the drug diffuses away from the site of injection and hence it seems probable that in all cases the time at which the effect is observed depends upon some diffusion process.

In this case conditions are favourable in that biological lag can be eliminated because the evidence of the human wheal shows that a local anaesthetic paralyses nerve endings very rapidly when it comes in contact with them.

The chief object in establishing time-concentration curves for local anaesthetics is to obtain a basis for the comparison of the activity of different drugs. In cases where two drugs follow approximately the formula $c^n t = $ constant and $n$ is a similar value in both cases, then it is easy to express the activity of one drug as a multiple of the other.

If however the values of $n$ are different it is not possible to state any definite ratio between their activities because the ratio obtained between the concentrations producing equal actions in equal time will be different for every time selected.

[1] Sollmann, T.: J. Pharmacol. Baltimore 10, 379 (1917).
[2] Schulz, L. W.: J. Labor. a. clin. Med. 11, 180 (1925/26).
[3] Gross, O.: Arch. f. exper. Path. 63, 80 (1910).
[4] Gross, O.: Arch. f. exper. Path. 67, 132 (1911).
[5] Meeker, W. R.: J. Labor. a. clin. Med. 11, 139 (1925/26).
[6] Gramaccioni, B.: Arch. int. Pharmacodyn. 40, 357 (1931).
[7] Uhlmann, F.: Arch. int. Pharmacodyn. 36, 253 (1930).
[8] Gessner, O., J. Klinke and F. R. Wurbs: Arch. f. exper. Path. 168, 447 (1932).
[9] Régnier, J.: Bull. Sci. pharmacol. 30, 580, 646 (1923).
[10] Schmitz, H. L., and A. S. Loewenhart: J. Pharmacol. Baltimore 21, 165 (1924).
[11] Cohen, S. J.: J. Labor. a. clin. Med. 11, 174 (1925/26).
[12] Sinha, H. K.: J. Pharmacol. Baltimore 57, 199 (1935).
[13] Copeland, A. J., and H. E. F. Notton: Brit. med. J. 1925 II, 457.
[14] Sollmann, T.: J. Pharmacol. Baltimore 11, 69 (1918).

There are various empirical methods for obtaining some sort of quantitative estimate of the intensity of local anaesthetic activity. RÉGNIER (1923)[1] and LEVY (1927)[2] have described a method which gives a combined expression of the intensity and duration of the action of local anaesthetics on the rabbit's cornea. The drug is applied under standard conditions and then at various intervals of time up to an hour the number of applications of a hair needed to produce a response is counted. This is done 12 times and the maximum number of applications each time is 100. The score can therefore vary from 12 to 1200 and depends upon how deeply the eye is anaesthetised and for how long the effect lasts. This method appears to give as good results in practice as any other.

In general the time concentration curves obtained with local anaesthetics provide little information regarding the mode of action of the drug. These measurements are not easy and small variations in technique may cause large errors. This is probably the reason for the divergent time-concentration relations that have been recorded.

## (3) Time-concentration Curves with Various Drugs.

In many cases the time until a drug produces an action on an isolated organ is the easiest of its effects to measure. In cases where the action is reversible this measurement can be used as a basis for biological standardisation, by applying various concentrations of the standard and of the unknown preparation, until concentrations producing an equal action in equal time are discovered. Provided that variations in concentration produce considerable variations in time ($t$ varies as $c$ or some power of $c$ more than one) this is a satisfactory method.

The exact balancing of two solutions has been found laborious and many attempts have been made to find expressions which will correlate concentration and time until action. It has been shown however that this relation varies widely with different drugs and hence such calculations are impossible unless the time-concentration relation of the system studied is known. The time-concentration curves obtained in most cases follow the formula $c^n t = \text{constant}$, and the value of $n$ usually is less than 1.

Experiments have been made on the rate of action of aliphatic narcotics on a wide variety of biological systems. It is interesting to note that in nearly all cases the time-concentration curves approximate to $ct = \text{constant}$, e.g. GROSS (1909)[3] paralysis of frog's sciatic by chloral hydrate and phenyl urethane ($n = 1.25$). HARTMANN (1918)[4] destruction of plankton by ethyl alcohol and by chloral hydrate ($n = 1.2$ and $0.75$). KUUESTO, SUOMINEN and RENQUIST (1925)[5] paralysis of frog's gastrocnemius by normal alcohols (methyl-octyl), ($n = 1$).

BLUME (1925)[6] measured the rate of paralysis by alcohols of nerve endings and of muscles of frogs. In the case of heptyl alcohol a graded time effect was obtained with concentrations varying from 0.006 to 0.04 p.c. and the figures approximated to a value of $n = 0.8$. In the case of ethyl alcohol 3 p.c. did not produce paralysis, 3.5 p.c. paralysed in 12 hours and 5 p.c. in 2 hours. This last result resembles the action of phenol on bacteria in that there is a high threshold concentration and further increases in concentration causes a great reduction in the time of action. The figures can

[1] RÉGNIER, J.: Bull. Sci. pharmacol. **30**, 580, 646 (1923).
[2] LEVY, J.: Essais de Substances médicamenteuses. Paris: Masson et Cie. 1927.
[3] GROSS, O.: Arch. f. exper. Path. **62**, 380 (1909).
[4] HARTMANN, O.: Pflügers Arch. **170**, 583 (1918).
[5] KUUESTO, P., Y. K. SUOMINEN and Y. RENQUIST: Skand. Arch. Physiol. **46**, 76 (1925).
[6] BLUME, W.: Arch. f. exper. Path. **110**, 46 (1925).

be fitted by the formula $c^5t =$ constant, but a more rational treatment is to subtract the threshold concentration and then the figures are fitted by the formula $(c - 3) t =$ constant. COLE and ALLISON (1930)[1] studied the stimulant action of alcohols (methyl-amyl) on Planaria. Their curves can fitted by the formula $c^3t =$ constant or alternatively by the formula $(c - c_m) t =$ constant.

The evidence in the case of the time-concentration curves obtained with alcohols and aliphatic narcotics shows in the first place a considerable variation in results obtained by different workers. This is an unfortunate general characteristic of time-concentration curves. The results vary however around the relation $ct =$ constant, and in cases where gross deviations are found, these can be accounted for by high threshold values for concentration. This suggests that the time measured in these cases is a fairly simple diffusion process, a result which is in accordance with what is known about the action of narcotics.

Table 16. Value of constant "$n$" expressing slope of time-concentration curves of various drugs (extracted from experimental results quoted).

| Drug-cell system | $n$ | Author |
|---|---|---|
| Oxytocin on guinea pig's uterus . . . . | 0,45 | LIPSCHITZ and HSING (1932)[2] |
| ditto . . . . . . . . . . . . . . . . . | 0.43 | LIPSCHITZ and KLAR (1933)[3] |
| Histamine on guinea pig's uterus . . . . | 0.15 | LIPSCHITZ and KLAR (1933)[3] |
| ditto . . . . . . . . . . . . . . . . . | 0.33 | WEBSTER (1935)[4] |
| Acetyl choline on guinea pig's ileum . . | 0.2 | BERNHEIM and GORFAIN (1934)[5] |
| Acetyl choline on guinea pig's uterus . . | 0.32 | WEBSTER (1935)[4] |
| Adrenaline on rabbit's uterus . . . . . . | 0.5 | BUTTLE and TREVAN (1928)[6] |
| Vibrion septique toxin on rabbit's uterus | 0.5 | BUTTLE and TREVAN (1928)[6] |

Table 16 shows the values of $n$ in the formula $C^nt =$ constant obtained with a variety of drugs acting on isolated tissues. In most cases the value of $n$ approximates to 0.5. The reason for this relation is not clear, but it is necessary to remember that the time elapsing between the introduction of a drug and the response of a sluggish tissue such as a plain muscle is most likely to be occupied firstly by diffusion into the tissue and secondly by the lag between the production of a chemical change and the appearance of the biological response. Hence the results appear to be of a limited theoretical value. The fact that the value of $n$ is low is of practical importance because it implies that large changes of concentration are required to produce small changes in time and consequently the method of measurement is unfavourable for biological standardisation in the cases shown in Table 16.

## (4) Time-concentration Relations in Disinfection.

These relations are of particular importance in the case of disinfection, firstly because it is necessary to know the duration of exposure which will produce disinfection and secondly because methods of biological standardisation of disinfectants are based on time-concentration relations.

A population of bacteria, other than spores, is either growing or dying and hence there are only two methods of obtaining a quantitative estimate of the action of a disinfectant; firstly the measurement of the minimum concentration effective in unlimited time and secondly the measurement of the concentration

[1] COLE, W. H., and J. B. ALLISON: J. gen. Physiol. 14, 71 (1930).
[2] LIPSCHITZ, W., and W. HSING: Pflügers Arch. 229, 672 (1932).
[3] LIPSCHITZ, W., and F. KLAR: Arch. f. exper. Path. 174, 223 (1933).
[4] WEBSTER, M. D.: J. Pharmacol. Baltimore 53, 340 (1935).
[5] BERNHEIM, F., and A. GORFAIN: J. Pharmacol. Baltimore 52, 338 (1934).
[6] BUTTLE, G. A., H., and J. W. TREVAN: Brit. J. exper. Path. 9, 182 (1928).

which will produce disinfection in some selected time. The former method is unsatisfactory because it is always difficult to measure exactly a minimum effective concentration, and this is particularly difficult in the case of a growing population.

Time-concentration curves for disinfectants show linear relations between the logarithms of the time and the concentration over very wide ranges of concentrations. Hence it is easy to determine the value of $n$ in the formula $c^n t = $ constant. CHICK (1930)[1] collected a large number of examples and found that in general they could be fitted with this formula but that the value of $n$ varied from 0.3 to 6.5.

Fig. 49 shows figures obtained by CHICK (1908)[2] for the rate of action of phenol and of mercuric chloride on *B. paratyphosus*. The mercuric chloride curve follows the formula $c^{0.95} t = $ constant (curve $B$) but the phenol curve follows the extraordinary formula $c^6 t = $ constant (curve $A$). There is however a high threshold concentration in the case of phenol and if a value of 3 per 1000 be subtracted then the curve (curve $A$) is fitted by the formula $(c - 3)^{3.3} t = $ constant, but even this modification does not reduce the concentration to a power that can be interpreted as an expression of any ordinary physico-chemical process.

The outstanding feature of the action of disinfectants, as in the case of lethal agents on small organisms, is the remarkable variation in the slope of the logarithmic relations, and this constitutes a difficult problem in relation to the standardisation of disinfectants.

The usual method of standardising disinfectants is based on time-concentration curves, for the method depends on the determination of the concentration ($c$) of

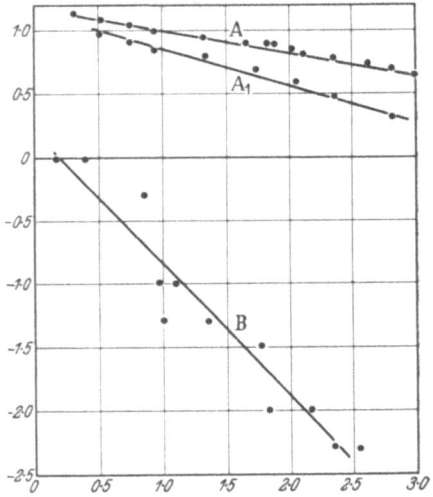

Fig. 49. Time-concentration curves of disinfection of *B. paratyphosus*. Abscissa:— log. time in minutes. Ordinate:— log. conc. per cent. (*A*) Phenol. (*A*¹) Curve $A$ corrected by subtraction of threshold concentration. (*B*) Mercuric chloride. (CHICK, 1908[2].)

disinfectant which produces disinfection in a measured time ($t$), and phenol is used as a standard for comparison.

In accordance with the general principles of biological standardisation the unknown and the standard are tested with all experimental conditions constant e.g. temperature, variety of organism used, amount of organism etc. A consideration of fig. 49 shows that phenol is very well suited for accurate measurement of the concentration needed to produce an action in equal time. The time-concentration curve follows the formula $c^6 t = $ constant and hence small variations in concentration make a great difference in the time.

This time-concentration relation, although exceptionally favourable for accurate measurements nevertheless makes phenol an unsuitable standard simply because the relation is exceptional and most other disinfectants have completely different time-concentration relations. Inspection of fig. 49 shows that it is, for example, impossible to state any definite relation between the disinfectant activity of mercuric chloride and of phenol because the ratio of concentrations needed

[1] CHICK, H.: Med. Res. Counc. System of Bacteriol. **1**, 179 (1930).
[2] CHICK, H.: J. of Hyg. **8**, 92 (1908).

to produce disinfection is different for every time limit chosen. This is an extreme example of the general rule that it is only possible to compare the activity of two drugs by measurements of concentrations which produce equal action in equal time, if the value of $n$ is similar in the relation $c^n t =$ constant. This question can be determined at once by plotting the logarithms of concentration against the logarithms of the time. If the slopes of the curves are parallel the values of $n$ are the same and the activities can be compared, but if the slopes are not parallel no valid comparison can be made. In some cases the two curves actually cross and then with one time limit one drug appears the stronger and with another time limit the other drug appears the stronger.

The standardisation of disinfectants is a matter of commercial importance and the "phenol coefficient" is widely used as a measure. It is however an arbitrary measure and cannot be made accurate. It is of practical value if the time limit chosen is one in which disinfection would need to be produced in practice. The only satisfactory way of obtaining a measure of disinfectant activity is to compare the activity of the disinfectant with the activity of a standard disinfectant, whose time-concentration curve has a similar slope.

Unfortunately it also is necessary to find by direct experiment the concentrations of the two drugs (unknown and standard), which produce equal actions in equal time. Only in the exceptional cases, where both drugs show the simple relation:— $c.t. =$ constant, is it possible to calculate the relative activities from simpler data, such for instance as the ratio between the times required by equal concentrations of the drugs to produce an equal action.

For example, if two drugs $a$ and $b$ show the time-concentration relation of $c^2 t =$ constant and if when applied in 2 p.c. solution, they produce equal effects after 10 and 20 min. respectively, this fact does not show that $a$ is twice as strong as $b$ because the respective concentrations of $a$ and $b$ which would produce the effect in 10 min. are 2 p.c. and 2.8 p.c. respectively which is a ratio of 1 to 1.4.

Similarly the relative activity of two drugs can only be determined by comparison of the amount of action produced after an equal time in the rare event of the time-action curve being linear.

In the case of disinfectants for example the rate of destruction approximates to a linear relation between log. survivors and time. Hence if the death curves of two different drugs are compared different proportions between the fractions of the population destroyed will be found at every time chosen.

HENDERSON SMITH (1923)[1] pointed out this source of error in the case of disinfectants, and the method is rarely suggested for the standardisation of these drugs. It is however sometimes suggested for other forms of biological standardisation but it is nearly always fallacious because the great majority of time action curves are either exponential or sigmoid.

The general principle, that should be followed in biological standardisation, is to determine the concentrations or doses of two preparations which produce the same effect on the same tissues under exactly similar conditions. A consideration of the complex relations that occur between concentration, time of action and amount of action shows that this is the only safe course and that all forms of short cuts are unsafe; such for example as calculating relative activities from relative rates of action, or relative actions produced in equal time.

## (5) Toxic Vapours.

The time relations of the effects produced by inhalation of toxic vapours are of great importance because when an animal is exposed to such vapours it is

---

[1] HENDERSON SMITH, J.: Ann. appl. Biol. **10**, 335 (1923).

impossible to measure the amount of toxic material absorbed and hence the only method by which the intensity of the toxic action can be expressed quantitatively is by some formula which expresses the concentration of the drug and the time needed to produce a toxic action. The subject is of practical importance in relation both to the chances of industrial poisoning and to the probable effects of war gases and it has been dealt with in a systematic manner in various monographs (HENDERSON and HAGGARD, 1927[1]; FLURY and ZERNIK, 1931[2]). No general survey of this extensive subject can be attempted in this article, but certain of the facts established regarding toxic vapours throw light on time-concentration relations in general.

Toxic gases may be divided into two classes:—

(a) Local poisons which produce a local action on the lungs.

(b) General poisons, which produce a toxic action after absorption.

The action of the former class depends on the following factors.

(1) Concentration of vapour.

(2) Amount of pulmonary ventilation.

(3) The manner in which the vapour is adsorbed by or dissolved in the cells on the surface of the respiratory tract.

The action of the latter class is more complex because it depends on the concentration attained by the drug in the blood stream.

Two degrees of complexity may be distinguished in this latter class. In the case of powerful poisons toxic effects arise before there is any large concentration in the blood and hence the rate of absorption from the lungs may be regarded as remaining constant during the exposure to a constant concentration of gas. In the case of drugs such as volatile anaesthetics the concentration attained by the drug in the blood is considerable and any calculation of rate of absorption must take into account the change in the concentration gradient between alveolar air and blood that occurs during exposure to the vapour.

**Deviation of Narcotics.** All time-concentration relations are calculated on the assumption that when organisms are exposed to varying concentrations of drugs, the appearance of the particular effect selected for measurement indicates the uptake by the organism of a certain quantity of drug. It is of interest to note that this assumption has been found to be untrue in the case of anaesthetics, an example in which it happens to be possible to measure the amount of drug taken up by the organism.

HENDERSON and HAGGARD (1927)[1] have worked out formulae for the absorption and elimination of non-reactive gases such as narcotics. These formulae are complex, since the number of factors influencing drug uptake are numerous. The theoretical value of such calculations is however greatly reduced by the fact that deviation of anaesthetic by inert tissues introduces an error, the effects of which are serious.

The narcotic action of an anaesthetic depends upon the concentration of drug in the blood passing through the central nervous system, but the drug also is absorbed and removed from the blood stream by many tissues, such as the subcutaneous fat, on which it exerts no action. These drugs therefore provide an example of the deviation of an active agent by inert material. The amount of deviation depends partly on the relative blood supply of the different tissues, because a tissue such as subcutaneous fat, which can absorb a large total quantity of narcotic, will absorb the narcotic very slowly on account of its relatively poor

---

[1] HENDERSON, Y., and H. W. HAGGARD: Noxious Gases. New York: Chem. Catalog. Co. 1927.

[2] FLURY, F., and F. ZERNIK: Schädliche Gase. Berlin: Julius Springer 1931.

circulation. The amount of narcotic taken up by a tissue appears indeed to depend more on the amount of blood passing through the tissue than upon the amount of narcotic the tissue can absorb when it attains equilibrium with the concentration of narcotic in the blood stream.

This deviation causes the narcotic action of an anaesthetic to be dependent on the rate at which the anaesthetic is administered. For example the total quantity of ether, that is absorbed before anaesthesia is produced, is smaller when the anaesthetic is given in high concentrations, than when it is given in low concentrations, because deviation is greater under the latter condition (HAGGARD, 1924[1]).

In the case of a volatile anaesthetic therefore the times needed by varying concentrations of vapour to produce an equal degree of anaesthesia do not provide a measure of the times needed for equal amounts of the vapour to be absorbed.

In the case of narcotics it has been found possible to measure the actual amount of narcotic taken up by the body, but in the case of most toxic gases

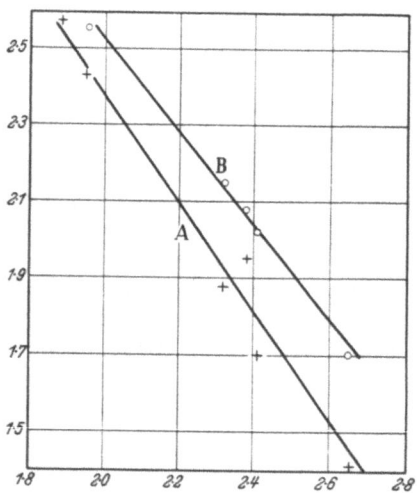

Fig. 50. Time-concentration curve of action of carbon tetrachloride vapour on cats. Abscissa:— log. conc. mg. per litre. Ordinate:— log. time in minutes. (*A*) Light narcosis. (*B*) Deep narcosis. (LEHMANN, 1911[1].)

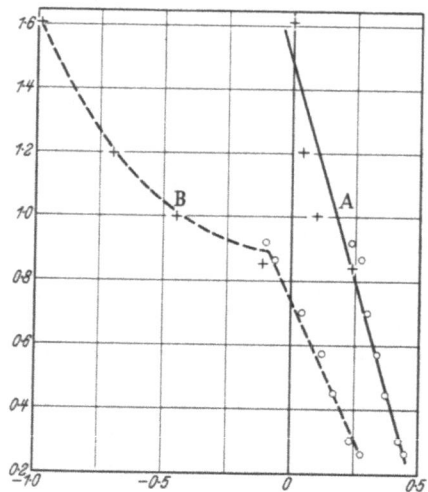

Fig. 51. Time-concentration curves of action of ether on mice. Abscissa:— log. m.mols per litre of air. Ordinate:— log. time. (*A*) Uncorrected figures. (*B*) Threshold conc. of 0.8 m. mols per litre subtracted. Crosses:— FÜHNER (1919)[3]. Circles:— KNOEFEL and MURRELL (1935)[4].

the only measurements available relate vapour concentration with the time needed to produce an equal biological response. In the case of drugs which produce a toxic effect after absorption, it therefore is quite uncertain whether the times of appearance of an equal biological response measure the times at which equal quantities of drug have been absorbed from varying quantities of vapour. Consequently the time-concentration relations are of empirical rather than theoretical value, and elaborate mathematical treatment seems inappropriate.

**Time-Concentration Curves of Anaesthetics.** The time-concentration relations for the anaesthetic activity of a number of halogenated hydrocarbons were worked out by LEHMANN (1911)[2] on cats. In most cases his results approximated to the very simple relation $ct =$ constant. Fig. 50 shows the results with carbon tetrachloride. In this case $c^{1.2}t =$ constant. The logarithmic method of plotting has

[1] HAGGARD, H. W.: J. of biol. Chem. **59**, 737, 753, 795 (1924).
[2] LEHMANN, K. B.: Arch. f. Hyg. **74**, 1 (1911).
[3] FÜHNER, H.: Biochem. Z. **115**, 241 (1919).
[4] KNOEFEL, P. K., and F. C. MURRELL: J. Pharmacol. Baltimore **55**, 235 (1935).

the advantage that it shows clearly the zones of action. The interval between curves $A$ and $B$ in this case shows the region between light and deep narcosis.

Fig. 51 shows the relation between concentration of ether and time until the production of anaesthesia in mice. The results are those obtained by KNOEFEL and MURRELL (1935)[1] and by FÜHNER (1919)[2]. Curve $A$ shows the combined figures of these authors and this follows the formula $c^{2.5}t = $ constant. FÜHNER showed however that a concentration of 0.8 m.mols per litre of ether did not anaesthetise mice however long the exposure. If this threshold concentration of 0.8 be subtracted then curve $B$ is obtained and in this case KNOEFEL and MURRELL's figures follow the relation $c^{1.5}t = $ constant, whilst FÜHNER's figures approximate to $ct = $ constant. A result such as this suggests that little theoretical significance can be attached in this case to the value of $n$ in the formula $c^{n}t = $ constant.

**Time-concentration Curves of Hydrocyanic Acid.** Hydrocyanic acid is an example of a gas which produces no local effects, but whose toxic action is so intense that the concentration in the blood is unlikely to rise to a figure which will modify the rate of absorption.

Fig. 52 shows results quoted by FLURY and ZERNIK (1931)[3] and other results obtained by BARCROFT (1931)[4]. They are shown on logarithmic scales. These results follow the formulae $c^{n}t = $ constant and $n$ lies between 1.5 and 1.8. The significance of this value is doubtful because in the case of mice for example the minimum lethal concentration of cyanide is known to be about 0.04 mg/L. If the quantity 0.03 be subtracted from the concentrations in the case of mice and cats the relation $ct = $ constant is obtained.

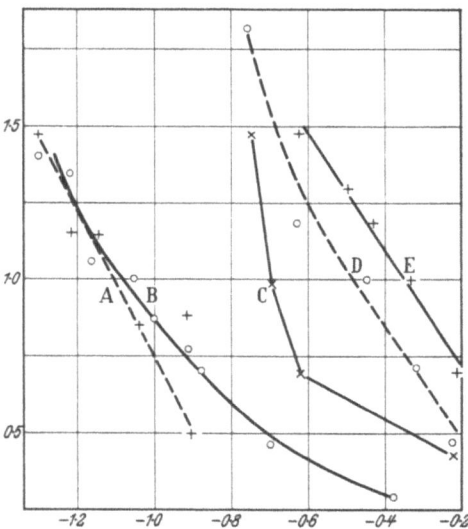

Fig. 52. Time-concentration curves for action of hydrocyanic acid. Abscissa:— log. conc. mg./litre. Ordinate:— log. time in minutes. ($A$) and ($B$) Time until paralysis of mice and of cats respectively. (FLURY and ZERNIK, 1931[3].) ($C$), ($D$) and ($E$) Duration of lethal exposure of cats, rabbits and goats respectively. (BARCROFT, 1931[4].)

Similarly a subtraction of 0.1 from the lethal concentrations for rabbits brings the results more nearly linear and the value of $n$ becomes 1.3.

It appears to the writer that it is not possible to attribute any theoretical significance to the value of $n$ obtained from these curves. It is however certain that the rate of action of cyanide must be influenced by a very large number of factors and it is interesting to find that the results approximate to the extremely simple formula $(c - c_m) t = $ constant. The chief value of the logarithmic method of plotting results is that, provided the slopes of the curves are not dissimilar, it permits the calculation of the relative susceptibility of animals. For example fig. 52 shows that the lethal concentration for goats (curve $E$) is about 1.5 times the lethal concentration for rabbits (curve $D$).

**Irritant Gases.** The factors influencing the action of irritant gases are considerably simpler than in the case of volatile narcotics or general poisons such

[1] KNOEFEL, P. K., and F. C. MURRELL: J. Pharmacol. Baltimore **55**, 235 (1935).
[2] FÜHNER, H.: Biochem. Z. **115**, 241 (1919).
[3] FLURY, F., and F. ZERNIK: Schädliche Gase. Berlin: Julius Springer 1931.
[4] BARCROFT, J.: J. of Hyg. **31**, 1 (1931).

as cyanide. FLURY and ZERNIK (p. 99) state that in the case of irritant gases the product $ct$ ($t$ = time till lethal action) is a constant, although as they point out, this is only occasionally true in the case of the gases with a general action.

The toxicity of an irritant gas for an animal can therefore be easily expressed quantitatively by the formula $ct$ = constant. The susceptibility of different animals for different gases varies widely, and hence only experiments made on the same species of animal can be directly compared.

**Discussion.** Time-concentration curves can be fairly easily obtained with toxic gases, and the results form the only practicable basis for the comparison of the relative toxicity of these substances.

In the case of irritant gases the curves follow the very simple formula $ct$ = constant, and hence are easy to compare.

In the case of gases with general toxic action the curves approximate to the formula $c^n t$ = constant. If the results are plotted on a logarithmic basis it is easy to obtain a measure of comparative toxicity, provided the slope of the curves (i.e. the value of $n$) is similar.

If the value of $n$ is markedly dissimilar it is impossible to state any comparative measure of toxicity because the ratio of toxicity will differ with every time chosen. In many cases the action of gases with a general toxic action approximates to the formula $ct$ = constant. The number of factors influencing the action must be very large and this provides another example of the fact that in the case of biological systems very complex relationships may often produce curves which can be fitted approximately by very simple formulae.

## Chapter 14
### Individual Variation of Response to Drugs.

**Methods of Measurement of Individual Variation.** One of the most familiar facts in medical practice is that no two persons respond in exactly the same manner to drugs. The use of biological methods for standardising drugs has necessitated the measurement of the extent and distribution of this individual variation in response to drugs, and in consequence a large literature has accumulated. Estimations of the distribution of individual variation of populations in respect of response to drugs are based on characteristic curves, which relate the dosage or concentration of a drug with the percentage of a population showing some selected response. The response which is usually chosen is death, but any other response can be used, provided that it permits the division of the population into two classes, those responding and those which fail to respond. In some cases the individual variation in response to drugs is distributed according to the normal curve of error, but in many cases skew distributions occur which cover very wide ranges of concentration.

An attempt will be made in this chapter to analyse some of the possible causes for this remarkable variety in the distribution of variation. The characteristic curves expressing distribution of variation are derived from various types of experiment.

(1) The most complete evidence is when the dosage required to produce an effect is determined for each individual in a large group of animals. In this case every individual response is known. The slow intravenous injection of tincture of digitalis into cats is a method of standardisation in which the exact dose needed to produce death can be measured for each individual. LIND VAN WIJN-

GAARDEN (1924)[1] measured the lethal dose in 573 cats and his results showed a symmetrical bell shaped distribution of variation. They ranged from −42 to +56 p.c. of the mean dose, and the standard deviation ($\sigma$) was about 12 p.c. of the median. These results require no discussion since the variation was measured directly in each individual, moreover the distribution of variation is symmetrical, follows the normal curve of error and shows a small scatter.

(2) In most cases however it is not possible to ascertain the dose needed by each individual, and hence it is necessary to use the group method. The population is divided into a series of groups and all members of a single group are given the same dose of drug. The percentage mortality for each of a series of doses is thus determined and the relation between dosage and incidence of death thus determined is termed a characteristic curve.

Fig. 53 shows the response of a population of rats to a series of doses of neoarsphenamine. In this case the standard deviation is 20 p.c. of the median. It will be seen that a frequency polygon can be integrated to form a characteristic curve or alternatively a characteristic curve can be analysed into a frequency polygon.

(3) In both the above cases the dose per individual is known but in the case of small organisms it is only possible to expose groups to a series of concentrations of a drug and to estimate the percentage incidence of response. In this case it is obvious that the variation in response may be due either to variation in drug uptake or to variation in regard to the effects produced in different individuals by different quantities of drug fixed. This method appears at first sight to be

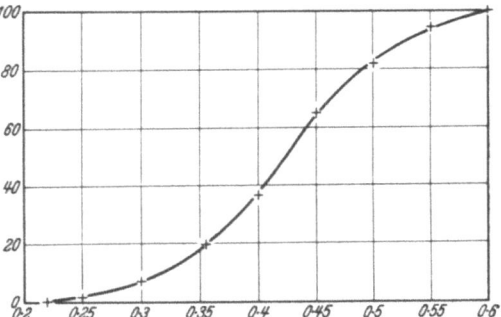

Fig. 53. Characteristic curve of neoarsphenamine injected intravenously into 1,331 rats. Abscissa:— dosage in mg./kg. Ordinate:— Per cent. mortality. (MORRELL and CHAPMAN, 1933[2].)

much less accurate than the former methods, but in reality there is not much difference, because when a drug is given to a mammal its action ultimately depends upon the amount taken up from the blood by the tissue upon which the drug exerts its action. Hence in all cases the individual variation observed may be caused by one or both of two factors, variation in uptake of drug by cells and variation in the cellular response when the uptake is equal.

(4) Individual variation also can be studied upon isolated organs and in this case two types of measurement are possible.

(a) Determination of the drug concentration needed to produce a selected effect on each of a series of preparations.

(b) Measurement in a series of groups of the amount of some graded action produced by a series of concentrations.

It may be stated at once that similar problems arise whichever method of estimation is chosen. With all the methods mentioned some drugs produce symmetrical sigmoid curves and other drugs produce markedly skew distributions of variation.

Fig. 53 shows a symmetrical distribution of variation over a moderate range. Such curves are easy to describe, because the median is equal to the mean in the case of symmetrical distribution of variation, furthermore the standard

[1] WIJNGAARDEN, L. VAN: Arch. f. exper. Path. **113**, 40 (1924).

[2] MORRELL, C. A., and C. W. CHAPMAN: J. Pharmacol. Baltimore **48**, 375, 391 (1933).

deviation can be estimated with approximate accuracy from the characteristic curve. The doses or concentrations of drug producing 16, 50 and 84 p.c. action ($C_{16}$, $C_{50}$ and $C_{84}$) can be read off from the characteristic curve, and $\dfrac{C_{84} - C_{16}}{2}$ gives an approximately accurate estimate of the standard deviation. The latter expressed as a percentage of $C_{50}$ gives the coefficient of variation.

In skew curves the median differs widely from the mean and the only way of obtaining the standard deviation is to analyse the characteristic curve into a frequency polygon, and estimate from this the mean and the standard deviation.

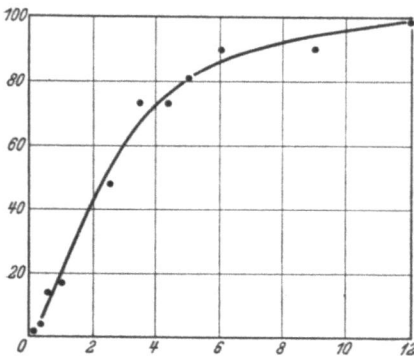

Fig. 54. Characteristic curve of nicotine spray on *Aphis rumicis* (1,700 individuals). Abscissa:— conc. in mol. per 1000 litres solvent. Ordinate:— per cent. population killed or moribund. (TATTERSFIELD and GIMINGHAM, 1927[1].)

This procedure is objectionable for various reasons. Firstly it is laborious, secondly the usual type of skew variation shows a "tail" of resistant individuals, and the squaring of the deviation from the mean, involved in the calculation of the standard deviation, gives these relatively few observations a predominant influence, but, unless very large populations are used, it is impossible to estimate accurately the true incidence of these rare individuals. Hence the least accurate estimations have the greatest influence in the estimation of the mean.

The systematic study of the distribution of individual variation in response to drugs was developed owing to the practical necessity of estimating the probable accuracy of bioassays of drugs. The bioassays of digitalis and of the organic arsenicals were the first to be studied carefully and it so happened that the responses to both these drugs show a relatively narrow range of individual variation which is distributed approximately symmetrically. Owing to this accident the narrow symmetrical distribution of variation was regarded as the normal and skew curves with wide distributions of variation were regarded as exceptions. A general survey of the distribution of individual variation in the responses to a wide range of drugs shows however that skew distributions are certainly as common if not commoner than symmetrical distributions. Fig. 54 shows an example of the type of skew distribution of variation that is commonly found in the response to drugs.

**Skew Variation in Biological Material.** FRANCIS GALTON (1879)[2] and DONALD McALISTER (1879)[3] have pointed out that GAUSS' formula $y = e^{-h^2 x^2}$ gave a fairly satisfactory expression for the distribution of instrumental errors but was unsatisfactory in relation to biological material. This formula assumes that errors in excess or in deficiency of the truth are equally probable and that, if two fallible measurements have been made of the same object, their arithmetic mean is more likely to be the true measurement than any other quantity. Even in the case of certain measurements these assumptions are untrue since the WEBER-FECHNER law applies in measurements which depend on the acuity of the special senses. For instance in the case of estimating a weight with a true measurement of 8, there is equal probability not of errors of −4 and of +4 but of errors of −4 and of +8. Hence the geometrical mean is nearer the thruth

[1] TATTERSFIELD, F., and C. T. GIMINGHAM: Ann. appl. Biol. **14**, 217 (1927).
[2] GALTON, F.: Proc. roy. Soc. **29**, 365 (1879).
[3] MACALISTER, D.: Proc. roy. Soc. **29**, 367 (1879).

than is the arithmetical mean. These authors pointed out the advantage of plotting the distribution of error against the logarithm of the measurements. These general arguments apply to the measurement of individual variation in response to drugs. If there is a geometrical relation between the dosage and the effect, the true median dose can best be found by plotting distribution against the logarithm of the dosage.

KAPTEYN (1916)[1] pointed out that in many cases it was impossible for two biological variations to be both distributed in a symmetrical bell shaped manner. For example if the diameter of peas were distributed in this manner, then the weight of the peas would of necessity show a skew distribution. Fig. 38 shows the difference in distribution of variation that occurs in a population when different characters are measured.

The normal bell shaped distribution of variation is in fact a mathematical conception. It expresses the distribution of a response when this is influenced by a number of independent factors, and when the possible range of variation is equal in the negative and in the position directions. Such a condition obtains when the scores are counted from each throw of a number of dice, or when small instrumental errors are compared.

In the case of biological material this method of calculation very frequently produces absurd results; for example GALTON showed that the GAUSS' formula applied to the variation in height of human beings led to the conclusion that occasionally adults would be found of impossible sizes.

GADDUM (1937)[2] has pointed out that in actual fact the commonest form of distribution of variation found, when the response of a population to drugs is measured, is a normal distribution in respect to the logarithm of the dosage or of the concentration of the drug. The most satisfactory method therefore of describing the distribution of variation in a population is to construct characteristic curves relating percentage incidence of response with the logarithm of the dosage or concentration. This procedure gives approximately symmetrical sigmoid curves in all cases. In the case of curves which show a symmetrical sigmoid relation between incidence and dosage it is of course impossible for the relation between incidence and log. dosage to be of the same shape, but in actual fact the variation in these cases is so small that the deviations from the symmetrical form are usually within the limits of error whether the incidence be plotted against dosage or against the logarithm of the dosage.

Many authors have shown the empirical advantage of plotting dosage (or concentration) on a logarithmic scale when describing variation. HEMMINGSEN and KROGH (1926)[3], TREVAN (1929)[4], BOURDILLON, BRUCE, FISHMANN and WEBSTER (1931)[5], COWARD, DYER, MORTON and GADDUM (1931)[6], GADDUM and HETHERINGTON (1931)[7]. The method has been discussed and described by CLARK (1933)[8], GADDUM (1933)[9] and BLISS (1935)[10].

---

[1] KAPTEYN, J. C.: Rec. Trav. bot. néerl. **13** (2), 105 (1916).

[2] GADDUM, J. H.: J. of Physiol. **89**, 7P (1937).

[3] HEMMINGSEN, A. M., and A. KROGH: League of Nations. Rep. Biol. Standards Insulin: C. H. **398**, 40 (1926).

[4] TREVAN, J. W.: J. of Path. **32**, 127 (1929).

[5] BOURDILLON, R. B., H. M. BRUCE, C. FISCHMANN and T. A. WEBSTER: Med. Res. Council. Spec. Report Ser. **158**. London 1931.

[6] COWARD, K. H., F. J. DYER, R. A. MORTON and J. H. GADDUM: Biochemic. J. **25**, 1102 (1931).

[7] GADDUM, J. H., and M. HETHERINGTON: Quart. J. Pharmacy **4**, 183 (1931).

[8] CLARK, A. J.: The Mode of Action of Drugs on Cells, Chapt. 6. London: Arnold and Co. 1933.

[9] GADDUM, J. H.: Med. Res. Council Spec. Report **183** (1933).

[10] BLISS, C. I.: Ann. appl. Biol. **22**, 134 (1935).

**Normal Equivalent Deviation.** The skew characteristic curves which are so frequently encountered are of a shape peculiarly inconvenient for comparison. The comparison of data can as a general rule be carried out most conveniently when relations are expressed in a linear form, and this form is particularly useful in the case of biological data which are so subject to casual errors. Characteristic curves whether symmetrical or skewed can be reduced to linear relations by the following method. The skewed characteristic curves can be reduced to symmetrical ogival or sigmoid curves by plotting incidence against the logarithm of the dosage or concentration.

The normal or ogival or sigmoid curve of error or variation can next be converted to a linear form if instead of plotting dosage against percentage of

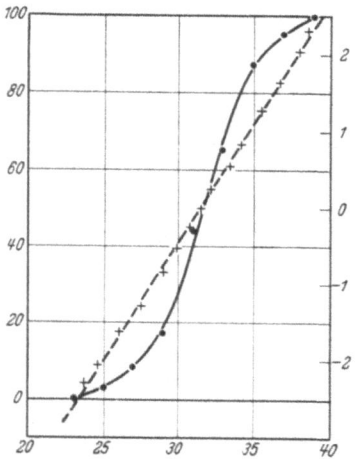

Fig. 55. Characteristic curve of ouabain and *Rana pipiens* (1440 individuals). Abscissa:— Dosage $y/100$ g. Ordinates:— Left:— per cent. mortality (dots). Right:— mortality expressed as multiples of standard deviation (crosses). (CHAPMAN and MORRELL, 1931[6].)

response the dosage is plotted against the response expressed in multiples of the standard deviation. Methods of this type were worked out by URBAN (1909)[1], by WHIPPLE (1916)[2], and by KAPTEYN and VAN UVEN (1916)[3]. The method has been elaborated for use in estimating variations in response to drugs by GADDUM (1933)[4] and by BLISS (1935)[5]. The present account of this method has been largely taken from GADDUM's paper.

A special form of graph paper known as probability or per mille paper is available on which the ordinates represent a scale of percentages so spaced that the actual distances on the paper are proportional to the corresponding values of the normal equivalent deviation. BLISS (1935)[5] has prepared tables for converting percentages into multiples of the standard deviation. Either of these methods can be conveniently used.

The following are certain of the relations between ($p$) percentage response and ($y$) multiple of standard deviation:—

| $p$ | 50 | 45 | 40 | 35 | 30 | 25 | 20 | 15.8 | 15 |
|---|---|---|---|---|---|---|---|---|---|
| $y$ | 0 | 0.126 | 0.253 | 0.385 | 0.524 | 0.674 | 0.842 | 1.00 | 1.036 |

| $p$ | 10 | 5 | 2.3 | 2 | 1 | 0.14 | 0.1 | 0.01 | |
|---|---|---|---|---|---|---|---|---|---|
| $y$ | 1.282 | 1.645 | 2.00 | 2.054 | 2.326 | 3.00 | 3.09 | 3.72 | |

Fig. 55 shows a characteristic curve obtained by CHAPMAN and MORRELL[6] for the action of ouabain on Rana pipiens and the manner in which the ogival curve is converted into a straight line when the dosage is plotted against multiples of the standard deviation. In the case shown in fig. 55 the characteristic curve was symmetrical and hence the theoretical course of the curve could be calculated from appropriate tables without any special method of treatment. The results recorded in fig. 54 show an extreme form of skew distribution of variation. This

[1] URBAN, F. M.: Arch. f. Psychol. **15**, 287; **16**, 168 (1909).
[2] WHIPPLE, G. C.: J. Franklin Instit. **18**, 237 (1916).
[3] KAPTEYN, J. C., and M. J. VAN UVEN: Skew Frequency Curves in Biology and Medicine 1. Groningen: Hortsema Bros 1916.
[4] GADDUM, J. H.: Med. Res. Council Spec. Report **183** (1933).
[5] BLISS, C. I.: Ann. appl. Biol. **22**, 134 (1935).
[6] CHAPMAN, C. W., and C. A. MORRELL: Quart. J. Pharmacy **4**, 195 (1931).

curve is however reduced to a linear relation between 2 and 98 p.c. action when log. concentration is plotted against the multiple of the standard deviation (fig. 56, curve $D$).

The plotting of dosage on the logarithmic scale and the plotting of response as the normal equivalent variation (N.E.D.) provides a method by which the scatter of the variation in the response of populations to drugs can be most easily compared, because approximately linear relations are obtained in all cases.

The standard deviation of the logarithms of the individual effective doses ($\lambda$) can be estimated directly from these curves, because this figure is the distance on the logarithmic scale corresponding to one normal equivalent deviation.

Fig. 56 shows a few examples of the results obtained by plotting log. dosage against the normal equivalent deviation.

Curves $A$, $B$ and $C$ are cases in which the scatter is small, and the results when plotted by the usual method (e.g. fig. 55) show approximately symmetrical sigmoid curves. In these cases the curves based either on dosage or on log. dosage are equally satisfactory. Curves $D$, $E$ and $F$ on the other hand express cases in which there is a wide scatter and an extreme skew distribution of variation. In these cases dosage plotted against incidence shows an extreme skew curve

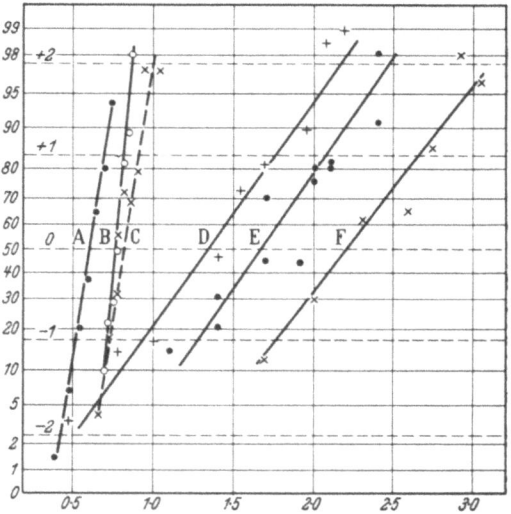

Fig. 56. Characteristic curves of various lethal actions. Abscissa:— log. dosage or concentration. Ordinate:— per cent. mortality and multiples of standard deviation (dotted lines). Number of experimental animals shown below in brackets. (A) Neoarsphenamine and rats (1331). Dosage, mg./10 kg. $\lambda = 0.08$. (MORRELL and CHAPMAN, 1933[1].) (B) Carbon bisulphide vapour on *Tribolium confusum* (480). Conc., mg./100 c.c. $\lambda = 0.07$. (STRAND, 1930[2].) (C) Hydrocyanic acid vapour on *Tribolium confusum* (450). Conc., mg./10 litres. $\lambda = 0.1$. (STRAND, 1930[2].) (D) Nicotine spray on *Aphis rumicis* (1700). Conc., mols/1000 litres. $\lambda = 0.44$. (TATTERSFIELD and GIMINGHAM, 1927[3].) (E) Dysentery toxin on mice. Dosage, $\gamma/200$ g. $\lambda = 0.4$. (TREVAN, 1929[4].) (F) Tetramethylammonium salts spray on *Aphis rumicis*. Conc., mols/1000 litres. $\lambda = 0.44$. (TATTERSFIELD and GIMINGHAM, 1927[3].)

(fig. 54) and the method employed in fig. 56 is the only one by which a linear relation can be obtained. This method therefore provides a common basis for the comparison of symmetrical and skew distributions of variation in response.

The contrast between the steep characteristic curves with a symmetrical variation (fig. 55) and the skew characteristic curves (fig. 54) is very striking, and it may be mentioned at once that this difference is not dependent on the form of population chosen. For example the responses of frogs' hearts to digitalis glucosides show a small and symmetrical variation whereas their responses to acetylcholine show an extreme example of skewed and widely scattered variation.

Similarly fig. 56 shows the actions of four insecticides on insect populations, which illustrate the gross differences that can occur in the scatter of the variation. Nicotine and the tetramethyl ammonium salts act over a wide range and the

[1] MORRELL, C. A., and C. W. CHAPMAN: J. Pharmacol. Baltimore **48**, 375, 391 (1933).
[2] STRAND, A. L.: Industr. Engineer., Chem. Analyt. Sect. **2**, 4 (1930).
[3] TATTERSFIELD, F., and C. T. GIMINGHAM: Ann. appl. Biol. **14**, 217 (1927).
[4] TREVAN, J. W.: J. of Path. **32**, 127 (1929).

value for $\lambda$ in these two cases is 0.44 whilst carbon bisulphide and hydrocyanic acid show a steep all or none effect and the value for $\lambda$ are 0.07 and 0.10 respectively.

The figure also shows that equally large differences in scatter may occur in the case of drugs given to mammals, for in the case of neoarsphenamine given to rats $\lambda = 0.08$, whilst in the case of dysentery toxin given to mice $\lambda = 0.44$. The last mentioned result also proves that a very extensive scatter may occur when a known dosage of drug is administered to each individual.

Inspection of fig. 56 shows that in order to obtain an accurate estimate of $\lambda$ in the case of drugs in which the response shows a relatively small scatter the logarithmic scale would need to be spread out so as to cover about $^1/_5$ of the range shown in the figure. It is easy to arrange a suitable scale for any particular case, and the only reason for plotting all the results shown in fig. 56 on a common scale was to demonstrate the contrast in the results with different drugs.

**Errors in Construction of Characteristic Curves.** Biological standardisation is an important pharmacological technique, and there is a considerable literature devoted to this subject. Most of this literature deals with the practical problem of how to obtain accurate estimations of the mean lethal doses of two preparations (unknown and standard preparations) with the minimum expenditure of material and of time.

This subject is discussed in the following papers. TREVAN (1927)[1], BURN (1930)[2], GADDUM (1933)[3], BEHRENS (1929)[4], KÄRBER (1931)[5], BEHRENS and KÄRBER (1935)[6].

In view of the detailed manner in which this subject has been dealt with it is unnecessary to review it here, but it is desirable to consider briefly the probable reliability of some of the data under discussion.

**Uniformity of Population.** All workers agree that the extent of the variation in the response to drugs can be reduced by obtaining as uniform a population as possible. WINTON (1927)[7] measured the lethal action of red squill on rats and found that females were twice as susceptible as males and that with males the standard deviation in stock rats was 67 p.c. of the mean, whilst this figure was reduced to 21 p.c. when inbred Wistar rats were used.

DURHAM, GADDUM and MARCHAL (1929)[8] found in the case of the bioassay of neosalvarsan on mice that a much smaller variation occurred with inbred stock than with ordinary stock.

The amount of information on this subject is limited because all persons making extensive experiments have endeavoured to obtain uniform populations. It is obvious that if diseased stock is used great variations are liable to occur. Moreover the susceptibility to drugs of animals of different ages varies greatly and there is also no satisfactory method of relating dosage to body weight when the latter varies extensively. All these sources of error can be avoided by using animals of inbred stock similar in respect of sex, age and weight, but even when these errors have been eliminated certain unknown causes of variation remain. In these cases where methods of bioassay have been carried out with particular

[1] TREVAN, J. W.: Proc. roy. Soc. B. **101**, 483 (1927).
[2] BURN, J. H.: Physiologic. Rev. **10**, 146 (1930).
[3] GADDUM, J. H.: Med. Res. Council Spec. Report **183** (1933).
[4] BEHRENS, B.: Arch. f. exper. Path. **140**, 237 (1929).
[5] KÄRBER, G.: Arch. f. exper. Path. **162**, 480 (1931).
[6] BEHRENS, B., and G. KÄRBER: Arch. f. exper. Path. **177**, 379 (1935).
[7] WINTON, F. R.: J. Pharmacol. Baltimore **31**, 123 (1927).
[8] DURHAM, F. M., J. H. GADDUM and J. E. MARCHAL: Med. Res. Council Spec. Rep. **128** (1929).

care it has been found that even when a uniform population is kept under strictly uniform conditions variations occur for which no obvious cause can be assigned.

CHAPMAN and MORRELL (1931)[1] measured the lethal dose of ouabain on 8 batches of 240 frogs each on different days. All the characteristic curves showed a similar slope (cf. fig. 55) but the median lethal dose found in different experiments varied from 28 to 33 $\gamma$ p. 100 g.

HEMMINGSEN (1933)[2] made an intensive study of insulin assay and found a number of unexpected causes of variation in response. The average sensitivity of batches of mice was found to vary from day to day, and mice with low body weight were found to be more susceptible in the evening than in the morning.

In general it would appear that our knowledge regarding the causes of variation in response to drugs is very imperfect, and that in the few cases where the subject has been studied carefully it has been found to be extremely complex.

**Errors of Sampling.** The author has mentioned the fact that the extremes of variation are of particular importance in determining the shape of the characteristic curve. The plotting of results according to the normal equivalent deviation accentuates the importance of these extremes. Fig. 56 demonstrates this fact very clearly for the height of the ordinate between 50 and 84 p.c. action is equal to that between 84 p.c. and 98 p.c. action or that between 98 p.c. and 99.85 p.c. action. The slope of the curve is therefore extensively influenced by the points representing actions outside the range of 16 p.c. to 84 p.c. action ($\pm 1\,\sigma$). These measurements of the extremes of action are however completely unreliable unless large populations of animals are used. The following argument applies (JACOBS, 1935[3]). If $n$ events be considered and if the probability of a success be represented by $p$ and of a failure by $q$ then the standard deviation is given by the formula

$$\sigma = \sqrt{n \cdot p \cdot q}.$$

When the number of successes (or failures) is small in comparison to the number of events, $\sigma$ is approximately equal to the square root of the number of successes (or failures).

Unless a figure is equal to at least twice its standard deviation it cannot be regarded as of great significance even in the case of biological data, where we are forced to be content with low standards of accuracy.

Hence in any experiment of this type the number of probable successes (or failures) should not be less than 4, and this means that a group of 400 animals is needed to establish the incidence of either a 1 p.c. mortality or a 1 per cent. survival. It is important to remember that if smaller groups are taken there is a serious chance of completely missing the presence of exceptional individuals. The size of sample needed to give a 20 to 1 chance against missing the presence of a small percentage of individuals can be easily calculated. If the sample is such that only 2 positive individuals are to be expected, then a negative result will be obtained once in 12 times, whereas if the expected occurrence is 3 a negative result will be obtained once in 23 times. A sample of 300 is therefore needed in order to establish with reasonable certainty whether 1 p.c. of exceptional individuals are or are not present; similarly a sample of 3000 is needed to exclude the presence of 1 in 1000 exceptional individuals. Samples of this magnitude can only be obtained in the case of small organisms and hence the results below 1 p.c. and above 99 p.c. response usually only indicate that some exceptional individuals are present but do not indicate their true number, whilst negative

[1] CHAPMAN, C. W., and C. A. MORRELL: Quart. J. Pharmacy **4**, 195 (1931).
[2] HEMMINGSEN, A. M.: Quart. J. Pharmacy **6**, 39, 187 (1933).
[3] JACOBS, M. H.: Erg. Biol **12**, 1 (1935).

results in these regions of dosage often do not establish even presumptive evidence for the absence of exceptional individuals.

The estimation of the frequency of the occurrence of exceptional individuals is of no great importance in biological standardisation, because in this case doses which produce a mortality around 50 p.c. are chosen. These considerations are however of great importance in relation to such problems as the estimation of the safety of large doses of drugs and the estimation of the chances of industrial poisoning.

## Chapter 15

## Relation Between Various Types of Curves Expressing Response of Cells to Drugs.

### (1) Concentration-action Curves as Expressions of Individual Variation.

GADDUM (1937)[1] has suggested that since skew variation is a natural characteristic of living tissues, therefore the shape of all the curves expressing pharmacological responses can be interpreted as expressions of variation. In support of this hypothesis it can be pointed out that growth must tend to produce skew variation in any population as regards many of its characteristics.

It was shown in the previous Chapter that the characteristic curves expressing the individual variation in a population showed forms ranging from a steep sigmoid curve to an extreme skew form, and that the skew forms can be transformed to sigmoid curves if the response is plotted against the logarithm of the concentration. It was shown in Chapter 8 that the curves relating the concentrations of drugs and the graded responses of tissues also showed a similar range of curves. The similarity between the two sets of curves is obvious. Furthermore there is an obvious correlation between the forms of the concentration-action and the characteristic curves obtained with any particular drug. For example both of these types of curve obtained with acetyl choline or nicotine approximate to a rectangular hyperbola. On the other hand phenol and its simpler derivatives show sigmoid curves in both cases.

This resemblance in the two different classes of curves can be explained in two ways, either by assuming that all curves are simply expressions of individual variation or that they express a chemical process which is distorted by individual variation.

The influence of growth is shown most clearly in the case of a population growing unchecked, e.g. a population of bacteria in a favourable medium. Suppose such a population varies in an arithmetic manner as regards its rate of growth, i.e. number of divisions in unit time. Then, if the standard deviation ($\sigma$) is 30 p.c. of the mean, and three samples of the population be considered which show the variations of $-1\sigma$, 0 and $+1\sigma$, after 10 units of time the number of divisions in the three samples will have been 7, 10 and 13 respectively and the population will be in the ratio of $2^7$, $2^{10}$ and $2^{13}$ or 1, 8 and 64.

Unchecked growth is a phenomenon which rarely occurs in nature and hence many characteristics (e.g. height of men) which depend on growth have an approximately symmetrical distribution of variation when measured arithmetically. It seems reasonable, however, to consider this an accident and to regard the logarithmic distribution of variation as the normal for characters resulting from growth.

---

[1] GADDUM, J. H.: Proc. roy. Soc. B. **121**, 598 (1937).

**Virus Infections.** Recent quantitative work on infection with the tobacco mosaic virus provides a striking example of the remarkable curves relating exposure and response which apparently are expressions of individual variation as regards a simple morphological character, namely, thickness of surface of leaf.

The tobacco mosaic virus has been shown to be a crystalline protein (STANLEY, 1935[1]). This virus when inoculated into tobacco leaves produces discrete lesions which can be counted. A considerable amount of quantitative work has been carried out on the infection of tobacco leaves with this virus, and this work is of interest, firstly because it demonstrates the influence of individual variations of living cells on the entrance of a chemical, and secondly because it forms an interesting link between the action of poisons and the action of infective agents.

The results of experiments in which the virus was inoculated with pin pricks or rubbed into the leaves of susceptible plants show a remarkable distribution of individual varia-tion. Two experiments by SAMUEL and BALD (1933)[2] are shown in fig. 57. The results show a very wide in-dividual variation with a markedly skew dis-tribution. In the case of curve $B$, the num-ber of lesions per half leaf varied from 15 to 215. If the distribu-tion is plotted against the logarithm of the number of lesions, ap-proximately symmetri-cal sigmoid curves are obtained (fig. 57 inset).

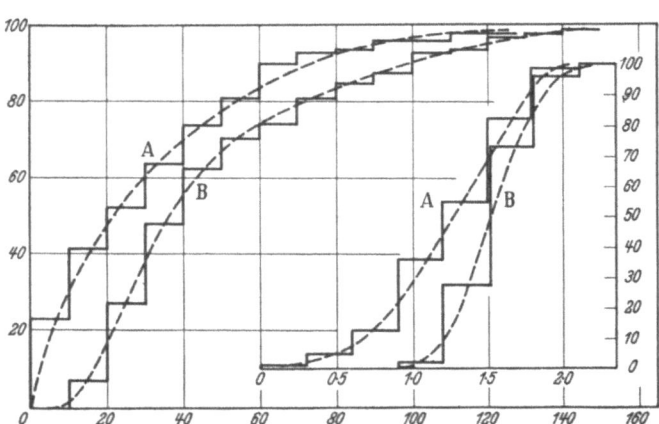

Fig. 57.  Action of tobacco mosaic on 100 tobacco leaves. Abscissa: — number of lesions per half leaf. Ordinate: — per cent. incidence. ($A$) Dilution of virus 1 in 3.3. ($B$) Dilution 1 in 100. Inset: — log. number of lesions and per cent. incidence. (SAMUEL and BALD, 1933[1].)

The question next arises as to the cause of the individual variation which has this curious distribution. Experiments were made on 100 half leaves, 10 taken from each of 10 plants, and the figures show that there was a marked individual variation in the resistance of different plants. For instance in one series the most resistant plant showed a total of 239 lesions, with a range of 15 to 32 lesions per half leaf, whereas in the least resistant plant the corresponding figures were 848 lesions, ranging from 30 to 215.

Furthermore the resistance of the plants could be reduced greatly by rubbing the leaves with fine sand. In one experiment the virus diluted to 1 in 10,000 produced 10 lesions in 10 half leaves, but when sand was added the same dilution produced 279 lesions. HOLMES (1929)[3] showed in pin prick experiments that with undiluted virus only 1 prick in 20 produced a lesion, a result which proves that the number of virus particles is very much greater than the number of lesions produced. The figures therefore express the variation in the powers of resistance of the plants, and cannot be interpreted as expressing any random error due to the varying chances of a virus particle entering a possible site of

[1] STANLEY, W. M.: Science (N. Y.) **81**, 644 (1935).
[2] SAMUEL, G., and J. G. BALD: Ann. appl. Biol. **20**, 70 (1933).
[3] HOLMES, F. O.: Bot. Gaz. **87**, 39 (1929).

infection. The figures show therefore that the leaves vary greatly in their susceptibility to infection.

It appears therefore that infection depends on the virus penetrating the surface of the leaf, and that this depends on some properties of the leaf of which thickness of the cuticle is probably the most important. The characteristic curves in fig. 57 show a variation of 100 fold in the effects produced in different individuals. The thickness of the cuticle cannot vary to this extent and hence the results indicate that the resistance of the leaf varies as some power of this thickness. This assumption is in accordance with the fact that the variation is nearly symmetrical when plotted against the logarithm of the number of lesions.

These results therefore provide fairly direct evidence that a simple morphological variation may cause a variation as regards the entrance of virus which is as extensive as any of the individual variations observed in the response to drugs. In the light of these results there seems to be no particular difficulty in assuming for example that different bacteria in a culture may vary over a similar range as regards the ease with which phenol penetrates their cell walls, and this removes the difficulty of assuming that curves recording the rate of death of bacterial populations exposed to disinfectants express variations in individual resistance.

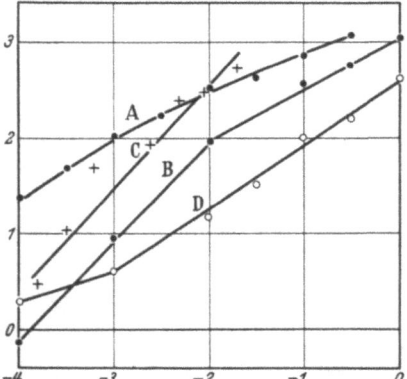

Fig. 58. Concentration-action relations of tobacco mosaic virus acting on tobacco leaves. Abscissa:— log. conc. Ordinate:— log. number of lesions per half leaf. (A) and (B) SAMUEL and BALD (1933)[3]. (C) CALDWELL (1936)[2]. (D) HOLMES (1929)[1].

The relation between the concentration of virus and the number of lesions has been determined by HOLMES (1929)[1], CALDWELL (1933)[2] and SAMUEL and BALD (1933)[3]. All these obtained curves (fig. 58) which show an approximately linear relation between log. concentration and log. effect, but the slope of the curves varies widely. CALDWELL (1936)[2] states that at low concentrations there is a linear relation between concentration and effect, but that at higher concentrations the curve becomes exponential. The concentration-action relations suggest therefore some form of adsorption regulating the relation between concentration and amount of virus fixed by the leaf.

The most remarkable feature about the curves in fig. 58 is that they show a graded response over a 10,000 fold range of concentration. This is in accordance with the hypothesis already advanced that the resistance is dependent on some power of the thickness of the surface layers for this would explain why relatively small variations in thickness in different portions of a leaf could make a very great difference in the chance of infection being produced in the different spots.

It appears to the writer that the most probable explanation for the shapes of the curves in figs. 57 and 58 is morphological variation in the leaf surface. Fig. 57 expresses this variation as regards different leaves and fig. 58 the variation as regards different patches on the same leaf.

[1] HOLMES, F. O.: Bot. Gaz. **87**, 39 (1929).
[2] CALDWELL, J.: Proc. roy. Soc. B. **119**, 493 (1936).
[3] SAMUEL, G., and J. G. BALD: Ann. appl. Biol. **20**, 70 (1933).

This example therefore shows that it is possible for individual variation to produce curves which show a striking resemblance to the extreme skew curves obtained with drugs. This fact can be taken as an argument in favour of GAD-DUM's hypothesis that all drug responses express individual variation, but it is equally in accordance with the line of argument adopted by the author. According to this view the skew characteristic curves of drugs express individual variation spread out over a wide range owing to a non-linear relation between drug concentration and drug fixation. Similarly in the case of the virus the variation is spread out owing to the non-linear relation between surface thickness of the leaf and the power of the virus to penetrate the leaf.

**Discussion.** The example of the tobacco mosaic virus indicates that individual variation can produce a highly skewed curve relating exposure to drug and response of tissues. The objection to the hypothesis that all drug response curves are primarily expressions of individual variation is that it assumes variation to be distributed in a similar manner in different forms of population. In the case of virus infection it is reasonable to suppose that the thickness of leaf surface varies both in different areas in a single leaf and in different leaves, and that this variation should produce somewhat similar results in both cases as regards variation in resistance to infection. If, however, this type of explanation be applied in the case of acetyl choline, difficulties at once arise. In this case the fact that requires explanation is that the concentration-action curve on a tissue such as the frog's heart follows a rectangular hyperbola, and that the same type of curve is obtained for the characteristic curve expressing the variation in a population of frogs' hearts as regards the concentration of acetyl choline needed to produce a similar action (e.g. 50 per cent. inhibition).

A frog's heart contains about $10^7$ cells and hence the measurement of the concentration of acetyl choline needed to produce a selected action (e.g. 50 per cent. inhibition) in a frog's heart expresses the average response of $10^7$ cells. A characteristic curve expressing the individual variation of different hearts therefore records the variations in the average response of huge populations.

If we try and explain the concentration-action relation found in a single heart as an expression of the individual variation of the cells, then it is necessary to assume that the distribution of variation of the cells is similar to the distribution of variation of the average response of aggregates each containing $10^7$ cells. The example of the tobacco virus shows us that such an assumption is not impossible. If the individual receptors in a frog's heart vary in some manner so that the most susceptible combine with acetyl choline at a concentration which is about $1/_{10,000}$ of the concentration needed to saturate the least susceptible, and if this factor varies from heart to heart so that the most susceptible receptors in the most resistant hearts are similar in character to the least susceptible receptors in the least resistant hearts, then the similarity of the concentration-action curve and the characteristic curve can be explained.

We are faced therefore with the difficulty that so frequently arises in quantitative pharmacology, namely the existence of alternative hypotheses which cannot be conclusively proved or disproved. The interpretation of the curves as expressions of individual variation is possible provided certain assumptions be made, but the author is not in favour of this form of explanation because it involves too many unproven assumptions and it provides a method of explaining any form of curve obtained, without however linking the reactions observed with any known physico-chemical process.

An attempt therefore will be made to interpret these curves on the basis of the hypothesis that the concentration-action curve is an expression of a chemical combination similar to that which occurs between drugs and active proteins such as haemoglobin or enzymes, and that other forms of curves such as characteristic curves are expressions of fundamental chemical processes modified by individual variation.

## (2) Characteristic Curves as Expressions of Chemical Processes.

This explanation was adopted in the case of the kinetics of drug action where it was assumed that the organisms or cells varied symmetrically as regards the lethal dose of drug needed to produce a given response, and that the rate of entrance of drug into the cell depended on diffusion and followed the monomolecular formula $kt = \log \dfrac{a}{a-x}$. It was shown (Chap. 11) that in this case the relation between the time ($t$) taken to produce a given internal concentration of drug ($x$) would result in a symmetrical variation in relation to the effects

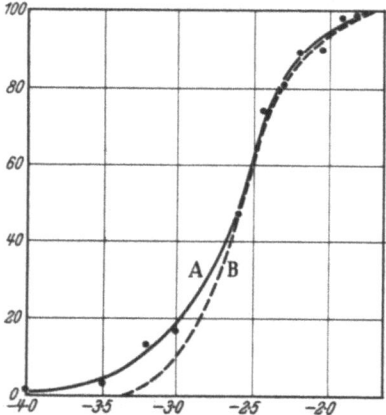

Fig. 59. Lethal action of nicotine spray on *Aphis rumicis*. Abscissa:— log. conc. Ordinate:— per cent. mortality. (*A*) Observed results. (*B*) Results as calculated in text.

produced by the amount fixed ($x$) becoming a skewed variation of incidence of effect in relation to time. This provided an explanation of the curious fact that the time-action curve expressing the rate of destruction of a population of small organisms often approximated to the curve expressing a monomolecular reaction.

A similar argument can be employed to explain the relation between concentration-action curves and characteristic curves.

The action of nicotine provides a convenient example. In the case of nicotine, two sets of observations are available. Firstly the concentration-graded action relation obtained with the rectus abdominis of the frog and secondly the characteristic curve of the lethal action of nicotine solutions sprayed upon *Aphis rumicis* (cf. fig. 54). If the logarithm of the concentration be plotted against the incidence of mortality, a nearly symmetrical sigmoid curve is obtained (fig. 59, Curve *A*). The results show that the most resistant individuals survived 100 times the concentration needed to kill the least resistant individuals.

The relation between concentration of nicotine and amount of concentration produced in the frog's rectus abdominis was determined by HILL (1909)[1], CLARK (1933)[2], and LAUBENDER and KOLB (1936)[3]. The data show an approximately linear relation between the logarithm of the concentration and the amount of action over a wide range, and also can be fitted by the formula $Kx = \dfrac{y}{100-y}$.

Analysis of the characteristic curve (fig. 59) shows the figures $C_{16} = 0.000,9$, $C_m = 0.002,8$ and $C_{84} = 0.005$, which gives a $C_{84}/C_{16}$ ratio of 5.5. The shape of the characteristic curve of nicotine may be regarded as well established, in view of the large population studied (1700 insects), and it therefore is worth while considering how it can be interpreted. Suppose the standard deviation of the individual variation of aphis in regard to the amount of drug that must be fixed

[1] HILL, A. V.: J. of Physiol. **39**, 361 (1909).
[2] CLARK, A. J.: The Mode of Action of Drugs on Cells. London: Arnold and Co. 1933.
[3] LAUBENDER, W., and H. KOLB: Arch. f. exper. Path. **182**, 401 (1936).

to produce a lethal effect be assumed to be equal to 30 p.c. of the median lethal dose, then the relation between drug fixed and individual response will be as follows:—

| (a) Amount of drug fixed as per cent. of median lethal dose | (b) Per cent. mortality of aphis | (a) Amount of drug fixed as per cent. of median lethal dose | (b) Per cent. mortality of aphis |
|---|---|---|---|
| 30 | 1 | 120 | 75 |
| 40 | 2.3 | 130 | 84 |
| 70 | 16 | 160 | 97.8 |
| 80 | 25 | 170 | 99 |
| 100 | 50 | | |

If the relation between nicotine concentration and nicotine fixation follows the formula $Kx = \dfrac{y}{100 - y}$, then the following relations will be obtained:—

| (x) Log. molar conc. nicotine | (y) Nicotine fixed as per cent. of that needed to produce half action | (x) Log. molar conc. nicotine | (y) Nicotine fixed as per cent. of that needed to produce half action |
|---|---|---|---|
| −3.6 | 18 | −2.3 | 130 |
| −3.3 | 33 | −1.8 | 180 |
| −2.8 | 80 | −1.6 | 200 |
| −2.6 | 100 | | |

A combination of these two sets of figures gives the results shown in Table 17.

Table 17. Calculated and observed concentration-mortality relations in the action of nicotine on Aphis rumicis.

| (a) Log. molar conc. nicotine | (b) Amount of drug fixed by organisms (as per cent. of median lethal dose) if reaction follows formula: $kx = y/100 - y$ | (c) Per cent. mortality of Aphis calculated from "b", when the individual variation is such that $\sigma = 30$ per cent. of median | (d) Per cent. mortality of Aphis as observed (fig. 59) |
|---|---|---|---|
| −3.6 | 18 | 0.4 | 3 |
| −3.3 | 33 | 1.0 | 8 |
| −3.2 | 40 | 2.3 | 12 |
| −2.9 | 70 | 16 | 24 |
| −2.8 | 80 | 25 | 30 |
| −2.6 | 100 | 50 | 50 |
| −2.4 | 120 | 75 | 76 |
| −2.3 | 130 | 84 | 84 |
| −2.0 | 160 | 97.8 | 96 |
| −1.9 | 170 | 99.0 | 98 |
| −1.8 | 180 | 99.5 | 99 |

The observed results (fig. 59, curve A) and the calculated results (fig. 59, curve B) agree exactly for mortalities between 40 and 100 per cent., but diverge in the case of mortalities below 40 per cent.

The agreement is, however, sufficiently good to suggest that the characteristic curve of nicotine can reasonably be explained as a combined effect of a hyperbola relating drug concentration and drug fixation and an individual variation in respect of the amount of drug needed to be fixed in order to produce a lethal effect.

The curious type of characteristic curve obtained with nicotine can therefore be explained as a moderate degree of variation exaggerated by the form of equilibrium between drug concentration and drug fixation.

### (3) Correlation Between Concentration-action Curves and Characteristic Curves.

The hypothesis outlined above can be tested to a certain extent by considering the correlation existing between different types of curves obtained with different drugs. Curves relating concentration and graded action fall into three chief classes: (a) hyperbolae, (b) linear relations, and (c) sigmoid or all-or-none relations.

If the hypothesis regarding the nature of characteristic curves is correct, then drugs of class (a) should show skewed characteristic curves, whilst drugs of classes (b) and (c) should show symmetrical characteristic curves.

In the case of class (b), if the cells vary symmetrically as regards the amount of drug fixed ($y$) and the relation between concentration ($x$) and drug fixed ($y$) is $Kx = y$, then the cells should vary symmetrically as regards $y$.

In the case of class (c) the concentration-graded action curves, which are of sigmoid type, are assumed not to measure a graded effect but to measure an all-or-none effect which is distorted by individual variation in the cells composing the tissue. In this case therefore the curves relating concentration with an action which can be graded and those relating concentration with a definite all-or-none effect should be of similar shape.

In order to discuss this problem it is necessary to adopt some method of describing the various curves. All forms of characteristic curves can be described by stating the normal equivalent deviation i.e. half the difference between the logarithm of the concentrations producing 84 and 16 per cent. action, or $\dfrac{\log. C_{84} - \log. C_{16}}{2}$. A similar and simpler method is to state the ratio between the concentrations producing 16 and 84 per cent. action ($C_{16}$ and $C_{84}$) and the symmetry of the curves can be tested by comparing the ratios between $C_{16}$ and $C_{84}$ and the median concentration ($C_{50}$) i.e. $C_{50}/C_{16}$ and $C_{84}/C_{50}$.

In the case of a symmetrical variation following a normal curve of error, with a moderate standard deviation such as 30 p.c. of the median, these quantities are in the proportion $C_{50} = 1.0$, $C_{16} = 0.7$ and $C_{84} = 1.3$, which gives a ratio for $C_{84}/C_{16}$ of 1.85. In the case of an action following the hyperbola expressed by the formula $Kx = \dfrac{y}{100 - y}$ the values are $C_{16} = 0.19$ and $C_{84} = 5.25$, which gives a ratio for $C_{84}/C_{16}$ of 27.5. In the case of a linear relation between concentration and action the values are $C_{16} = 0.32$ and $C_{84} = 1.68$ and the ratio $C_{84}/C_{16}$ is 5.25.

These ratios differ so widely in the case of the three different forms of curves that they provide an easy method of indicating the form of curve to which any particular group of results approximates.

A general consideration of the forms of characteristic curves shows that a number of these curves are nearly symmetrical and approximate to the normal curve of error, but that an equally large number show a skewed variation covering a remarkable range of dosage or concentration of drug. These latter curves only occur with drugs in which the concentration-graded action curves follow a hyperbola, but, on the other hand, steep symmetrical characteristic curves are sometimes obtained with this same class of drugs, and a single drug occasionally shows a symmetrical sigmoid characteristic curve with one population and a skewed curve with another. In such cases, skew variation is usually seen with simple cell systems and symmetrical variation with more complex systems (e.g. mammals), hence it appears probable that the latter form is produced by an increase in the number of independent variables.

**Examples of Skewed Characteristic Curves.** The case of nicotine has already been considered and acetylcholine and adrenaline are two other drugs which show highly skewed characteristic curves. In both cases the concentration-action relation with a wide variety of tissues has been shown to follow a hyperbola, whilst all workers who have studied the action of acetylcholine on the frog's heart have been struck by the remarkable range of individual variation in respect of the concentration of drug needed to produce a given effect (e.g. 50 p.c. inhibition).

FÜHNER (1923)[1] found that some hearts responded to 0.001 $\gamma$ per litre and others required 1.0 $\gamma$ per litre of acetylcholine. BEZNAK (1934)[2] described an even more remarkable range of variation in the study of 1000 frogs' hearts. He found that variations from $10^{-5} \gamma$ per c.c. to $50 \gamma$ per c.c. were common, but stated that occasionally responses were found far below this range.

The author (CLARK, 1927[3]) measured the concentration of acetylcholine needed to produce 50 p.c. inhibition in the hearts of 70 frogs and found these to be distributed as follows:—

| Molar conc. acetylcholine producing response $\times 10^9$ | 3—30 | 30—300 | 300—3,000 | 3,000—30,000 | >30,000 |
|---|---|---|---|---|---|
| Per cent. of population of frogs' hearts responding | 21 | 33 | 34 | 7 | 3 |

These figures when integrated show a symmetrical sigmoid distribution when the incidence is plotted against log. concentration and the ratio $C_{84}/C_{16}$ is about 40.

WHITE and STEDMAN (1931)[4], however, found that the characteristic curve for the lethal action of acetylcholine measured on 450 mice followed an ordinary curve of variation; the lethal doses (mgm. acetylcholine, intravenous, per 20 gm. mouse) were $C_{16}$ 0.47, $C_M$ 0.66, $C_{84}$ 0.9. The curve is not markedly asymmetrical and the ratio $C_{84}/C_{16}$ is 2, which corresponds to a standard deviation of 30 p.c. of the median lethal dose. It is therefore necessary to assume that the lethal action of acetylcholine on mice is produced by some action completely different in its nature from the inhibitory action of the drug on the heart.

In the case of adrenaline there is a large amount of evidence to show that the concentration-graded action relation follows a hyperbola similar to that found with acetylcholine. LANGECKER (1926)[5] measured the concentration of adrenaline needed to produce a selected amount of contraction in the isolated uteri of 172 rabbits. He obtained the following figures:—

| Molar conc. of adrenaline $\times 10^6$. | 0.05 | 0.15 | 0.3 | 0.6 | 1.2 | 2 | 3 | 6 |
|---|---|---|---|---|---|---|---|---|
| Per cent. of population of uteri showing contraction . . . . . | 5 | 9 | 27 | 59 | 85 | 94 | 97 | 100 |

These figures follow a hyperbola drawn to the formula $Kx^2 = \dfrac{y}{100-y}$, and the ratio $C_{84}/C_{16}$ is 6.

The characteristic curve of the lethal action of adrenaline on mice follows a similar curve to the above, as is shown by the figures obtained by SCHULTZ (1909)[6]:—

| Dose of adrenaline subcutaneous mgm. per mouse. . . . . . . | 0.5—1 | 2—4 | 5—6 | 8 | 10 | 12—20 | 20—35 |
|---|---|---|---|---|---|---|---|
| Deaths . . . . . . . . . . . . | 0/4 | 4/19 | 2/17 | 12/21 | 12/21 | 25/34 | 6/6 |
| Per cent. response . . . . . . . | 0 | 21 | 12 | 57 | 57 | 74 | 100 |

The results when plotted indicate the following values $C_{16} = 4$, $C_m = 8$, $C_{84} = 22$. The curve is not symmetrical and the ratio $C_{84}/C_{16}$ is 5.5.

[1] FÜHNER, H.: Heffters Handb. exper. Pharmakol. 1, 640 (1923).
[2] BEZNAK, A. B. L.: J. of Physiol. 82, 129 (1934).
[3] CLARK, A. J.: J. of Physiol. 64, 123 (1927).
[4] WHITE, A. C., and E. STEDMAN: J. Pharmacol. Baltimore 41, 259 (1931).
[5] LANGECKER, H.: Arch. f. exper. Path. 118, 49 (1926).
[6] SCHULTZ, W. H.: U. S. Hyg. Labor. Bull. 55 (1909).

The concentration-action curve of adrenaline acting upon the rabbit's uterus (GADDUM, 1926[1]) and upon arterial strips (WILKIE, 1928[2]) follows the formula $Kx = \dfrac{y}{100 - y}$ $(C_{84}/C_{16} = 25)$, whilst the concentration-action curve of adrenaline acting upon the dog's blood pressure (HUNT, 1901[3]; MOLINELLI, 1926[4]) follows the formula $Kx^2 = \dfrac{y}{100 - y}$ $(C_{84}/C_{16} = 5)$.

In the case of adrenaline, therefore, the evidence suggests that in the case of the simplest tissues the concentration-action curve expresses a monomolecular reaction. This relation is partially distorted both in the case of the concentration-action measured on the rise of dog's blood pressure and also in the case of the characteristic curves obtained with the isolated rabbits' uteri and with mice. In these latter cases, however, a markedly skew distribution of variation is found.

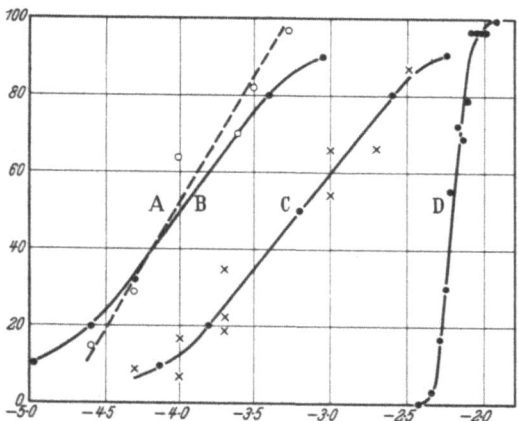

Fig. 60. Concentration-action relations of hydrocyanic acid. Abscissa:— log. molar conc. Ordinate:— action as per cent of maximum. (A) Inhibition of oxygen consumption of isolated frog's ventricle. (WEIZSÄCKER, 1912[5].) (B) Curve drawn to formula $kx = y/100 - y$. (C) Depression of mechanical response of isolated frog's ventricle. (PICKFORD, 1927[6].) (D) Lethal action of vapour on *Tribolium confusum*. (STRAND, 1930[7].)

Fig. 60 shows a case in which there is a striking difference between the form of the concentration-action and the characteristic curves. The action of hydrocyanic acid in inhibiting both the respiration and the mechanical response of the frog's heart follows a hyperbola and can be satisfactorily explained as a reaction between HCN and a tissue receptor. The toxic action of HCN vapour on *Tribolium confusum* (confused flour beetle) shows, however, a fairly symmetrical characteristic curve with a narrow range of variation $(C_{84}/C_{16} = 1.6)$. Hydrocyanic acid may be assumed to produce a similar fundamental toxic effect on all forms of living tissue, and the steep characteristic curve obtained with the beetles suggests that in some cases the characteristic curve is not affected by the nature of the fundamental chemical process.

Characteristic curves which express either the lethal action of bacterial toxins or their antagonism by antitoxins usually show a highly skewed distribution of variation.

TREVAN's (1929[8]) figures for the lethal action of dysentery toxin on mice show a ratio for $C_{84}/C_{16}$ of 9.5. HARTLEY et al. (1933)[9] measured the power of pneumococcus antiserum to antagonise a fixed dose of pneumococcus toxin and in this case (fig. 61) the $C_{84}/C_{16}$ ratio was 12.5.

[1] GADDUM, J. H.: J. of Physiol. **61**, 141 (1926).
[2] WILKIE, D.: J. Pharmacol. Baltimore **34**, 1 (1928).
[3] HUNT, REID: Amer. J. of Physiol. **5**, 7 (1901).
[4] MOLINELLI, E. A.: Tésis, Buenos Aires (1926).
[5] WEIZSÄCKER, V.: Pflügers Arch. **147**, 135 (1912).
[6] PICKFORD, L. M.: J. of Physiol. **63**, 19 (1927).
[7] STRAND, A. L.: Industr. Engineer., Chem. Analyt. Sect. **2**, 4 (1930).
[8] TREVAN, J. W.: J. of Path. **32**, 127 (1929).
[9] HARTLEY, P., H. J. PARISH, G. E. PETRIE and W. SMITH: Lancet **1933 II**, 91.

In the case of pneumococcus antibody, the curve expresses experiments on 880 mice. It will be seen (fig. 61) that the shape of the extremes of the curve are uncertain, a fact which indicates the enormous populations required to establish with certainty characteristic curves which spread over a wide range of concentration. The wide spread of the results is in this case explained by the fact that the relation between concentration ($x$) and fixation ($y$) of antibodies and toxins follows approximately FREUNDLICH's adsorption formula $K x^{0.66} = y$ (ARRHENIUS, 1915[1]). Such a relation between concentration and fixation could cause a spread of the relation between concentration and individual variation in response to drug fixed in the same manner as do the concentration-action relations which follow a hyperbola.

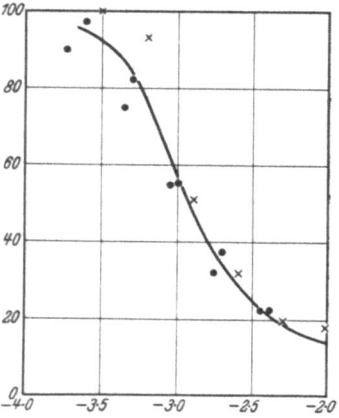

Fig. 61. Protective action of antipneumococcal serum on 800 mice given standard dose of toxin. Abscissa:— log. dose serum in c.c. per mouse. Ordinate: — per cent. mortality. (HARTLEY, PARRISH, PETRIE and SMITH, 1933[2].)

The characteristic curve of insulin has been studied intensively and it has been shown clearly that the variation is symmetrical to the logarithm of the dosage and not to the dosage. The ratio $C_{84}/C_{16}$ is about 2 and this would be produced by a standard deviation of 33 p.c. of the median; hence in this case it is the skew variation rather than the extent of the variation that requires explanation. The concentration-action relation of insulin has been shown to approximate to the relation:— effect varies as log. dosage, and this will explain the asymmetry of the characteristic curve.

Similar arguments apply to the characteristic curves of the sex hormones. In the case of oestrin, the ratio $C_{84}/C_{16}$ varies from 2 (MARRIAN and PARKES, 1929[3]) to 5.5 (COWARD and BURN, 1927[4]). In the case of the ovulation substance of the anterior pituitary, the ratio $C_{84}/C_{16}$ lies between 2 and 4 (HILL, PARKES and WHITE, 1934[5]) and in this case the authors' figures also prove that the graded response of mouse ovaries shows a linear relation between log. dosage and effect. This same relation has been found between the dosage of male hormone and the action as estimated by the increase in size of the capon's comb (GALLAGHER and KOCH, 1935[6]).

Similar arguments apply to other hormones such as thyroxine and to vitamins. In all cases the relation between log. concentration or dosage and effect is approximately linear and in all cases the characteristic curves are skewed and spread over a wide range (CLARK, 1933[7]).

*Narcotics.* The exact relation between concentration-action and characteristic curves has been demonstrated by SHERIF (1936)[8] in the case of ether acting upon a large population of isolated frogs' hearts.

[1] ARRHENIUS, S.: Quantitative Laws in Biological Chemistry. London: Bell and Sons 1915.
[2] HARTLEY, P., H. J. PARISH, G. E. PETRIE and W. SMITH: Lancet **1933 II**, 91.
[3] MARRIAN, G. P., and A. S. PARKES: J. of Physiol. **67**, 389 (1929).
[4] COWARD, K. H., and J. H. BURN: J. of Physiol. **63**, 270 (1927).
[5] HILL, R. T., A. S. PARKES and W. E. WHITE: J. of Physiol. **81**, 335 (1934).
[6] GALLAGHER, T. F., and F. C. KOCH: J. Pharmacol. Baltimore **55**, 97 (1935).
[7] CLARK, A. J.: The Mode of Action of Drugs on Cells. London: Arnold and Co. 1933.
[8] SHERIF, M. A. F.: J. pharmacol. Baltimore **56**, 1 (1936).

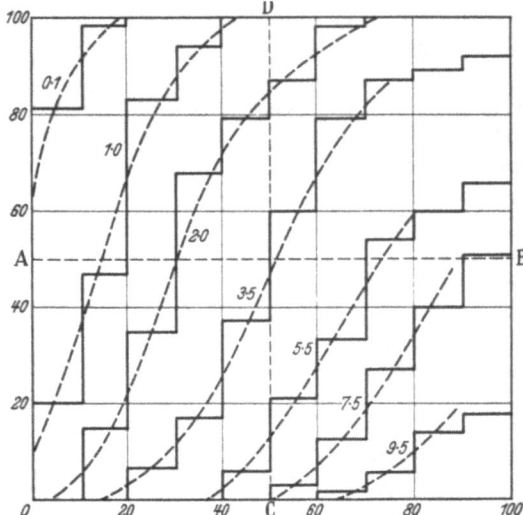

Fig. 62. Action of ether on population of 537 frog's hearts. Abscissa: — Per cent. inhibition of mechanical response. Ordinate: — Per cent. of individuals showing a given percentage of inhibition. The curves show the effects of seven concentrations of ether (0.1—9.5 per mille wt./vol.). (SHERIF, 1936[1].)

Fig. 62 shows characteristic curves obtained with a series of different concentrations of ether. Since ether produces a graded effect it was possible to measure quantitatively the response of each heart and the figure shows the responses of 527 hearts. The general shape of these curves is sigmoid; they are nearly but not exactly symmetrical. From these curves it is simple to read off the median response produced by each concentration of ether measured (line $A-B$). These figures are:

| Conc. ether . . . | 0.1 | 1.0 | 2.0 |
|---|---|---|---|
| Median response . | 0.5 | 15 | 30 |

| Conc. ether . . . | 3.5 | 5.5 | 7.5 |
|---|---|---|---|
| Median response . | 51 | 73 | 93 |

These results show a curve relating ether concentration and response (fig. 63) which is just the same as the relation between concentration of narcotic (ethyl urethane) and percentage depression produced that is found when a series of concentrations are measured on a single heart (fig. 15).

Alternatively we can regard the production of 50 p.c. inhibition (fig. 62,

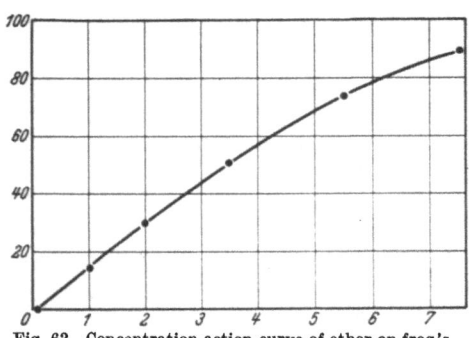

Fig. 63. Concentration-action curve of ether on frog's hearts. Abscissa: — conc. ether. Ordinate: — median response of population. (Taken from fig. 62, line $A-B$.)

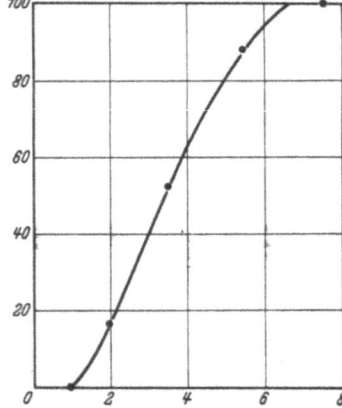

Fig. 64. Characteristic curve of action of ether on frog's hearts. Abscissa: — conc. ether per mille. Ordinate: — per cent. of population showing 50 per cent. inhibition. (Taken from fig. 62, line $C-D$.)

line $C-D$) as an all-or-none effect for each dose, and divide the population into those in which the response is less than or more than 50 p.c. inhibition: —

| Conc. ether . . . . | 1.0 | 2.0 | 3.5 | 5.5 | 7.5 |
|---|---|---|---|---|---|
| Response < 50 p.c. | 100 | 84 | 48 | 12 | 0 |
| > 50 p.c. | 0 | 16 | 52 | 88 | 100 |

The result is a characteristic curve relating concentration and per cent. of effect (fig. 64). This curve is essentially similar to the characteristic curves

[1] SHERIF, M. A. F.: J. pharmacol. Baltimore **56**, 1 (1936).

relating concentration of narcotic and the production of some obligatory all-or-none effect such as the inhibition of cell division.

The characteristic curve derived from SHERIF's figures is essentially similar to the characteristic curve obtained by KNOEFEL and MURRELL (1935)[1] for the action of ether on mice, and it may be said that as a general rule symmetrical characteristic curves showing a relatively small scatter of variation are obtained with aliphatic narcotics. This result is in agreement with the general theory that a wide scatter is caused by a logarithmic relation between drug concentration and drug fixation and when this relation is a simple linear one the scatter is relatively small.

SHERIF's figures provide an interesting example of the manner in which both a concentration-action curve and a characteristic curve can be obtained from a single set of curves. Such examples are naturally uncommon because of the laborious nature of the work involved in obtaining the primary curves.

**All-or-None Effects.** Steep symmetrical sigmoid curves are common types of characteristic curves; moreover they are obtained with certain important drugs such as the cardiac glucosides and the organic arsenicals which are standardised biologically.

In many cases the form of the curve can be explained by the fact that the concentration-graded action curve of the drug is an all-or-none effect. Caffeine provides a simple example of this fact. The author (CLARK, 1933[2], Table 14 and fig. 30) measured the amount of contraction produced by varying concentrations of caffeine on 73 pairs of frogs' muscles and his results show the relations $C_{16} = 0.05$ and $C_{84} = 0.07$ p.c. which gives a $C_{84}/C_{16}$ ratio of 1.4 and this indicates a sharp all-or-none action. TAKAHASHI (1925)[3] measured the effect of caffeine on isolated frogs' muscles and his results show that 0.029 p.c. produced histological change in 16 p.c. of the muscles ($C_{16}$) and that $C_{84} = 0.035$, which is a ratio of 1.2. The two curves are therefore essentially similar in type and both are due to the same fact namely that up to a certain concentration caffeine produces no change and that a slight increase in concentrations produces a nearly maximum change. In this case the concentration-action curve does not measure the uptake of drug but only expresses the fact that at a certain concentration a biological response is produced.

Phenol and the substituted phenols such as dinitrophenol are another group of drugs which show an all-or-none effect under all conditions. The inhibition of yeast fermentation and respiration (fig. 10) and the stimulation of oxidation of arbacia eggs (fig. 11) which are potentially graded actions, show an all-or-none response to dinitrophenol and the same type of curve is seen in characteristic curves, e.g. inhibition of cell division (fig. 11), lethal action on yeast (fig. 9) destruction of *aphis rumicis*, $C_{84}/C_{16} = 2.2$ (TATTERSFIELD et al., 1925[4]).

In the case of digitalis, a similar condition obtains, since up to a certain concentration it produces no measurable action on the heart whilst a relatively small increase causes systolic arrest.

In a large number of other cases drugs show steep characteristic curves although they show concentration-action relations ranging over a wide range of concentrations. For example, heavy metals and arsenicals inhibit ferments and there is an approximately linear relation between log. concentration and amount of inhibition, nevertheless the characteristic curves for the lethal action of these drugs are steep and fairly symmetrical ($C_{84}/C_{16} = 1.5—2.0$. cf. fig. 53 and GADDUM, 1933[5], Table 1).

[1] KNOEFEL, P. K., and F. C. MURRELL: J. Pharmacol. Baltimore **55**, 235 (1935).
[2] CLARK, A. J.: The Mode of Action of Drugs on Cells. London: Arnold and Co. 1933.
[3] TAKAHASHI, Y.: Okayama-Igakkai-Zasshi No. **429**, 1020 (1925).
[4] TATTERSFIELD, F., C. T. GIMINGHAM and H. M. MORRIS: Ann. appl. Biol. **12**, 218 (1925).
[5] GADDUM, J. H.: Med. Res. Council Spec. Report **183** (1933).

Certain alkaloids such as cocaine and aconitine show similar characteristic curves, although in this case also it is highly probable that the action varies as the log. of the concentration.

**Discussion.** The examples given in this section show that the strongly skewed characteristic curves which occur with certain drugs can be satisfactorily explained as an expression of individual variation distorted by the non-linear relation between concentration and drug fixation.

The most difficult point to explain is why the same drug sometimes shows skewed characteristic curves with one population and symmetrical curves with another population. It must, however, be remembered that reliable characteristic curves can only be obtained if the drugs are tested on a homogeneous population of adequate size. The middle portion of a curve can be determined by the use of one or two hundred animals, but at least 1000 animals are needed to establish the full course of the curve. Consequently although the data regarding characteristic curves are very extensive, yet the data suitable for theoretical discussion are relatively scanty. The conception that the shape of characteristic curves is determined fundamentally by the physico-chemical nature of the reaction between drug and population is supported by the following facts:—

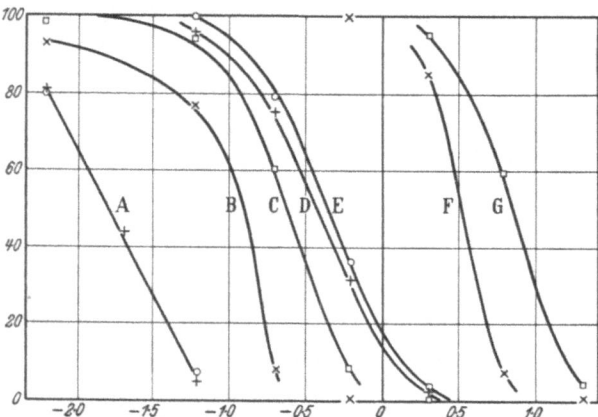

Fig. 65. Action of sulphuretted hydrogen spores of on eight different species of fungi. Abscissa:— log. conc. H₂S (mg./litre). Ordinate:— per cent. of spores germinating. (A) *Venturia inequalis* and *Uromyces caryophyllinus.* (B) *Puccinia antirhini.* (C) *Sclerotina americana.* (D) *Macrosporidium sarcinaeforme.* (E) *Pestalotia stellata.* (F) *Glomerella cingulata.* (G) *Botrytis.* (McCALLAN and WILCOXON, 1931[1].)

(1) A single drug usually shows characteristic curves of a similar shape when tested on a variety of different populations.

(2) A single population tested with different drugs may show a very wide variety of characteristic curves.

The first point is illustrated by the experiments of McCALLAN and WILCOXON (1931)[1] who measured the action of solutions of sulphuretted hydrogen upon the spores of 8 species of fungi. Their results which are shown in fig. 65 record the effects of the poison over a 1400 fold range of concentration. The figures deal with large numbers, since 2000 spores were counted for each point. Except in the cases of curves B and F a fairly exact linear relation was found between the logarithm of the concentration and the standard equivalent deviation. Curve C is of interest since it shows that a small mortality was produced by 0.06 mgm. H₂S per litre whilst 1 p.c. of the spores survived a concentration 30 times as great. The drug was allowed to act for 22 hours and hence rate of entrance can scarcely have played a part in causing this remarkable scatter. It can also be concluded that the scatter is due to the nature of the action of the drug on the spores since other drugs acting on similar spores showed much less scatter. The slope of these curves is relatively constant as is seen from inspection of the figure. The values of (log. $C_{50}$—log. $C_{16}$) for curves $A$—$G$ are

[1] McCALLAN, S. E. A., and F. WILCOXON: Contrib. Boyce Thompson Instit. **3**, 13, 31 (1931).

as follows:— 0.4, 0.25, 0.3, 0.5, 0.4, 0.23 and 0.3. This relative uniformity is remarkable since the median lethal concentration for *Venturia inequalis* (curve *A*) is $^1/_{1400}$ of the corresponding concentration for *Botrytis* (curve *G*).

This similarity of distribution of variation in the different forms of spores, suggests a common type of chemical action. The spores of the different species might vary either (a) as regards the amount of drug fixed or (b) the amount of drug needed to be fixed in order to produce an action.

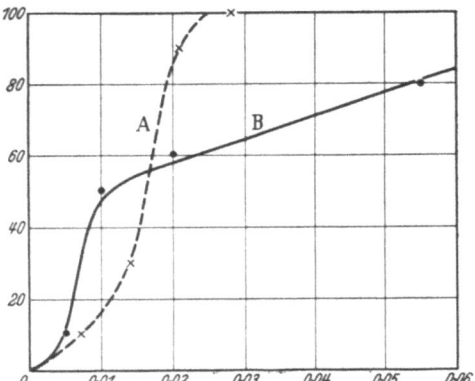

It is improbable that there should be a 1400 fold variation as regards the latter factor, and therefore it is more probable that there is a wide variety in the dissociation constant of the receptors in the spores and the drug. The wide individual variation in the spores of a single species also can most easily be explained by the same hypothesis.

The fact that different drugs acting on the same species may give widely different forms of characteristic curves is exemplified by fig. 66 which shows the actions of different drugs on aphis. The same fact has been observed with all

Fig. 66. Characteristic curves of destruction of *Aphis rumicis*. Abscissa:— concentration. Ordinate:— per cent. mortality. (*A*) Dichlorobenzene, mols per 100 c.c. (TATTERSFIELD et al., 1925[1].) (*B*) Tetra methyl ammonium sulphate, mols per 1000 c.c. (TATTERSFIELD et al., 1927[1].)

populations that have been used extensively for drug standardisation. For example every form of characteristic curve has been obtained with mice from the highly skewed curves with dysentery toxin ($\lambda = 0.48$) to the steep symmetrical curves such as are obtained with neoarsphenamine ($\lambda = 0.084$).

### (4) Drug Responses and Individual Variation.

There are five types of curves which express the response of cell populations to drugs, namely:—

(1) Time-action curves. (a) Graded action. (b) All-or-none action. — (2) Time-concentration curves. — (3) Concentration-action curves. — (4) Characteristic concentration-action curves.

All these curves can be obtained with a single drug, although such data are rarely complete.

For example, the following actions can be recorded with nicotine:—

1. (a) Course of response of rectus abdominis.

1. (b) Course of destruction of an insect population such as *Aphis rumicis*.

2. Relation between concentration and time of response until some selected response is produced on rectus abdominis.

3. Relation between concentration and response of rectus abdominis.

4. Relation between concentration and per cent. mortality in *Aphis rumicis*.

The possible influence of individual variation varies in these different cases.

It has been shown that time-action curves measuring all-or-none effects and characteristic concentration-action curves must to a large extent express individual variation in a population of cells.

It has been shown that the shape of concentration-action curves can reasonably be considered as being expressions of physico-chemical processes.

---

[1] TATTERSFIELD, F., C. T. GIMINGHAM, and J. M. MORRIS: Ann. appl. Biol. **12**, 218 (1925).
[2] TATTERSFIELD, F., and C. T. GIMINGHAM: Ann. appl. Biol. **14**, 217 (1927).

The time-graded action curves appear to the author to be of subsidiary importance. The significance of these curves is less certain than that of any other class of curve because in most cases they express chiefly the biological lag in the response of the tissue to the stimulus of the drug.

If there happens to be a linear relation between the time and the amount of drug entering the cell, then the time graded-action curves should show the same shape as the concentration curve obtained with the same system. A linear relation in such a complex process as drug uptake is extremely unlikely, and if the relation is not linear the course of the curve is very difficult to predict. One generalisation is, however, true, namely, that if the concentration-action curve shows an all-or-none response, then the time graded action curve will show the same response. In both cases no response is obtained until a certain threshold concentration has been produced in the cells and then a small increment of concentration is sufficient to produce a maximum response.

In general it would appear that the effects of increasing uptake of drug as measured in the time-graded action curves are similar to the effect of increasing concentrations as measured in the concentration-action curves. The essential difference is that in the latter case time for equilibrium is allowed at each concentration, and hence a very large number of casual errors are eliminated. For these reasons it seems unnecessary to discuss time graded-action curves in detail because they can be interpreted as special examples of concentration-action curves.

In favourable cases time-concentration curves measure the time required for the uptake of equal amounts of drug at different concentrations. Since it is often possible to repeat a series of these observations on a single population and the same end point is taken in each case, individual variation does not greatly affect the shape of these curves. The difficulty about time-concentration curves is that they express the time occupied by a whole chain of processes and only in favourable cases is it possible to correlate the time measured with any particular process. In general it may be said that, if the interval between drug uptake and cell response is a small fraction of the time, then the time-concentration curve indicates the relation between concentration and rate of uptake of drug.

If $ct = $ constant then the rate of uptake of drug is proportional to the concentration. If a relation such as $c^{0.3}t = $ constant is obtained, then this suggests that the rate of uptake is dependent on an initial adsorption process.

The time-graded action curves and the time-concentration curves appear therefore to be of subsidiary importance for the purposes of the present discussion and attention can be directed to the remaining three classes of curves, namely, concentration-action, characteristic concentration-action and characteristic time-action curves.

The highly skewed characteristic concentration-action curves present the most obvious problem and it is of interest to note that extreme skew variation distributed symmetrically as regards the logarithm of the function studied is met with occasionally in physical chemistry. For example a distribution of this type has been postulated for the receptors on the surface of charcoal. In this case it has been suggested that the activity of the surface molecules varies over an enormous range. A similar type of skew variation has been postulated by Sheppard for the sensitivity of the grains in photographic plates (TRIVELLI and LOVELAND, 1930[1]).

Physical chemistry does not however provide much assistance in the solution of the problem of the limits of cell variation because both the nature of the

---

[1] TRIVELLI, A. P. H., and P. R. LOVELAND: J. Franklin Instit. **209**, 639 (1930).

surface of charcoal and the nature of the action of light on emulsions of silver bromide are matters of controversy. In the latter case there are two alternative explanations for the relation between exposure and effect, one based on the individual variation of the grains and the other on the chances of the hitting of a sensitive spot in the grains.

The interpretation of the significance of the quantitative data in pharmacology really depends on the interpretation of the relation between concentration-action and characteristic curves.

This problem has been discussed at length and it has been shown that it is possible to relate the concentration-action curves obtained with cell populations with chemical processes occurring between drugs and active processes. If such chemical relations are assumed to occur in drug-cell systems then it is possible to show that these will distort curves expressing individual variation so that this appears to be spread out over a very wide range.

The time-characteristic action curves can be explained by a similar method. The advantages claimed for this explanation are as follows:—

(1) It relates the action of drugs on cells with simple chemical processes.

(2) It does not assume properties for living cells that are unknown in non-living matter.

(3) It does not assume any unusual distribution of variation.

This theory of drug action cannot be regarded as proved. A consideration of the doubts and uncertainties existing regarding the nature of reactions in the much simpler heterogeneous systems studied by physical chemists shows the absurdity of talking of proof in relation to chemical processes in which living cells are involved.

All the curves expressing drug response can be attributed to individual variation, but the objection to this mode of explanation is that it involves unproven and improbable assumptions and does not relate the action of drugs on cells with reactions occurring in simpler systems.

Chapter 16

## Special Problems Relating to Variation of Populations.

Many points regarding the variation of populations have been discussed in previous chapters, but the variation of individuals in response to drugs is a problem of such great theoretical and practical importance that certain points deserve a more detailed consideration.

**Uniformity of Population.** The normal curve of error represents the resultant of a large number of random causes of variation and it is conceivable that the introduction of additional errors into a series of experiments intended to determine a characteristic curve might merely bring the curve closer to the theoretical normal curve of error. In practice however no such fortunate result ensues, and inaccurate experimental technique usually results in an increased spread in the distribution of variation.

One important source of error in such experiments is inadequate uniformity in the biological material. WINTON (1927)[1] determined the lethal action of squills on rats; with ordinary stock animals he found a variation with a standard deviation as high as 67 per cent. of the mean, but when male rats of inbred stock were used the standard deviation fell to 21 per cent. of the mean. This

---

[1] WINTON, F. R.: J. Pharmacol. Baltimore **31**, 123 (1927).

difference implies that ten times more rats of mixed than of inbred stock would be needed in order to obtain equally accurate results. DURHAM, GADDUM and MARCHAL (1929)[1] found a similar difference between mixed and inbred stock of mice in the case of neoarsphenamine standardisation. The use of uniform stock is therefore of great importance for the determination of the true shape of characteristic curves. This fact is so widely recognised that it is difficult to find many examples of large scale experiments carried out on populations in which obvious causes of variation have not been eliminated. This is somewhat unfortunate because the most important use of medicinal drugs is their application to a population subject to gross causes of variation, namely diseased human beings of varying ages, sex and size. The extent of variation in a population of inbred rats uniform in all these respects is likely to give an uncertain indication of the amount of variation that will be encountered when a drug is administered to a diseased population.

A knowledge of the probable extent of variation in response that is likely to occur in human populations is an obvious necessity for estimating the probable safety of drugs which require to be given in doses sufficient to produce a definite response. The essential difficulty of this subject is that naturally there are no extensive data regarding the effects of drugs given in doses beyond the limits of safety and hence all the evidence is indirect. The writer dealt with this subject a few years ago (CLARK, 1935[2]), but since then has collected additional data.

**Influence of Sex, Age and Weight on Response to Drugs.** It is impossible to obtain a population of animals of exactly uniform size and hence it is necessary to provide some correction of the dosage for variations in weight. The usual method is to calculate the dosage per unit of weight but this is known to be unsatisfactory. Two causes of difference in weight are sex and age. Females in many species are smaller than males, but in addition sex differences in susceptibility to drugs occur in some cases. WINTON (1927)[3] found in the case of squills that female rats were twice as susceptible as males. KISSKALT (1915)[4] found however that the lethal dose of caffeine was the same in male and female rats. HANZLIK (1913)[5] measured the amount of sodium salicylate taken by patients with rheumatic fever before the first toxic symptoms appeared, and his figures show that the mean toxic doses of sodium salicylate for men and women were 10.7 g. and 8.7 g. respectively; a difference which is roughly proportional to the average difference in body weight. These examples show that the influence of sex on susceptibility to drugs differs in the case of different drugs.

The influence of age on susceptibility to drugs is well known to be complex. For example children are susceptible to morphine but tolerant to atropine. FALCK (1884, 1885)[6] studied the influence of age on the minimal lethal dose per kilo of strychnine. He found that the new-born rabbit had the same sensitivity as an adult, but that young animals (7 to 20 days) were nearly twice as susceptible as adults. A similar variation was seen in mice, whilst guinea pigs showed a maximum sensitivity at birth and adults were twice as resistant. His figures for the period during which the sensitivity decreases with increasing age and weight suggest the relation that the dose needed varies as $\sqrt{\text{body weight}}$.

---

[1] DURHAM, F. M., J. H. GADDUM and J. E. MARCHAL: Med. Res. Council Spec. Rep. **128** (1929).

[2] CLARK, A. J.: Edinburgh med. J. (N. S. IV) **42**, 1 (1935).

[3] WINTON, F. R.: J. Pharmacol. Baltimore **31**, 123 (1927).

[4] KISSKALT: Biochem. Z. **71**, 468 (1915).

[5] HANZLIK, P. J.: J. amer. med. Assoc. **60**, 957 (1913).

[6] FALCK, A.: Pflügers Arch. **34**, 525, 530 (1884); **36**, 285 (1885).

Various attempts have been made to establish some definite relation between dosage and body weight in adult animals. MOORE (1909)[1] suggested that the dosage did not vary as the body weight but as the body surface, i.e. the two thirds power of the body weight. This is a plausible suggestion because drugs act on the viscera rather than on the skeletal muscles, skeleton and fat, and the weight of the viscera and also the blood volume is more nearly proportional to the body surface than to the body weight, facts pointed out by BISCHOFF (1863)[2] and by DREYER and WALKER (1914)[3]. Another relevant fact is that the metabolic rate varies approximately as the body surface. Most authors who have studied the influence of body weight on dosage agree that dosage is not proportional to the body weight, but it is difficult to draw any general conclusions from the results.

BAZETT and ERB (1933)[4] measured the narcotic dose of nembutal given by intraperitoneal injection to cats and dogs of varying size and found the following median doses:—

Small cats of 2 kilo:— . . . . . . . . 37—62 mg. p. kilo
Thin cats and thin dogs of 4 kilo:— . . 45 mg. p. kilo
Thin dogs of 26 kilo:— . . . . . . . . 22 mg. p. kilo

These results follow the formula dosage varies as (body weight)$^{\frac{2}{3}}$. This formula can be transposed to the form:—

$$(\text{dosage per unit weight}) \times \sqrt[3]{\text{body weight}} = \text{constant}$$

and this gives the following relations:—

| | | | | |
|---|---|---|---|---|
| (a) Body weight . . . . . | 1 | 10 | 100 | 1000 |
| (b) $\sqrt[3]{\text{Body weight}}$ . . . . | 1 | 2.15 | 4.6 | 10 |
| (c) Dosage per unit of body weight . . . . . | 1 | 0.47 | 0.22 | 0.1 |

Wide specific differences exist as regards susceptibility to drugs and hence the comparison of the dosage of drugs needed to produce equal effects on animals of different species provides information of doubtful significance. It is however of interest to note that the narcotic doses of hypnotics for animals of widely different size do not vary as widely as is suggested by this formula.

For example the subcutaneous narcotic doses of chloral hydrate in g. per kilo is 0.1 in the mouse and 0.4 in the rabbit (MUNCH and SCHWARTZE, 1925[5]); whilst the oral narcotic dose is 0.25 to 0.3 in the cat and dog and between 0.3 and 0.5 in the horse (WOOLDRIDGE, 1934[6]). Similarly in the case of nembutal the intraperitoneal dose in the rat is 0.05, whilst the intravenous dose in man, cattle and horses is about 0.01. These results do not show as extensive a difference in dosage per unit weight between small animals and large animals as is indicated by the formula dosage varies as (body weight)$^{\frac{2}{3}}$.

The necessity for accurate standardisation of digitalis has caused careful attention to be paid to all factors likely to increase the variation in response. BEHRENS (1929)[7] found that the individual variation in frogs was the same whether the drug was given intravenously or into the lymphatic sacs, a fact which shows that the rate of absorption is not an important factor in producing

[1] MOORE, B.: Biochemic. J. **4**, 323 (1909).
[2] BISCHOFF: Z. rationelle Med. **1863**.
[3] DREYER, G., and E. W. A. WALKER: Proc. roy. Soc. B. **87**, 320 (1914).
[4] BAZETT, H. C., and W. H. ERB: J. Pharmacol. Baltimore **49**, 352 (1933).
[5] MUNCH, J. C., and E. W. SCHWARTZE: J. Labor. a. clin. Med. **10**, 985 (1925).
[6] WOOLDRIDGE, G. H.: Encyclop. Veterin. Med. **1**, 816. Oxford: Univ. Press 1934.
[7] BEHRENS, B.: Arch. f. exper. Path. **140**, 237 (1929).

variation. BEHRENS and REICHELT (1933)[1] found that when the same dose of gratus strophanthin per unit weight was given to frogs the mortality with small frogs (20 g.) was least (4 p.c.) and the mortality rose steadily with increasing weight until a mortality of 88 p.c. was obtained with 50 g. frogs. These authors found that the heart ratio was nearly the same for all sizes of frogs (0.42 p.c. of body weight). They also (1934)[2] gave 1100 frogs of varying weight the same dose of g. strophanthin making no allowance for variation in weight, and in this case the mortality varied from 100 p.c. with the smallest frogs (14 g.) to 0 p.c. with the largest frogs (52 g.). The authors concluded that it was not possible to calculate the relation between dosage and body weight and that for accurate standardisation it was necessary to use frogs of uniform weight.

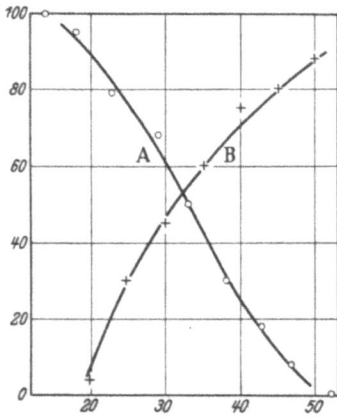

Fig. 67. Influence of body weight on lethal action of g-strophanthin on frogs. Abscissa:— body weight in g. Ordinate:— per cent. mortality. (A) Mortality in 1100 frogs divided into groups according to weight and all given the same dose (13.5 γ) of g-strophanthin. (B) Mortality in 864 frogs divided as in (A) but dosed according to body weight (0.95 γ per g.). (BEHRENS and REICHELT, 1933 and 1934[2].)

Their results are shown in fig. 67 and if it be assumed that the characteristic curve is such that mortalities of 16 and 84 p.c. correspond to dosages 20 p.c. below and above the median, then these results suggest that the dosage varies approximately as (body weight)$^{\frac{2}{3}}$. This relation is however very uncertain, but the figures show with certainty that the dosage calculated per unit weight gives results which are nearly as inaccurate as when a uniform dosage per frog is given. This point is important because the massive method of digitalis dosage introduced by EGGLESTON (1915, 1917)[3] assumes that in man variations in weight can be corrected for by calculating the dosage per unit of body weight. This method has been criticised by REID (1923)[4] and LUTEN (1925)[5] on account of its danger. The results quoted above suggest that there is little justification in assuming that in any animal there is a simple linear relation between body weight and dosage of digitalis.

The convulsive dose of strychnine given subcutaneously has been measured on a number of animals and the following results indicate that the dosage per kilo falls as the body weight increases.

Mouse . . . . 0.6 mg. p. kilo (FALCK, 1884[6])
Rabbit. . . . 0.3 mg. p. kilo
Dog . . . . . 0.1 mg. p. kilo (HATCHER and EGGLESTON, 1917[7])

KISSKALT (1915)[8] found on the other hand that the mean lethal dose of caffeine (intraperitoneal) for rats was nearly the same for small animals (< 40 g.) as for large animals (> 120 g.).

Finally in some cases the dosage needed to produce an equal action is actually greater in large than in small animals. BLISS (1936)[9] analysed the results obtained

[1] BEHRENS, B., and E. REICHELT: Z. exper. Med. 91, 417 (1933).
[2] BEHRENS, B., and E. REICHELT: Z. exper. Med. 94, 130 (1934).
[3] EGGLESTON, C.: Arch. int. Med. 16, 1 (1915) — J. amer. med. Assoc. 69, 951 (1917).
[4] REID, E.: J. amer. med. Assoc. 81, 435 (1923).
[5] LUTEN, D.: Arch. int. Med. 35, 74, 87 (1925).
[6] FALCK, A.: Pflügers Arch. 34, 525, 530 (1884).
[7] HATCHER, R. A., and C. EGGLESTON: J. Pharmacol. Baltimore 10, 281 (1917).
[8] KISSKALT: Biochem. Z. 71, 468 (1915).
[9] BLISS, C. I: J. of exper. Biol. 13, 95 (1936).

by CAMPBELL (1926)[1] for the toxic action of arsenic upon silkworm larvae and concluded that dosage varied as (body weight)$^{1.5}$. Similarly large mice are less susceptible than small mice to both neoarsphenamine (DURHAM, GADDUM and MARCHAL, 1929[2]) and to aconite (BROOM et al., 1932[3]). In the latter case the median lethal doses were for small mice 0.14 c.c. of tincture of aconite per 100 g. and for large mice 0.21 c.c. per 100 g.

These examples suffice to show that at present it is impossible to enunciate general laws regarding the relation between dosage and body weight, since completely different relations appear to be obtained with different drugs.

**Seasonal Variations in Sensitivity.** Many workers who have extensive experience of biological standardisation have noted seasonal variations in sensitivity to drugs. ROSENKRANZ (1933)[4] and LENDLE (1935)[5] found that winter frogs were from one and a half to two times as sensitive as summer frogs to digitalis CHAPMAN and MORRELL (1932)[6] on the other hand found only a difference of 18 p.c. between summer and winter. MUNCH (1931[7], Table 145) quotes results by VANDERKLEED and PITTINGER (1913)[8] who found that the minimal lethal dose of ouabain was ten times as great for winter as for summer frogs. These results appear very discrepant and agree only in showing that wide seasonal variations may occur in the susceptibility of frogs to digitalis and strophanthin.

MUNCH (1931)[7] quotes other results such as the lethal action of ouabain and of aconitine on guinea pigs which show no seasonal variation throughout the year.

Finally it is interesting to note that in many cases different median lethal doses have been found with a single drug in different groups of the same animal for which no cause can be assigned. BROOM et al. (1932)[3] noted differences in susceptibility of different colonies of mice to tincture of aconite due to unknown causes. HEMMINGSEN (1933)[9] noted shifts of sensitivity of a single colony of mice to insulin which occurred from day to day even though the animals were kept under apparently identical experimental conditions. In this case the median convulsive doses varied from 0.006 to 0.014 international units of a standard preparation of insulin within a fortnight.

These various and largely unknown causes of variation in populations are a considerable embarrassment in the biological standardisation of drugs. Fortunately they can be eliminated by comparing the activity of the unknown and a standard preparation of drug simultaneously upon two groups of animals as nearly similar as possible as regards weight, age, sex, etc.

**Variation in Human Populations.** The wide variations in response to drugs that have been revealed by accurate quantitative work upon large populations of animals, which are as nearly uniform as is possible, naturally raises the question as to the variations in response that may be expected in the case of ordinary patients, i.e. human beings of varying age and sex suffering from disease of varying intensity.

[1] CAMPBELL, F. L.: J. gen. Physiol. **9**, 433, 727 (1926).
[2] DURHAM, F. M., J. H. GADDUM and J. E. MARCHAL: Med. Res. Council Spec. Rep. **128** (1929).
[3] BROOM, W. A., J. H. GADDUM, J. W. TREVAN and S. W. F. UNDERHILL: Quart. J. Pharmacy **5**, 33 (1932).
[4] ROSENKRANZ, S.: Arch. f. exper. Path. **172**, 18 (1933).
[5] LENDLE, L.: Heffters Handb. exper. Pharmakol. Ergänzbd. **1**, 1 (1935).
[6] CHAPMAN, C. W., and C. A. MORRELL: J. Pharmacol. Baltimore **46**, 229 (1932).
[7] MUNCH, J. C.: Bioassays. London: Baillière, Tyndall and Cox 1931.
[8] VANDERKLEED, C. E., and P. S. PITTINGER: J. amer. pharmaceut. Assoc. **2**, 558 (1913).
[9] HEMMINGSEN, A. M.: Quart. J. Pharmacy **6**, 39, 187 (1933).

It has been shown that the various types of characteristic curves can be converted to approximately linear relations by plotting the incidence expressed as a multiple of the standard deviation against the logarithm of the dosage.

This method greatly simplifies the comparison of characteristic curves of varying shape and will be employed in this section. The spread of variation will be expressed as the normal equivalent deviation (N.E.D.).

Data regarding the variation of patients suffering from rheumatic fever have been collected by MURRAY LYON (1936)[1] and some of these are shown in fig. 68. Curve $A$ shows the variation in duration of disease in untreated cases, whilst $B$ and $C$ show the corresponding durations in cases treated with sodium salicyl-

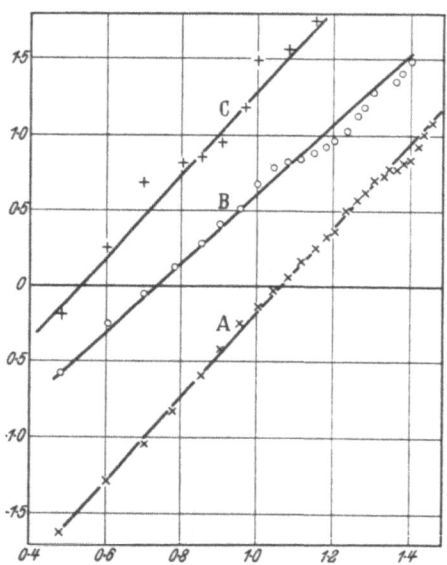

Fig. 68. Variation of duration of rheumatic fever and influence of sodium salicylate treatment. Abscissa:— log. of duration of fever in days. Ordinate:— incidence expressed as multiples of standard deviation. ($A$) No salicylate given. 338 cases (1881). ($B$) Medium dosage of salicylate. 355 cases (1881). ($C$) Full salicylate treatment. (MURRAY LYON, 1936[1].)

ate. The treatment was more intense in the cases shown in curve $C$ than in those shown in curve $B$. The fact that curve $A$ is approximately linear is a surprising fact. The duration of disease in an untreated patient must depend on two factors, namely intensity of infection and resistance of the patient. The result is a skew distribution of variation in respect of the duration of the disease, which shows a striking resemblance to the distribution of response of animals to varying doses of certain drugs (cf. fig. 56).

The chief theoretical importance of this result is to prove that this form of linear relation may be the result of all kinds of different causes. Curves $B$ and $C$ show that, when rheumatic fever is treated with sodium salicylate, the distribution of variation is not altered since the slope of the three curves is similar, but the general effect is to cause a shortening of the duration of the disease. As a general average the duration of disease in slope $B$ was one half of that of the untreated cases, and in slope $C$ one third of that of the untreated cases. The actual values for $\lambda$ in the three curves are $A$ 0.34, $B$ 0.42 and $C$ 0.34. HANZLIK (1913)[2] measured the amount of salicylate taken by patients before they showed toxic symptoms such as vomiting, etc. His results, which are recorded in fig. 69, show a normal equivalent deviation of 0.17, which is half that shown in fig. 68 for the duration of the disease. The appearance of toxic effects may be assumed to be a more direct consequence of the drug than the time until reduction of fever, and in the former case the response is much more uniform than the latter.

PAXSON (1932)[3] gave 55 cases intravenous amytal and measured the dose needed in each case to produce anaesthesia. In this case the median dose was 11 mg. per kilo and $\lambda = 0.12$. These cases were women in child birth and therefore were uniform as regards sex, were all adults in the first half of life and were presumably healthy individuals. It is interesting to note that with a selected

[1] MURRAY LYON, R. C.: Edinburgh med. J. **43**, 84 (1936).
[2] HANZLIK, P. J.: J. amer. med. Assoc. **60**, 957 (1913).
[3] PAXSON, N. F.: Anesth. Analges. **11**, 116 (1932).

group of patients of this kind the scatter of the individual variation in response to a narcotic was not greatly different from that shown in animal experiments.

The skin is notoriously a variable organ, and PERCIVAL (1934)[1] who studied the response of a group of skin sensitive patients to skin irritants obtained results which showed a surprising range of variation. Fig. 70 shows the results when plotted log. conc. × results as multiples of standard deviation. The results indicate the value $\lambda = 0.45$.

The writer has observed for some years the effects produced by the subcutaneous injection of atropine (0.5—1.0 mg.) into healthy students. The average effect is a slowing of the pulse for ten minutes, which is followed by an increase of frequency up to about 90 per min. The individual variation in response ranges from a slowing without subsequent quickening to a violent acceleration up to 120 per min.

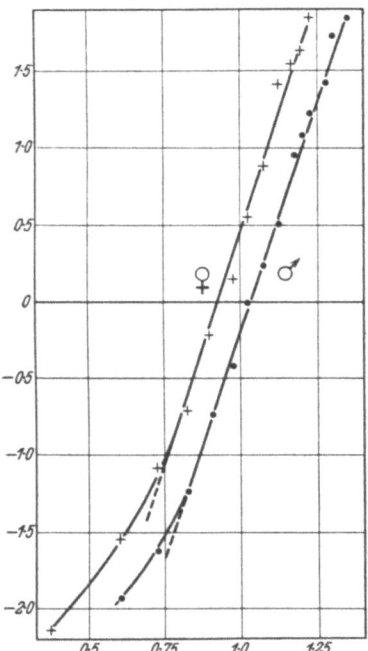

Fig. 69. Variation of cases of rheumatic fever as regards quantity of sodium salicylate taken before toxic symptoms produced. Abscissa:— log. dose of sodium salicylate (g.). Ordinate:— incidence measured as multiples of standard deviation. (A) 301 male patients. (B) 181 female patients. (HANZLIK, 1913[2].)

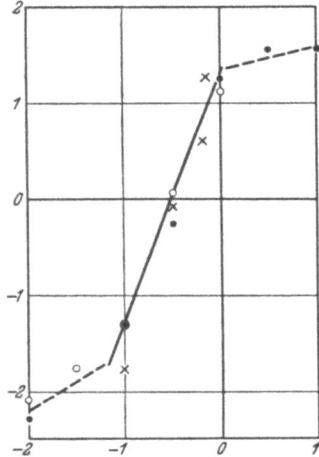

Fig. 70. Variation of response of patients to skin irritants. Abscissa:— log. conc. per cent. Ordinate:— incidence of response expressed as multiples of standard deviation. Dots = chrysarobin. Circles = mercuric chloride. Crosses = mercuric iodide. (PERCIVAL, 1934[1].)

FREEMAN and CARMICHAEL (1936)[3] have reported experiments made under more accurate conditions. They gave 1.0 mg. atropine intravenously to healthy fasting subjects at rest in bed. The average effect was to change the pulse rate from 61 to 85 per min. but the standard deviation of each figure was 9, which implies a variation in response similar to that described above.

They also made similar measurements of the action of adrenaline (0.05 mg.), ergotamine (0.375 mg.) and physostigmine (1.0 mg.). All the drugs were given intravenously. In all cases a very wide individual variation was observed in the responses measured (blood pressure and pulse rate).

**Hypersensitivity and Idiosyncrasy.** Modern methods of treatment have tended to favour the administration of drugs in doses sufficient to produce a full physio-

[1] PERCIVAL, G. H.: Edinburgh Med. J. **41**, Chir. 177 (1934).
[2] HANZLIK, P. J.: J. amer. med. Assoc. **60**, 957 (1913).
[3] FREEMAN, H., and H. T. CARMICHAEL: J. Pharmacol. Baltimore **58**, 409 (1936).

logical effect, and hence it is of importance to consider the chances of meeting individuals at the lower extremes of the curve of variation. The data obtained with large populations ($>$1000) of animals suggests that the distribution of individual variation does follow GAUSS' formula provided that the incidence is plotted against the logarithm of the dose, and hence it seems permissible to calculate the probability of occasional positive responses by extrapolation of the known curves of variation. When the logarithm of the dose is plotted against the multiple of the standard deviation (figs. 55, 56, 68, 69, 70), the normal equivalent deviation ($\lambda$) can be measured directly from the linear relation obtained. The chances of rare events can be easily estimated if this figure is known.

Table 18. Calculation of chance of occurrence of rare events from the normal equivalent deviation ($\lambda$).

| Chance | Multiple of standard deviation ($\sigma$) | Fraction of median dose which produces effect |
|---|---|---|
| 1 in 100 | 2.326 | Log. median dose $-2.326\,\lambda$ |
| 1 in 1000 | 3.09 | ditto $-3.09\,\lambda$ |
| 1 in 10,000 | 3.72 | ditto $-3.72\,\lambda$ |

Table 18 shows the manner in which the chance of a rare event occurring can be calculated if the value of $\lambda$ is known for the action of the drug on the population, whilst Table 19 shows the chances of rare events occurring with different values of $\lambda$.

Table 19. The fractions of the median lethal dose ($=1$) which produce occasional deaths with various values of the normal equivalent deviation ($\lambda$).

| Normal equivalent deviation ($\lambda$) | One death per 100 (2,32 $\sigma$) | One death per 1000 (3,09 $\sigma$) | One death per 10,000 (3,72 $\sigma$) |
|---|---|---|---|
| 0.05 | 0.77 | 0.70 | 0.65 |
| 0.1 | 0.59 | 0.49 | 0.42 |
| 0.2 | 0.34 | 0.24 | 0.19 |
| 0.3 | 0.20 | 0.12 | 0.076 |
| 0.4 | 0.12 | 0.058 | 0.033 |

Table 19 shows that in cases when the response is very uniform ($\lambda = 0.05$) a dose as large as $^2/_3$ of the median lethal dose will only kill one animal in 10,000. Uniformity of this character is only likely to be found with populations of experimental animals such as inbred Wistar rats of uniform age and sex. Values of $\lambda$ between 0.1 and 0.2 are common under experimental conditions and it is wise to assume that diseased human beings will vary twice as much as experimental animals and hence we may assume that in human beings the value for $\lambda$ is likely to fall between 0.2 and 0.4. In the latter case a dose equal to $^1/_{30}$ of the median lethal dose may be expected to kill one individual in 10,000.

The influence of the extent of the scatter in response on the safety of a drug can be calculated from the experimental results shown in figs. 55 and 56.

Fig. 55 shows the response of frogs to ouabain and the scatter is very small. The dosage is expressed in natural numbers, but when plotted on a logarithmic scale $\lambda = 0.07$. The mean lethal dose is 31.5 $\mu$.g. ouabain per 100 g. Each point in the figure represents about 200 animals and no deaths were found with a dose of 23 $\mu$.g. This dose corresponds to 2.505 times the standard deviation and this implies a mortality of 6 per 1000. Even though the population used (200) was exceptionally large, it was not large enough to establish with certainty the absence or presence of a mortality as small as 1 in 166. Application of the figures given above shows that one animal in 10,000 would be killed by 19 $\mu$.g. These results show that in a population of frogs 19 $\mu$.g. ouabain p. 100 g. would represent a safe therapeutic dose and this is 60 per cent. of the mean lethal dose.

On the other hand a drug such as dysentery toxin (fig. 56, curve $E$) gives a completely different result since in this case 1 individual per 100 would be killed by 38 per cent. of the median lethal dose, 1 in 1000 by 18 per cent. and 1 in 10,000 by 10 per cent.

These examples shows the manner in which the requisite margin of safety for drugs varies in the case of different drugs. They also indicate the huge populations that are required if it is desired to demonstrate by direct experiment the chance of occurrence of rare events.

Statistical studies of the effect of drugs on thousands of persons are rarely made and hence the usual type of evidence available is that a certain dosage of drug has been given in safety a large number of times and that a few cases have shown undesirable effects. These occasional results are sometimes termed cases of idiosyncrasy. It seems to the writer that this is an undesirable use of this term, which should be reserved for cases which show a wholly abnormal response to a drug.

Acetyl salicylic acid (aspirin) provides a convenient example of the difference between hypersensitiveness and idiosyncrasy. Sufficiently large doses of this drug will cause gastric disturbance in most persons and in a few cases this effect is produced by a small therapeutic dose (0.5 g.). Such cases may be termed sensitives and if a person suffered gastric disturbance from a dose of 0.1 g. it would be reasonable to term him hypersensitive in that a common response was produced by an abnormally small quantity of drug. A few persons (about 1 in 10,000) show quite a different response, for in these a small dose of aspirin may produce urticaria, an effect which the drug does not produce on a normal person. This type of response may be termed idiosyncrasy, the term being reserved to denote cases which show a response which is of an abnormal character in addition to being provoked by a very small dose.

**Margin of Safety with Massive Doses.** The data from experimental animals supplemented by the scanty data regarding human beings permit a few rough calculations regarding the probable dangers attending massive dosage.

The study of characteristic curves informs us of the amount of variation in response to a drug that will occur when all variables have been reduced to a minimum. If this variation is small, then the response of human patients may be fairly uniform, but if the variation under optimum conditions is still large, then extensive variation in human response must be expected and it is highly unlikely that any form of massive dosage will be safe.

In actual fact the drugs which are used in therapeutics in massive doses show small ranges of variation under experimental conditions. This is shown by the examples of neoarsphenamine, digitalis and basal narcotics.

In the case of neoarsphenamine the characteristic curves for the lethal action of neoarsphenamine on rats shows values of $\lambda$ of 0.04 (MORRELL and CHAPMAN, 1933[1]) and of 0.084 (DURHAM, GADDUM and MARCHAL, 1929[2]). Both these results show a narrow range of variation and even the latter less favourable figure implies that half the mean lethal dose would only kill one individual in 10,000.

The dangers associated with administration of organic arsenicals would appear therefore to be due chiefly to the fact that the population to which they

[1] MORRELL, C. A., and C. W. CHAPMAN: J. Pharmacol. Baltimore **48**, 375, 391 (1933).
[2] DURHAM, F. M., J. H. GADDUM and J. E. MARCHAL: Med. Res. Council Spec. Rep. **128** (1929).

are administered varies widely as to the extent to which the internal organs are injured by disease.

Similarly in the case of the cardiac glucosides, a number of workers have produced characteristic curves for digitalis, strophanthin and ouabain, and their results show values of $\lambda$ varying from 0.04 to 0.13 (GADDUM, 1933[1]). A value of 0.1 may be taken as an average and this indicates an amount of scatter similar to that of neoarsphenamine. In this case it is known that, even with healthy animals, when the drug is given in repeated doses, so that cumulative effects are produced, the variation in response is much greater than that observed after a single dose.

The aliphatic narcotics also are characterised by a narrow range of variation in their action. The following values for $\lambda$ are shown by the characteristic curves obtained by various workers. Ethyl urethane on division of sea urchin eggs $\lambda = 0.115$ (SCOTT quoted by CLARK, 1933[2], Fig. 29); ethyl alcohol on snails $\lambda = 0.052$ (SHACKELL, 1924[3]). PAXSON (1932)[4] measured the amount of sodium amytal needed to anaesthetise 55 women and his figures show a value of $\lambda = 0.12$. TUNGER (1931)[5], avertin on rats; lethal action; $\lambda = 0.04$; light narcosis; $\lambda = 0.06$. KNOEFEL and MURRELL (1935)[6], ether on mice; $\lambda = 0.11$. These results suggest an upper limit of $\lambda = 0.12$ for the scatter of the action of anaesthetics on healthy individuals. This implies that a dose equal to 0.35 times the median lethal dose would kill one individual in 10,000. The figures suggest that the scatter in the case of lethal and of the narcotic actions is similar and hence the results indicate that in order to use a basal narcotic with safety even on healthy individuals the median narcotic dose should not be more than $1/_3$ of the median lethal dose. The following figures show the values for this ratio obtained with rats in the case of avertin.

| Mode of Administration | Median narcotic dose / Median lethal dose | Ratio | Author |
|---|---|---|---|
| Intraperitoneal Injection. . . | 0.11/0.42 | 1/3.8 | LENDLE and TUNGER, 1930[7] |
|  | 0.13/0.55 | 1/4.2 | TUNGER, 1931[5] |
| Subcutaneous Injection . . . | 0.18/0.73 | 1/4 | TUNGER, 1931[5] |
|  | 0.21/0.52 | 1/2.5 | TOBERENTZ, 1933[8] |
| Rectal Injection . . . . . | 0.20/0.63 | 1/3.1 | TUNGER, 1931[5] |

These results suggest that the ratio between narcotic and lethal dose in the case of avertin is adequate to provide complete safety in the case of healthy animals but there seems very little margin to allow for variation in patients due to disease.

The response of healthy animals to insulin has been studied extensively in relation to its biological standardisation. Various values obtained for $\lambda$ in the case of the production of insulin convulsions in mice are 0.143 (HEMMINGSEN and KROGH, 1926[9]), 0.182 (TREVAN, 1927[10]), 0.22 (HEMMINGSEN, 1933[11]). If we

---

[1] GADDUM, J. H.: Med. Res. Council Spec. Report **183** (1933).
[2] CLARK, A. J.: The Mode of Action of Drugs on Cells. London: Arnold and Co. 1933.
[3] SHACKELL, L. F.: J. Pharmacol. Baltimore **25**, 275 (1924).
[4] PAXSON, N. F.: Anesth. Analges. **11**, 116 (1932).
[5] TUNGER, H.: Arch. f. exper. Path. **160**, 74 (1931).
[6] KNOEFEL, P. K., and F. C. MURRELL: J. Pharmacol. Baltimore **55**, 235 (1935).
[7] LENDLE, L., and H. TUNGER: Klin. Wschr. **9**, 1293 (1930).
[8] TOBERENTZ, H.: Arch. f. exper. Path. **171**, 346 (1933).
[9] HEMMINGSEN, A. M., and A. KROGH: League of Nations. Rep. Biol. Standards Insulin: C. H. **398**, 40 (1926).
[10] TREVAN, J. W.: Proc. roy. Soc. B. **101**, 483 (1927).
[11] HEMMINGSEN, A. M.: Quart. J. Pharmacy **6**, 39, 187 (1933).

take 0.2 as an average value for $\lambda$ this implies that in healthy animals $^1/_4$ of the median effective dose will produce convulsions in 1 animal in 1000. This result shows a very much wider individual variation than was found in the favourable cases previously discussed and indicates that occasional unexpected results are likely to be obtained if large doses of insulin are given to human patients.

The individual variation of the cardiac inhibition produced by acetylcholine shows an extraordinarily wide scatter ($\lambda = 0.91$; CLARK, 1927[1]), but on the other hand the lethal action of acetylcholine on mice is relatively uniform ($\lambda = 0.15$; WHITE and STEDMAN, 1931[2]). In the case of adrenaline its action on the isolated uterus shows a wide scatter ($\lambda = 0.43$; LANGECKER, 1926[3]) and the lethal action of adrenaline on mice shows a similar scatter ($\lambda = 0.37$; SCHULTZ, 1909[4]). In the case of a drug in which $\lambda = 0.4$, one eighth of the median lethal dose would kill one person in 100 and one thirtieth would kill one person in 10,000, and hence it is obvious that drugs, which show this amount of scatter in response in experimental animals, could never be used with safety in full doses on human patients.

A study of characteristic curves shows therefore that some drugs are inherently unsafe, and that others may be safe, when given in massive dosage to human patients. In the latter case, however, it is always necessary to remember the wide difference between the homogeneity of populations of experimental animals and the variability of human patients.

**Disinfection, etc.** The distribution of individual variation in response to drugs is important in relation to the destruction of organisms by drugs for in this case it is important to know the chances of occasional survivors. In such cases large numbers are involved and hence the possibility of the survival of one parasite in 10,000 is a serious matter. The evidence put forward in previous chapters shows that micro-organisms vary as extensively as do higher animals and that the variation of micro-organisms usually shows a skew distribution.

As regards bacteria it is difficult to obtain satisfactory evidence of individual variation because bacteria usually are in the form of a multiplying population. It is therefore more satisfactory to consider evidence obtained with spores. The evidence available shows that the spread of individual variation differs very greatly in the case of different drugs. The action of phenol on micro-organisms is of an all-or-none character, for there is a relatively narrow range between the minimum effective concentration and concentrations which produce rapid destruction. For example HENDERSON SMITH's (1921)[5] figures for the killing of Botrytris spores by phenol show that 0.5 p.c. phenol killed 16 p.c. whilst 0.6 p.c. killed 96 p.c. in 30 min. at $25°$ C. These results indicate a value for $\lambda$ of less than 0.03, which is an unusually uniform effect. Fig. 71 shows the effect of mercuric chloride on anthrax spores (KRÖNIG and PAUL, 1897[6]). McCALLAN and WILCOXON (1931)[7] measured the incidence of death in various species of macrosporidia when exposed for a uniform time to varying concentrations of sulphuretted hydrogen. Their results show a distribution similar to that represented in fig. 71. In both these cases the value of $\lambda$ is about 0.5.

[1] CLARK, A. J.: J. of Physiol. **64**, 123 (1927).
[2] WHITE, A. C., and E. STEDMAN: J. Pharmacol. Baltimore **41**, 259 (1931).
[3] LANGECKER, H.: Arch. f. exper. Path. **118**, 49 (1926).
[4] SCHULTZ, W. H.: U. S. Hyg. Labor. Bull. **55** (1909).
[5] HENDERSON SMITH, J.: Ann. appl. Biol. 8, 27 (1921).
[6] KRÖNIG, B., and T. PAUL: Z. Hyg. **25**, 1 (1897).
[7] McCALLAN, S. E. A., and F. WILCOXON: Contrib. Boyce Thompson Instit. **3**, 13, 31 (1931).

DREYER and CAMPBELL-RENTON (1936)[1] measured the incidence of destruction in bacteria exposed for 22 hours to various concentrations of disinfectants. Their results show the following values for $\lambda$. Formalin on B. coli, $\lambda = 0.53$; formalin on Staph. aureus, $\lambda = 0.7$; lysol and phenol on B. coli and Staph. aureus, $\lambda = 0.1$ to $0.14$.

These results show clearly that the amount of spread of individual variation depends chiefly on the drug used. The variation is small with phenol both in the case of spores and of B. coli and it is large with mercuric chloride, sulphuretted hydrogen and formalin. In these latter cases where $\lambda = 0.5$, it is of interest to note that according to the laws of probability one organism in 10,000 would survive 70 times the concentration needed to kill 50 per cent. This wide variation also indicates how unlikely it is for complete destruction of organisms *in vivo* to be achieved by a single dose of a disinfectant or chemotherapeutic agent.

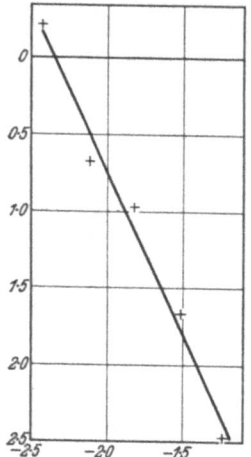

Fig. 71. Action of phenol on anthrax spores. Abscissa:— log. conc. phenol. Ordinate:— incidence of mortality expressed as multiples of standard deviation. (10 min. exposure at 25° C.) (KRÖNIG and PAUL, 1897[2].)

## Chapter 17

## Quantitative Aspects of Drug Antagonism and of Drug Synergism.

(1) **Introduction.** It was shown in the last chapter that, in populations of animals, changes in sensitivity to drugs can be produced by a wide variety of causes, and that in some cases variations in sensitivity occur for which the causes are unknown. It seems justifiable to assume that if the condition of organisms is altered by the administration of one drug, then this change will probably alter the sensitivity of the organism to other drugs. According to this view almost any pair of drugs are likely to show either antagonism or synergism to a greater or less extent.

The study of a field of this extent would be of little value and therefore it is necessary to confine attention to certain particular forms of antagonism and synergism.

The three chief forms of drug antagonism are as follows:—

(a) *Chemical antagonism in vitro.* In this case the antagonists react together to form a product of reduced activity.

(b) *Physiological antagonism.* In this case two drugs produce opposite but independent effects on cells or organs.

(c) *Specific antagonism.* This term is reserved for cases in which one drug inhibits the action of another drug on living cells, although no reaction between the drugs occurs in vitro.

This classification is not exact, but a large proportion of cases of antagonism fall definitely into one of these classes.

Drug synergisms can be divided into similar classes.

The general subject of drug antagonism has been discussed fully by LOEWE (1927, 1928)[3] and by ZUNZ (1930)[4] and attention therefore will be confined

[1] DREYER, G., and M. L. CAMPBELL-RENTON: Proc. roy. Soc. B. **120**, 447 (1936).
[2] KRÖNIG, B., and T. PAUL: Z. Hyg. **25**, 1 (1897).
[3] LOEWE, S.: Klin. Wschr. **6**, 1077 (1927) — Erg. Physiol. **27**, 47 (1928).
[4] ZUNZ, E.: Eléments de Pharmacodynamie Générale. Paris: Masson et Cie. 1930.

chiefly to certain cases in which the occurrence of specific antagonism or synergism appears to throw some light on the nature of the reaction between the drug and the cells.

The general aim of the author in this article has been to consider the simplest systems. The study of the simultaneous action of two drugs is far more difficult than the study of a single drug, and hence the only forms of antagonism worth considering are those in which the effects are both obvious and easily measurable.

Although drug antagonism is a difficult and complex subject, yet its importance is very great. Modern theories of enzyme structure are to a large extent based on the manner in which the action of enzyme poisons can be inhibited by other changes. Similarly the theory of humoral transmission of nerve impulses is partly based on the acetyl choline-atropine antagonism.

The classes of chemical and physiological antagonisms or synergisms are of minor interest for the purposes of this article. There are an indefinitely large number of toxic substances which react in vitro to form inert compounds. The complexity of the reactions varies from the neutralisation of acids by alkalies to the neutralisation of toxins by antitoxins. Although reactions such as the last mentioned are of great practical importance, yet they do not provide much indication of the manner in which drugs act on cells and therefore will not be considered.

The same argument applies to physiological antagonisms. For example atropine dilates the pupil, whereas morphine causes constriction, but since the one effect is peripheral and the other central, this antagonism is not of importance to general pharmacology. The antagonisms of strychnine by narcotics and of cocaine by barbiturates are of therapeutic importance, but from the point of view of this article, they are of subsidiary interest because too little is known regarding the manner in which these actions are produced. The antagonism between monovalent and divalent cations is of greater interest because analogies can be found between the balanced actions of these ions upon living cells and upon colloidal systems. It is, however, important to note that even the well known antagonism that can be demonstrated on many tissues between calcium and potassium salts is only effective over a relatively narrow range of concentrations (CLARK, 1926[1]). It is probable that this effect depends on the ions altering the condition of the cell surface, and CLOWES (1916)[2] put forward the attractive hypothesis that the action of these ions on the cell surface resembled their action in changing the condition of a water/oil emulsion. This subject is, however, of more interest to general physiology than to general pharmacology.

The antagonisms which appear to the writer to be of chief interest are, firstly, the antagonism between narcotics and other drugs, and secondly, the specific antagonisms, such as the antagonism of acetyl choline by atropine and of adrenaline by ergotoxin, and the special interest of these systems is that analogies can be found between the phenomena observed in living cells and those observed with simpler systems such as the poisoning of purified enzymes.

**(2) The Antagonism of Cyanides by Narcotics.** WARBURG (1911 and 1921)[3] showed that oxidations produced by blood charcoal could be inhibited both by cyanides and by aliphatic narcotics, but that the combination of a narcotic with cyanide reduced the action of the latter. He concluded that the oxidation in this case was due to an active group containing iron and that the iron was inactivated by combination with cyanides. The group also could be inactivated

---

[1] CLARK, A. J.: J. Pharmacol. Baltimore **29**, 311 (1926).
[2] CLOWES, G. H. A.: J. physic. Chem. **20**, 407 (1916).
[3] WARBURG, O.: Hoppe-Seylers Z. **76**, 331 (1911) — Biochem. Z. **119**, 134 (1921).

by being covered with an aliphatic narcotic, but this also prevented access of cyanide and at certain concentrations the latter effect outweighed the former effect. WARBURG showed that the same effects could be observed in cells and concluded that the oxygen uptake of cells was dependent on an iron containing compound. The action of cyanides and of narcotics on enzymes and their mutual interference is therefore a problem of general physiological interest, and hence it is worth considering some of the outstanding facts relative to this problem.

A general theory widely accepted regarding the action of aliphatic narcotics is that these drugs cover the cell surfaces with an inert layer of hydrocarbon radicals and thereby interfere with all processes occurring at the cell surface.

In the case of other drugs, it may be assumed that in a large number of cases the first stage of their action is either adsorption on the cell surface or chemical combination with some specific receptor.

These two theories imply that the presence of narcotics ought to interfere with the action of many other drugs on cells.

A consideration of the action of narcotics on the simplest contact catalysts, i. e. polished metal surfaces, shows that the view outlined above is improbably simple because a contact catalyst may be poisoned by a quantity of narcotic only sufficient to cover a small fraction of the surface, and hence even in this simple system a selective adsorption of the narcotic must occur.

Similarly the action of narcotics on purified ferments shows complexities that are not easy to explain as effects due to non-specific adsorption forming an inert layer. For example MEYERHOF (1914)[1] found that saccharase was inhibited by narcotics but SCHÜRMEYER (1925)[2] showed that highly purified saccharase, which he claimed was protein-free, was not inhibited by phenyl urethane, although, when globulin was added to the saccharase, phenylurethane produced a powerful inhibition. This result suggests that the action of narcotics is on the carrier rather than on the prosthetic group of the ferment.

These results indicate the improbability of any single simple hypothesis explaining all the antagonisms occurring between narcotics and other drugs.

The action of enzyme poisons can in general be regarded as a form of antagonism in which the poison prevents the substrate being acted upon by the active group of the enzyme. In some cases the action of narcotics on enzymes can be related to simple physico-chemical processes. It has already been shown (fig. 12) that the inhibitory action of alcohol on invertase in vitro follows the same concentration-action curve as does its action on cellular metabolism, and this concentration-action curve can be related to the action of narcotics on the air/water surface tension.

The manner in which the activity of various members of any homologous series of narcotics varies in proportion to their action on surface tension is very striking (cf. fig. 14) and the inhibition of enzymes by narcotics usually follows the same general law.

WERTHEIMER (1934)[3] studied the action of the enzymes in living yeast cells on sucrose, and concluded that the initial process was a highly specific combination between the sugar and the protoplasmic cell membrane, which could most conveniently be termed specific adsorption. He showed that this fixation of sugar was inhibited to an approximately equal extent by isocapillary concentrations of different alcohols. Some of his results are shown in Table 20. WERTHEIMER also found that the initial adsorption of sugar was followed by a specific activation

---

[1] MEYERHOF, O.: Pflügers Arch. **157**, 251, 307 (1914).

[2] SCHÜRMEYER, A.: Pflügers Arch. **208**, 595 (1925).

[3] WERTHEIMER, E.: Protoplasma (Berl.) **21**, 521 (1934).

and that this process also was inhibited by narcotics. In this relatively simple case, therefore, the narcotics acted at two stages in the chain of reactions. This illustrates the general principle that non-selective drugs such as narcotics are likely to act at all stages in chain processes and hence their effects are likely to be more complex than the effects produced by more selective drugs.

Table 20. Action of alcohols on yeast fermentation. (WERTHEIMER, 1934[1].)

| (a) Alcohol | (b) Molar conc. producing 75 to 100 per cent. Inhibition of sugar fixation by yeast cells | (c) Relative capillary depression produced by concentration shown in column b |
|---|---|---|
| Methyl . . . | 5.0 | 31 |
| Ethyl . . . | 1.5 | 28 |
| n-Propyl . . | 0.8 | 35 |
| iso-Butyl . . | 0.15 | 28 |
| iso-Amyl . . | 0.045 | 28 |

This point is of importance in relation to the antagonism between narcotics and cyanides. WARBURG demonstrated this antagonism in the case of blood charcoal and also showed that although cyanides and narcotics both diminished the uptake of oxygen by sea urchin eggs, yet the addition of narcotics to cyanide reduced rather than increased the action produced by the latter. LIPSCHITZ and GOTT-SCHALK (1921)[2] showed the same effect in the case of the action of narcotics and cyanides upon the power of minced frog's muscle to reduce dinitrobenzole. COOK, HALDANE and MAPSON (1931)[3] found, however, that a concentration of phenyl urethane which produced a slight inhibition of the oxygen uptake of B. coli potentiated the inhibitory action produced by cyanides, a result which is the reverse of those previously quoted.

The work of KEILIN (1925)[4] appears to provide a possible explanation for the fact that cyanide and a narcotic together may produce no more effect than either does alone. KEILIN showed that cyanide inhibited the uptake of oxygen by cytochrome, whereas aliphatic narcotics did not interfere with the oxygenation of cytochrome but inhibited the activity of dehydrogenase and thereby prevented the utilisation by the cell of the oxygen combined with cytochrome. In such a case if half the dehydrogenase were inactivated by narcotic, then inhibition of the cytochrome by cyanide would not affect the rate of oxygen uptake until the amount of oxygen in the cytochrome was reduced to a point at which it no longer sufficed to supply the reduced amount of dehydrogenase. The inhibition of the activity of living tissues by cyanides and narcotics is therefore likely to show considerably more complex relations than are found when these drugs act on inorganic systems.

In the case of the frog's heart poisoned with iodoacetic acid, cyanide produces a rapid inhibition, which can reasonably be attributed to arrest of oxygen uptake. Cyanides, however, also depress the mechanical response of the normal frog's heart perfused with alkaline Ringer's fluid (DE, 1928[5]) and this effect is produced far more rapidly than is the depression produced under these conditions by total deprivation of oxygen. Hence in this latter case the depressant effect of cyanides cannot be due to asphyxia, but is probably due to the cyanides inhibiting glycolysis in addition to inhibiting oxygen uptake. Hence the depression of the normal

[1] WERTHEIMER, E.: Protoplasma (Berl.) 21, 521 (1934).
[2] LIPSCHITZ, W., and A. GOTTSCHALK: Pflügers Arch. 191, 1 (1921).
[3] COOK, R. P., J. B. S. HALDANE and L. W. MAPSON: Biochemic. J. 25, 534 (1931).
[4] KEILIN, D.: Proc. roy. Soc. B. 98, 312 (1925).
[5] DE, P.: J. Pharmacol. Baltimore 33, 115 (1928).

and of the I.A.A. poisoned frog's heart by cyanide is due to depression of different enzyme systems.

PICKFORD (1927)[1] found that the combination of cyanides and narcotics was · not a simple addition, and indeed showed a certain resemblance to the effects described by WARBURG. The following is a typical example of her results:—

| Drug | Per cent. inhibition of mechanical response of frog's heart |
|---|---|
| (a) NaCN 0.000,3 molar . . . . . . . | 21 |
| (b) $C_2H_5OH$ 0.2 molar . . . . . . . . | 38 |
| (c) Combination of a + b . . . . . . . | 47 |

This is an example of a result which appears to be in fair accordance with a simple physico-chemical explanation, but which on detailed analysis is found to depend on factors so complex that any attempt at analysis seems unprofitable.

**(3) Selective Antagonisms with Haemoglobin.** Haemoglobin provides a model of unique value for the study of drug actions because it is an active protein and the amounts of chemical combining with it can be measured directly. The manner in which carbon monoxide interferes with the uptake of oxygen by haemoglobin is therefore of special interest, because the reactions can be followed by direct quantitative measurements, whereas in the case of drugs acting on enzymes and cells, the amounts of drug taking part in the reaction can only be estimated indirectly.

It is generally agreed that carbon monoxide and oxygen unite with a common receptor in the haemoglobin molecule. The haemoglobin is equally distributed as HbCO and $HbO_2$ when the relative pressures of $O_2$ and CO are about 200 to 1. ROUGHTON (1934)[2] has shown that although Hb combines with CO about ten times more slowly than it does with $O_2$, yet the dissociation of HbCO proceeds far more slowly than does the dissociation of $HbO_2$, and this accounts for the great difference in pressures at which equilibrium occurs between the two gases.

The complexity of the reactions between oxygen and haemoglobin in its natural state has been discussed already, but old haemoglobin in dilute watery solution provides an artificially simplified system. In this case the distribution of the haemoglobin between the two gases is expressed by the simple formula

$$\frac{Pco}{Po} = K \cdot \frac{x}{100 - x}.$$

In this case $x$ = percentage of haemoglobin combined with carbon monoxide, and for any particular value of $x$, the ratio Pco/Po is constant (BOCK, 1923[3]).

This result can be interpreted by the simple assumption that the two gases combine with the same prosthetic group, that both form a reversible compound and that in both cases one molecule of gas combines with one receptor.

The competition of carbon monoxide and oxygen for combination with a watery solution of haemoglobin provides therefore an extremely simple model of the antagonism between two drugs which combine with an active protein, and the antagonism can be interpreted in this case by the simplest laws of mass action. It is, however, important to remember that if haemoglobin under natural conditions be studied, the relations become more complex.

1 PICKFORD, L. M.: J. of Physiol. **63**, 19 (1927).
2 ROUGHTON, F. J. W.: Proc. roy. Soc. B. **115**, 473 (1934).
3 BOCK, J.: Heffters Handb. exper. Pharmakol. **1**, 1 (1923).

In the case of haemoglobin the reactions can be measured quantitatively, but in all the other cases of drug antagonisms that will be considered, no quantitative measurements of drug uptake can be made. The measurements made tell us that drug $A$ at a given concentration causes a certain change in activity in an enzyme solution or cell population, and that the introduction of drug $B$ changes this response. It is obvious that a formidable series of unproven assumptions must be made before such events can be linked with any physico-chemical process.

It will be shown that in many cases antagonisms observed with enzymes and cells show a striking resemblance to the antagonisms found with haemoglobin. This fact is in accordance with the hypothesis that the reaction between drugs and cells is of a nature comparable to that which occurs in the simpleᵢ system, but it must not be forgotten that in the more complex systems there is no direct evidence regarding the nature of the reactions.

(4) **Antagonism in Enzyme Poisoning.** The interpretation generally accepted for the phenomena of enzyme poisoning is that the enzymatic activity is dependent upon active groups and that enzyme poisons combine with these active groups and thereby prevent access of the substrate.

Most forms of enzyme poisoning can therefore be regarded as antagonism or competition between substrate and poison for occupation of the active group.

Researches on the influence of $p_H$ on the action of enzyme poisons have shown certain antagonisms between the hydrogen ion concentration $(H)$ and the drug concentration $(D)$, which have an interesting resemblance to the antagonism between drugs such as acetyl choline and atropine.

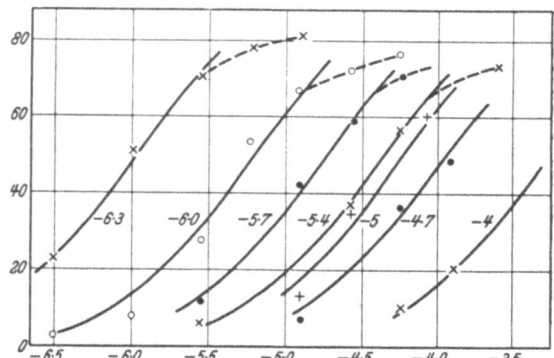

Fig. 72. Influence of $p_H$ on inhibition of saccharase by silver nitrate. Abscissa:— log. $C_H$. Ordinate:— per cent, inhibition of saccharase. The curves show the actions of different concentration of silver nitrate (log. molar conc. (MYRBÄCK, 1926[2].)

EULER and MYRBÄCK (1922)[1] showed that when saccharase was poisoned by silver, the concentration-inhibition curve was of the simple type which occurs when one molecule of a drug forms a reversible compound with an active group.

MYRBÄCK (1926)[2] measured the relation between $(H)$ and the action of silver on saccharase. Fig. 72 shows an example of some of the results he obtained. In this case, when the inhibition produced is equal to more than 20 per cent. of the total activity, the relation between concentration $(x)$ and inhibition $(y)$ follows the dissociation formula $Kx = \dfrac{y}{100 - y}$. Alterations of $(H)$ alter the value of $K$, and hence a series of parallel curves are obtained with different values of $(H)$.

If any particular action be selected (e.g. 50 per cent. inhibition), then the concentration of silver (Ag) and of hydrogen ion (H) which produce this effect show approximately the relation (Ag)/(H) = constant. The actual relation

[1] EULER, H. VON, and K. MYRBÄCK: Hoppe-Seylers Z. **177**, 182 (1922).
[2] MYRBÄCK, K.: Hoppe-Seylers Z. **158**, 160 (1926).

between (Ag) and (H) is shown in fig. 73, and the more exact interpretation of this curve will be discussed later. MYRBÄCK showed that these results could be interpreted on the simple assumption that both the silver and hydrogen ions competed for a common receptor, namely a carboxyl group. He also found that copper, lead, zinc and cadmium salts behaved similarly to silver, in that their inhibitory action was influenced in the same manner by change in $p_H$. Aniline

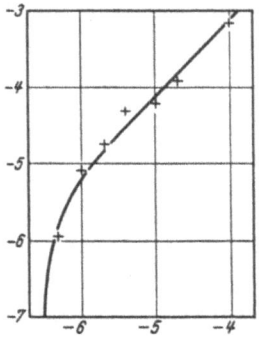

Fig. 73. Molar concentrations of silver nitrate and of hydrogen ion which together produce 50 per cent. inhibition of saccharase (cf. fig. 72). Abscissa:— log. (Ag). Ordinate:— log. (H). The curve is drawn to the formula:—
$k_1$ (Ag) $= 1 + k_2$ (H)
($k_1 = 10^{6.5}$ and $k_2 = 10^{5.89}$).

and related compounds also were influenced in a similar manner, but in this case the interpretation of the curves was more difficult because increase in $p_H$ not only altered the dissociation of the active group of the enzyme, but also changed the dissociation of the aniline and hence reduced the concentration of active base.

MYRBÄCK showed that the activity of another group of enzyme poisons was increased by increase in hydrogen ion concentration. Such compounds were picric acid, phosphotungstic acid, osmic acid and mercury salts. These results were interpreted by the hypothesis that the poisons combined with amino groups in the enzyme and hence there was competition between these poisons and the hydroxyl ions.

QUASTEL and YATES (1936)[1] studied the effect of changes in $p_H$ on the poisoning of invertase by a number of basic and acid dyes. Their results confirm and extend the observations of MYRBÄCK. They found the same relation between dye concentration $[D]$ and percentage action $(y)$, namely, $K[D] = \dfrac{y}{100 - y}$. In the case of the basic dye safranine, they obtained the results shown in Table 21 for the concentrations of hydrogen ion and dye resulting in 50 per cent. inhibition of invertase activity. They interpreted their results by the formula $p_H - \log. 1/[D]$ $=$ constant, and this can be transposed to the formula $[H]/[D] =$ constant. This formula gives a fair approximation to the observed results, but shows a definite deviation with the lowest concentration of dye.

Table 21. Concentrations of hydrogen ion and safranine producing 50 per cent. inhibition of invertase. (QUASTEL and YATES, 1936[1].)

| Log $(H)$ | −3.67 | −4.02 | −4.35 | −4.73 | −5.32 |
|---|---|---|---|---|---|
| Log. molar conc. Safranine $(D)$ | | | | | |
| (I) Observed | −2.11 | −2.60 | −3.07 | −3.55 | −4.02 |
| (II) Calculated | | | | | |
| (a) $(H)/(D) = k = 0.05$ | −2.37 | −2.72 | −3.05 | −3.43 | −4.02 |
| (b) $k_1(D) = 1 + k_2(H)^{1.4}$ | −2.10 | −2.58 | −3.02 | −3.49 | −4.03 |

The author has plotted these results in fig. 74. He found that the results could be interpreted more accurately by the formula

$$k_1[D] = 1 + k_2[H]^{1.4}.$$

The theoretical justification for this formula will be discussed later; it is preferable to the previous formula because it shows a lower limit for the active concentration of dye producing 50 per cent. inhibition, even when the $p_H$ is optimal for its action.

---

[1] QUASTEL, J. H., and E. D. YATES: Enzymologia 1, 60 (1936).

In the case of acid dyes, the action was increased by increase in $[H]$, but the relation between $[D]$ and $[H]$ was complex. The authors expressed it by the formula

$$p_H + {}^1/_n \log. \frac{1}{[D]} = \text{constant.}$$

This can be transformed to $[H] \cdot [D]^{\frac{1}{n}} = \text{constant}$. They found that the value of $n$ usually lay between 2 and 3.

The relation between $[H]$ and $[D]$ is shown in fig. 75. The result can be regarded as a synergism between enzyme poison (acid dye) and the hydrogen ions, but it can equally well be regarded as an antagonism between the enzyme poison and the hydroxyl ions. It will be seen that a considerable portion of the curve follows the formula $[D]/[OH] = \text{constant}$. The curve is difficult to analyse because it does not indicate any minimum effective concentration of dye at a low $p_H$.

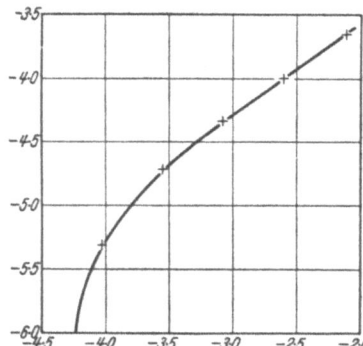

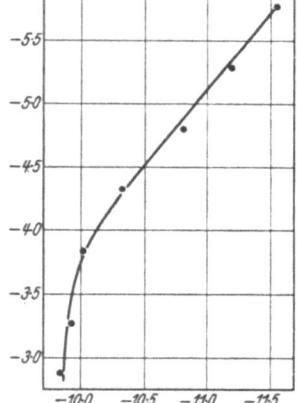

Fig. 74. Concentrations of safranine (basic dye) and of hydrogen ions which together produce 50 per cent. inhibition of invertase activity. Abscissa:— log. conc. safranine (Sa). Ordinate:— log. (H). Curve drawn to formula:— $k_1(\text{Sa}) = 1 = k_2(\text{H})n \cdot (\log. k_1 = 4.25, \log. k_2 = 7.3$ and $n = 1.4$). (QUASTEL and YATES, 1936[1].)

Fig. 75. Concentrations of Bordeaux red (acid dye) and of hydroxyl ions which together produce 50 per cent. inhibiton of invertase. Abscissa:— log. (H). Ordinate:— log. conc. of dye. (QUASTEL and YATES, 1936[1].)

These studies of the inhibition produced on invertase activity by varying the concentration of two substances constitute a valuable introduction to the study of the antagonism and synergism of drugs on cells, because they indicate the probable order of complexity likely to be found.

The enzyme studies show that in some cases the actions can be interpreted as simple examples of dissociation. It is, however, necessary to assume that some poisons combine with carboxyl groups and some with amino groups, and that in either case the combination can cause inhibition of enzymatic activity.

An examination of the extensive data provided by MYRBÄCK and by QUASTEL and YATES shows that only in a few cases do the results fit the simplest formulae, and that in many cases the results have to be fitted by formulae with empirical modifications which have a doubtful theoretical significance.

In the case of drug antagonisms observed on cells, it is therefore unreasonable to hope always to find results which can be fitted by the simplest formulae. When such results are obtained they are of great interest, but it is not a matter for surprise if a simple relation found with one cell-drug system disappears when other systems are examined.

---

[1] QUASTEL, J. H., and E. D. YATES: Enzymologia **1**, 60 (1936).

The inhibition of acetyl choline esterase by physostigmine is an example of enzyme poisoning which illustrates another point of considerable theoretical interest.

STEDMAN and STEDMAN (1931)[1] showed that the inhibition of this esterase by both physostigmine and by synthetic muscarine could be accounted for on the hypothesis that these drugs occupied the same receptor on the esterase as did acetyl choline, but, since they could not be destroyed by the esterase, they inhibited its activity by occupying the active group. The esterase activity was therefore inhibited by drugs which resembled acetyl choline in that they were fixed by a similar receptor, but differed from it in that fixation by the enzyme did not result in their being split. In the case of drug antagonisms on cells, examples are found of drugs with related chemical structure acting as antagonists, and the above provides a simple model of this effect.

**(5) Acetyl Choline-Atropine Antagonism.** The examples given above show that in some cases when two drugs compete for the same receptor, the result can be expressed in a simple manner.

The writer (1926)[2] measured the response of the frog's heart and rectus abdominis to acetyl choline in the presence of various concentrations of atropine. The concentration-action curves of acetyl-choline in the presence of varying concentrations of atropine resembled those shown in fig. 72. A series of parallel curves were obtained, all following the general formula $K x = \dfrac{y}{100 - y}$, but the value of $K$ varied from 1,000,000 in the absence of atropine to 20 in the presence of $N/_{1000}$ atropine.

The author at first (1926)[2] interpreted these results as showing that $[Ac]/[At] = $ constant. Further work on the ergotamine-adrenaline antagonism showed that this formula did not interpret the results obtained with very low concentrations of antagonist and the formula was modified (CLARK, 1933[3]) to the form

$$([Ac_2] - [Ac_1])/[At] = \text{constant}.$$

In this case $[Ac_1]$ and $[Ac_2]$ represent the concentrations of acetyl choline which produce a selected action respectively in the absence of atropine and in its presence at the concentration $[At]$.

GADDUM (1937)[4] has pointed out that this formula is incorrect because the concentration-action curves of acetyl choline with varying concentrations of atropine follow a parallel course. When no atropine is present $K_1[Ac_1] = \dfrac{y}{100 - y}$ ($y = $ percentage action) and when atropine is present $K_2[Ac_2] = \dfrac{y}{100 - y}$. Hence the relation between $[Ac_2]$ and $[At]$ should show the same constant whatever intensity of inhibition be chosen as the basis for comparison, and this cannot occur if

$$\frac{[Ac_2] - [Ac_1]}{[At]} = \text{constant}.$$

GADDUM has put forward the following solution.

Let drug $B$ be an antagonist to drug $A$, when both drugs compete for the same receptors, and let $y$ and $z$ be the percentages of the receptors occupied respectively by $A$ and $B$. Then when both drugs are present the number of free receptors equals $100 - y - z$.

[1] STEDMAN, E., and E. STEDMAN: Biochemic. J. **25**, 1147 (1931).
[2] CLARK, A. J.: J. of Physiol. **61**, 547 (1926).
[3] CLARK, A. J.: The Mode of Action of Drugs on Cells. London: Arnold and Co. 1933.
[4] GADDUM, J. H.: J. of Physiol. **89**, 7P (1937).

The rate of association of a drug is proportional to its concentration and to the number of free receptors. The rate of dissociation is proportional to the amount of drug fixed, or to the number of receptors occupied by the drug. Equilibrium occurs when the rate of dissociation equals the rate of association. Hence

$$K_1[A] \cdot (100 - y - z) = y$$

and

$$K_2[B] \cdot (100 - y - z) = z.$$

Elimination of $z$ gives the equation

$$K_1[A] = (1 + K_2[B]) \cdot \frac{y}{100 - y}.$$

This formula only covers the simplest cases where one molecule of drug unites with one receptor. A formula which covers a larger range of results is as follows:

$$K_1[A] = (1 + K_2[B]^n) \cdot \frac{y}{100 - y}.$$

This formula has an additional important advantage over the writer's formula in that the ratio $K_2/K_1$ indicates the intensity of the antagonism exerted by one drug upon the other.

In the case of acetyl choline acting on the frog's heart $n = 1$ and when 50 per cent. inhibition is the action chosen $\frac{y}{100 - y} = 1$. Hence the formula in this case can be simplified to

$$K_1[Ac] = 1 + K_2[At].$$

The figures in Table 22 show the observed values of acetyl choline needed to produce 50 per cent. inhibition of the mechanical response of the frog's heart in the presence of atropine in varying concentrations (CLARK, 1926)[1], together with the values calculated according to the above formula with the constants $K_1 = 10^6$ and $K_2 = 3 \times 10^7$.

Table 22. Antagonism of Acetyl choline by Atropine (CLARK, 1926[1]).

| Molar. conc. Atropine sulphate ($\times 10^6$) | 0 | 0.01 | 0.1 | 1.0 | 10 | 100 | 1000 |
|---|---|---|---|---|---|---|---|
| Molar. conc. Acetyl choline ($\times 10^6$) producing 50 p.c. inhibition | | | | | | | |
| (a) observed | 1 | 1.6 | 3.6 | 25 | 300 | 3,500 | 47,000 |
| (b) calculated | 1 | 1.3 | 4.0 | 31 | 300 | 3,000 | 30,000 |

The agreement between the calculated and observed figures is good except in the case of the highest concentrations of atropine, but the fact that the formula does account for the results obtained over a huge range of concentrations, is a very remarkable fact.

When the same two drugs were tested on the rectus abdominis of the frog, a more complex relation was obtained. In this case the figures for 50 p.c. inhibition can be fitted by the formula

$$K_1[Ac] = 1 + K_2[At]^{1.3}.$$

COOK (1926)[2] measured the antagonism of acetyl choline by methylene blue. In this case the results are fitted by the formula given above and the value of $n$ lies between 1 and 1.3.

[1] CLARK, A. J.: J. of Physiol. 61, 547 (1926).
[2] COOK, R. P.: J. of Physiol. 62, 160 (1926).

HUNT (1934)[1] measured the antagonism of acetyl $\beta$-methyl choline by atropine when injected intravenously into cats. Estimations made of the doses resulting in an equal fall in blood pressure show in this case a value of $n = 1$ and $K_2/K_1 = 2$. The absolute values of $K_1$ and $K_2$ in this case are of little significance because the actual concentrations of the drugs in the blood are unknown.

The values of these constants in the case of acetyl choline as calculated from various experiments are shown in Table 23.

Table 23. Constants found in Acetyl choline antagonisms.

| System | $n$ | $k_1$ | $k_2$ | Ratio $k_2/k_1$ |
|---|---|---|---|---|
| Acetyl choline-Atropine | | | | |
| Frog's Heart (CLARK, 1926[2]) . . . . . . . | 1.0 | $10^6$ | $3 \times 10^7$ | 30 |
| Rectus abdominis (CLARK, 1926[2]) . . . . . | 1.8 | $5 \times 10^5$ | $2 \times 10^7$ | 40 |
| Acetyl choline-Methylene Blue | | | | |
| Frog's Heart (COOK, 1926[3]) . . . . . . . . | 1.25 | $3 \times 10^6$ | $8 \times 10^7$ | 25 |
| Acetyl $\beta$-Methyl choline-Atropine | | | | |
| Cat's Blood Pressure (HUNT, 1934[1]) . . . . | 1.0 | — | — | 2 |

These results show that in the case of a single pair of drugs (acetyl choline and atropine) $n$ is not constant. In the case of the isolated tissues shown above, the ratios between $K_1$ and $K_2$ are similar with the different systems, but it will be shown later that this ratio is not constant in the case of the adrenalin-ergotoxine antagonism on isolated tissues, and hence the apparent constancy shown above for this ratio has no certain significance, a fact which indeed is indicated by the completely different value of the ratio in the case of doses producing an equal fall of blood pressure in cats.

(6) **Adrenaline-Ergotoxine Antagonism.** GADDUM (1926)[4] first studied this antagonism quantitatively. He used the isolated rabbit's uterus and found a linear relation between the ergotoxine concentration and the multiple of the adrenaline concentration needed to produce a constant effect. The results follow the formula already given. MENDEZ (1928)[5] measured this antagonism on the rabbit's uterus and on the vas deferens of the guinea pig. NANDA (1930)[6] made similar experiments on the antagonism of these drugs on the rabbit's gut. He found striking differences in the intensity of the antagonism occurring in the ileum, duodenum and colon.

MENDEZ and NANDA both used the formula

$$[A\,d_2] - [A\,d_1] = K\,[E\,t]^n$$

but their results are fitted equally well by the formula

$$K_1\,[A\,d] = (1 + K_2\,[E\,t]^n)\frac{y}{100 - y}.$$

The author has extracted from their results the values for these constants shown in Table 24.

The figures for the colon are incomplete and not very accurate, but they show that the constants in this case are quite different from the constants in the other cases, and apart from these figures, the table shows wide variations in all the constants.

[1] HUNT, REID: J. Pharmacol. Baltimore **51**, 237 (1934).
[2] CLARK, A. J.: J. of Physiol. **61**, 547 (1926).
[3] COOK, R. P.: J. of Physiol. **62**, 160 (1926).
[4] GADDUM, J. H.: J. of Physiol. **61**, 141 (1926).
[5] MENDEZ, R.: J. Pharmacol. Baltimore **32**, 451 (1928).
[6] NANDA, T. C.: J. Pharmacol. Baltimore **42**, 9 (1931).

Table 24. Constants found in antagonism of Adrenaline by Ergotamine.

| System | $n$ | $k_1$ | $k_2$ | Ratio $k_2/k_1$ |
|---|---|---|---|---|
| Motor response | | | | |
| Rabbit's uterus (MENDEZ, 1928[1]) . . . . . | 1 | $5.6 \times 10^5$ | $2.7 \times 10^7$ | 48 |
| Guinea pig vas deferens (MENDEZ, 1928[1]) . . | 0,48 | $5 \times 10^4$ | $7 \times 10^3$ | 0.14 |
| Inhibitor response | | | | |
| Rabbit's gut (NANDA, 1931[2]) | | | | |
| Ileum. . . . . . . . . . . . . . . . . . | 1 | $8 \times 10^6$ | $3.8 \times 10^7$ | 4.8 |
| Duodenum . . . . . . . . . . . . . . | 1 | $2 \times 10^7$ | $10^8$ | 5.5 |
| Colon. . . . . . . . . . . . . . . . . . | 0.25 | $10^7$ | $10^2$ | 0.00001 |

The antagonism of adrenaline by other drugs than ergotamine shows similar quantitative relations. For example BACQ and FREDERICQ (1935)[3] obtained the results shown in fig. 76 for the antagonism of the action of adrenaline on the nictitating membrane of the cat by piperido-methyl-benzo-dioxane (933. Fourneau). These results show that the antagonist drug shifts the concentration-action curve of adrenaline and that the curves are approximately parallel. These experiments are of interest since they show that the general laws of antagonism are followed in the case of drugs administered to the intact animal.

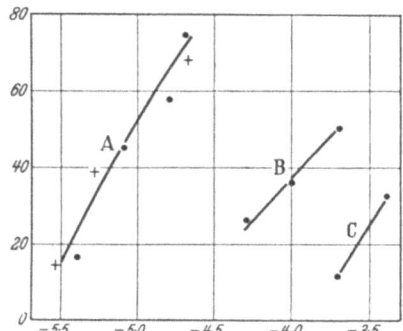

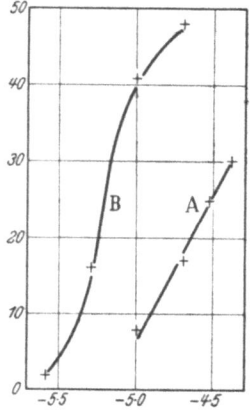

Fig. 76. Action of adrenaline on the nictitating membrane of cat's eye and antagonism by 933 Fourneau. Abscissa: − log. dose adrenaline in g. Ordinate: − response as per cent. of maximum. (A) Adrenaline alone. (B) Adrenaline after 10 mg. 933 F. (C) Adrenaline after 30 mg. 933 F. (BACQ and FRÉDERICQ, 1935[3].)

Fig. 77. Action of adrenaline on nictitating membrane of cat's eye and synergism by hydroxy-hydroquinone. Abscissa: − log. dose adrenaline in g. Ordinate: − response. (A) Adrenaline alone. (B) Adrenaline after 300 mg. hydroxy-hydroquinone. (BACQ, 1936[4].)

**(7) Synergists of Adrenaline.** The potentiation of synergism of drugs is in general a much weaker effect than is drug antagonism.

Quantitative data are available for the synergism between adrenaline and cocaine. Fig. 28 shows the results obtained by BACQ and FRÉDERICQ (1935)[5] for the action of adrenaline in the absence and presence of cocaine on the nictitating membrane of the cat. The figure shows that the two concentration-action curves are parallel and that, as a first approximation the effect of cocaine is to increase six fold the value of $K$ in the formula $Kx = \dfrac{y}{100 - y}$, where $x =$ adrenaline concentration.

Fig. 77 shows a similar synergism found by BACQ (1936)[4] in the case of adrenaline and hydroxy-hydroquinone.

[1] MENDEZ, R.: J. Pharmacol. Baltimore **32**, 451 (1928).
[2] NANDA, T. C.: J. Pharmacol. Baltimore **42**, 9 (1931).
[3] BACQ, Z. M., and H. FRÉDERICQ: Arch. int. Physiol. **40**, 454 (1935).
[4] BACQ, Z. M.: Arch. int. Physiol. **42**, 340 (1936).
[5] BACQ, Z. M., and H. FRÉDERICQ: Arch. int. Physiol. **40**, 297 (1935).

Similarly RAVENTOS (1936/37 and 1937)[1] found that the action of acetyl choline on the frog's heart was potentiated by certain quaternary ammonium salts, and that in this case the effect of the synergist drug was to displace the concentration-action curve, without altering its shape.

The quantitative results of drug synergism are not complete enough for exact analysis, but they indicate that synergists alter the value of $K$ in the formula $Kx = \dfrac{y}{100 - y}$, and hence displace the concentration-action but do not alter its shape.

In the case of antagonists, this effect can be readily interpreted as being due to competition of drugs for a common receptor, but this explanation cannot hold in the case of synergic drugs.

In the case of adrenaline, it is fairly certain that hydroxy-hydroquinone and certain other reducing substances act by preventing the oxidation of adrenaline. The duration of action of adrenaline on isolated tissues is limited by its oxidation (PRASAD, 1936[2]). In the case of intact animals, as used in BACQ's experiments, it seems probable that the concentration of adrenaline at the site of action is largely determined by the rate at which it is oxidised during its passage to the site of action.

The simplest explanation of the synergism between reducing substances and adrenaline is to suppose that the former increases the concentration of drug attained around the responding tissue after the injection of a given quantity of adrenaline.

This explanation will not hold, however, in the case of the adrenaline-cocaine synergism, and the simplest explanation in this case is the assumption that the cell receptor is a complex structure and that cocaine alters it in some manner so that either the rate of association of adrenaline is increased or its rate of dissociation is decreased.

The results with synergistic drugs can therefore only be partially explained, but this is not surprising in view of the fact that many of the phenomena associated with synergisms in relatively simple inorganic systems, e. g. the activation of inorganic catalysts, are only partially understood.

**(8) Comparison of Antagonisms found with Enzymes and with Hormones.** The two cases of drug antagonism that have been considered are remarkable in that powerful antagonistic actions can be measured quantitatively over a remarkable range of concentrations. For example an isolated frog's heart in the presence of $N/1000$ atropine sulphate functions normally except that the concentration of acetyl choline needed to produce 50 per cent. depression is nearly 50,000 times as great as that required by the normal heart.

This remarkable antagonism can be expressed quantitatively by a formula based on the simple assumption that the two drugs compete for a common receptor in the same manner as carbon monoxide and oxygen compete for the active group in haemoglobin.

The antagonism of enzyme poisons by hydrogen ions or hydroxyl ions shows similar quantitative relationships, and it is of interest to note that these antagonisms can be expressed accurately by the formula introduced by GADDUM.

MYRBÄCK's results shown in fig. 73 can be expressed approximately by the formula $[Ag]/[H] = $ constant, but the result with the lowest concentration of silver shows a clear deviation from this linear relation.

[1] RAVENTOS, J.: J. of Physiol. 88, 5P (1936/37) — Quart. J. exper. Physiol. 26, 361, 375 (1937).
[2] PRASAD, B. N.: J. of Physiol. 86, 425 (1936).

The results can, however, be expressed accurately by the formula $K_1[Ag] = 1 + K_2[H]$ as is shown by the curve drawn in the figure.

Fig. 74 shows that the antagonism of safranine by increasing hydrogen ion concentration can be expressed by a similar but slightly more complex formula $K_1[Sa] = 1 + K_2[H]^{1.4}$ and in this case also the formula expresses accurately the results obtained with the lowest concentration of dye.

Fig. 75 which shows the antagonism of Bordeaux red by hydroxyl ions cannot be fitted easily with a formula because the results show no lower limit for the active concentration of dye in strongly acid solutions, but show that the dye becomes nearly inert when the $p_H$ rises above 4.

The antagonism with both enzyme poisons and drugs agree in showing that when substance $B$ antagonises substance $A$, the antagonism can be expressed by the formula $K_1[A] = 1 + K_2[B]^n$, and that in some cases $n = 1$ but that it may be either less or more than unity.

LANGMUIR's formulae for specific adsorption provide such a wide variety of curves following the general formula $Kx^n = \dfrac{y}{100 - y}$, that it would probably be possible with a little ingenuity to explain all these results. The number of unknown factors is, however, so great that this exercise seems profitless.

Examination of the other constants obtained with the specific drugs acting on isolated organs, shows that $K_1$ and $K_2$ vary widely. This merely expresses the well known fact that the sensitivity of tissues to the drugs in question varies widely. The ratio between $K_2$ and $K_1$ also varies widely in the case of a single pair of drugs. This fact also accords with the common knowledge that in the case, for example, of adrenaline, some of its actions (e.g. augmentor effects) are more easily inhibited by ergotamine than are other actions (e.g. inhibitor effects). The ratio $K_2/K_1$ provides, however, a simple quantitative expression for the intensity of inhibition.

The irregularities observed in the antagonism of the action of drugs on both enzymes and cells suggest to the writer that probably the receptors on which the drug acts are complex structures whose activity can be modified in a graded manner.

This view is supported by the fact that the antagonism of acetyl choline and of atropine cannot be explained as a simple displacement such as occurs with the system haemoglobin-oxygen-carbon monoxide.

Atropine is removed slowly from the frog's heart and this rate of removal is not accelerated by exposure to high concentrations of acetyl choline (CLARK, 1926[1]). Hence the latter drug does not displace the atropine in the manner that high concentrations of oxygen displace carbon monoxide.

Another important point is that the theoretical basis for the formula applied is that both of two antagonistic drugs form a reversible compound with some receptor. The rate of wash-out of the various drugs varies, however, over a very wide range and in some cases is so slow that the reversibility is actually doubtful.

In the case of acetyl choline and atropine, the acetyl choline is removed by washing out so quickly that any delay observed may reasonably be attributed to the time taken to change the fluid at the cell surface. Atropine, on the other hand, takes about 20 min. to wash out. This contrast in rates of wash-out is even more marked in the case of adrenaline and ergotamine. The former drug is very quickly removed, whilst the latter drug is only partially removed by washing for an hour. Several authors have indeed stated that the action of ergotamine on isolated organs is irreversible.

[1] CLARK, A. J.: J. Physiol. **61**, 530 (1926).

On the other hand, each of the constants $K_1$ and $K_2$ represents the ratio between the rate of combination and the rate of dissociation of a drug. It is true that the rate of dissociation of ergotamine is very slow, but the rate of combination also is slow, whilst both dissociation and combination are rapid in the case of adrenaline.

Hence the gross differences observed in the rate of wash-out of antagonistic drugs do not disprove the theoretical validity of GADDUM's formula.

It is of course improbable that actions of drugs on living cells should be of a simplicity comparable to the fixation of gases by metal surfaces, and it is probable that future investigations will show that the processes described are in reality more complex than is indicated by the formulae adopted.

In spite of these difficulties, however, the outstanding fact remains that it is possible to express by a simple formula the antagonism between two such drugs as acetyl choline and atropine, over enormous ranges of concentrations.

This fact indicates that the antagonism depends fundamentally on some relatively simple physico-chemical process.

The study of the quantitative aspects of drug antagonism shows, therefore, that there is a very striking resemblance found between the competition of gases for haemoglobin, the antagonism of enzyme poisons by alteration in $p_H$, and the antagonism of specific drugs.

This similarity is at once explained if it be assumed that in all cases the substances compete for common receptors in active groups on proteins. It is, however, extremely difficult to explain these results on any other theory, and the author considers this to be a strong argument for the hypothesis that drugs act in this manner.

## Chapter 18

## Qualitative Aspects of Drug Antagonism.

**(1) Introduction.** The relation between chemical structure and pharmacological action is a subject of notorious difficulty. It may be said that there are scarcely any general rules discernible and that every cell-drug system appears to be a law unto itself. In the case of drugs which have sharply specific actions, it is common to find that the activity even of optical isomers differs widely, but on the other hand, drugs of widely different structure may have a similar action.

Although it is very difficult to formulate any general laws, yet those engaged in the production of new synthetic drugs for any purpose recognise empirical laws regarding the types of structure which are worth investigating. The fragmentary character of present knowledge is, however, indicated by the fact that the history of new synthetic drugs often shows that these were produced with the intent of obtaining a therapeutic action totally different from the one for which they were finally employed. For example, the search for new anti-malarial drugs in one case resulted in the discovery of a new and powerful local anaesthetic.

The writer felt that it was hopeless to attempt to deal with a field of this magnitude and complexity in the limits of the present monograph.

The study of the structure of certain drugs which produce antagonism to other drugs is, however, a limited field which is of interest because it provides a means of testing the general theory that drugs act on cells by combining with specific receptors in a manner similar to the action of enzyme poisons.

In the case of drugs such as acetyl choline and adrenaline, the author postulates the following general theory. The drugs combine with specific receptors on the cell surface. The selective action of the drugs depends on two factors, firstly, the power to combine with the receptor, and secondly, the power to produce an effect after they have combined. The intensely selective action of the drugs is presumed to depend upon the configuration of the drug molecule fitting exactly some configuration of the cell surface.

This hypothesis is similar to modern views regarding the action of enzymes. QUASTEL and YATES (1936)[1], for example, conclude that invertase acts as a zwitter ion, whose oppositely charged groups are bridged by sucrose. They suggest that the glucose moiety of sucrose is attached to the anion of the enzyme and the fructose moiety to the kation of the enzyme. This assumption explains why the enzyme is poisoned by either basic or acid dyes which combine respectively with the anion and the kation of the enzyme. Presumably the most effective of all enzyme poisons would be one which accurately bridged the zwitter ion but which was not acted on by the enzyme.

STEDMAN and STEDMAN (1931)[2] put forward a similar theory to account for the poisoning of acetyl choline esterase. Effective poisons were those which were sufficiently like acetyl choline in structure to combine with the active group, but which were not acted on by the esterase.

According to this theory, drug antagonists should show a certain resemblance in structure to the drugs which they antagonise, and it is of interest to consider whether the evidence available supports this hypothesis.

(2) Antagonism of Adrenaline. The quantitative evidence regarding the antagonism of adrenaline by ergotoxine shows at once that the intensity of the antagonism varies enormously with different tissues. For example ergotoxine has a powerful antagonistic action when tested on the rabbit's ileum, but scarcely any such action when tested on the rabbit's colon.

Hence if the receptor theory of drug action be adopted, it is necessary to assume that the form of the receptors with which adrenaline combines differs in different tissues.

This assumption makes it easier to understand the unexpected forms of drug antagonism which occasionally occur. For example, atropine inhibits a certain number of adrenaline actions.

The general hypothesis that a drug is most likely to be antagonised by drugs which have a similar molecular configuration is supported by the work of LOEWE (1927)[3] who tested the pharmacological actions of thirty-three new cycloethane amines on isolated tissues. He found that two thirds of these compounds produced interference with adrenaline action and one third produced adrenaline reversal. MODERN and THIENES (1936)[4] investigated 40 compounds of a similar type and found that 35 of these antagonised adrenaline.

The antagonism of adrenaline is therefore an effect produced by many substances other than ergotoxine, although curiously enough it is not produced by ergometrine.

(3) Chemical Structure of Acetyl Choline Antagonists. The antagonism of acetyl choline can be investigated in two ways, firstly by considering the effects on acetyl choline action of the presence of drugs which show certain resemblances

---

[1] QUASTEL, J. H., and E. D. YATES: Enzymologia 1, 60 (1936).
[2] STEDMAN, E., and E. STEDMAN: Biochemic. J. 25, 1147 (1931).
[3] LOEWE, S.: Z. exper. Med. 66, 271 (1927).
[4] MODERN, F. S., and C. H. THIENES: Arch. int. Pharmacodyn. 53, 413 (1936).

in structure, and secondly by considering the antagonisms observed when the same pair of drugs are tested on a number of different tissues.

Acetyl choline is a relatively simple compound ($OHMe_3NCH_2CH_2OCOCH_3$). It is a strong base, but is not readily adsorbed and hence it is probably fixed by combination of the substituted ammonium group with carboxyl radicles in the cell protoplasm. This hypothesis suggests that the action of acetyl choline is likely to be influenced by the reaction of the fluid bathing the cells. The author (1927)[1] found that increased alkalinity antagonised the action of acetyl choline in a curious manner in that it reduced the maximum effect that the drug could produce, but did not change markedly the concentration needed to produce half the maximum possible effect. ANDRUS (1924)[2] also found that acetyl choline produced less action on the frog's heart at $p_H$ 8 than at $p_H$ 7, but he found the reverse to be true in the case of the action of acetyl choline on the rabbit's gut. DAVIS (1931)[3] also found that acetyl choline produced less action on the frog's heart when the fluid was strongly alkaline.

These results show that the influence of $p_H$ on acetyl choline action is not very definite, and hence do not provide any certain evidence for or against the hypothesis outlined above.

The simple quaternary ammonium salts are fairly closely related to acetyl choline in their structure, and hence their influence on acetyl choline action is of interest. These compounds are best known on account of their power to paralyse motor nerve endings, but in addition they produce many acetyl choline-like actions.

KÜLZ (1923)[4] made a sytematic investigation of the pharmacological actions of these compounds and showed that the series $Me_3NMe$ to $Me_3NBu$ produced contracture of the rectus abdominis of the frog with an intensity that increased with increasing length of chain. He also showed that $Me_3NOct$ and $Et_3NEt$ did not produce contracture but antagonised the action of the series $Me_3NMe$ to $Me_3NBu$.

RAVENTOS (1937)[5] has repeated and confirmed this work and also has studied the combined action of quaternary ammonium salts and acetyl choline. Table 25 shows some of his results which were obtained with the isolated frog's heart. Experiments with the rectus abdominis and with the isolated rat's gut showed that these substituted ammonium salts potentiated or antagonised the action of acetyl choline in the same manner in all three tissues.

Table 25. Actions of quaternary Ammonium Salts on frog's auricle.
(KÜLZ, 1923[4]; RAVENTOS, 1936/37 1937[5].)

| | Action of salt. | Influence on acetyl choline action |
|---|---|---|
| Series—$Me_3NR$ | | |
| R = Me to Bu . . | Depressant action increasing with length of chain | Addition or Potentiation |
| R = Oct. . . . . | Nil | Powerful Antagonism |
| Series—$(Et)_3NR$ | | |
| R = Me—Oct. . . | Nil | Antagonism |
| $Me_3N$ . . . . . . | Feeble depressant action | Addition or Potentiation |
| $Et_3N$ . . . . . . | Nil | Antagonism |

[1] CLARK, A. J.: J. of Physiol. **64**, 123 (1927).
[2] ANDRUS, E. C.: J. of Physiol. **59**, 361 (1924).
[3] DAVIS, E.: J. of Physiol. **71**, 431 (1931).
[4] KÜLZ, F.: Arch. f. exper. Path. **98**, 339 (1923).
[5] RAVENTOS, J.: J. of Physiol. **88**, 5P (1936/37) — Quart. J. exper. Physiol. **26** (1937).

The reversal of action that occurs in the $Me_3NR$ series between the butyl and the octyl compound is similar to results that have been obtained with more complex series.

In the case of choline esters, REID HUNT (1910)[1] noted that when the length of chain of the acyl radicle was increased, the activity diminished. BLANKART (1936)[2] observed a reversal of action on the isolated gut. Acetyl homocholin ($CH_3COOCH_2CH_2CH_2NMe_3OH$) had an excitant action, whilst allyl isopropyl homocholine (substitution of methyl group by $C_7H_{13}$) antagonised the action of acetyl choline on the gut.

These reversals of action within homologous series are of considerable interest. The results obtained by RAVENTOS with the MeNR series can most simply be explained on the assumption that the drugs are anchored by the $Me_3$-N group and that the intensity of adsorption increases with increasing length of chain. This point is indicated by the fact that the action of these drugs in paralysing motor nerve endings increases steadily from the $Me_3NEt$ to $Me_3NOct$ (ING and WRIGHT, 1932[3]). It would appear that when the side chain contains not more than four carbon atoms, the drug can produce a depressant action, but that when the side chain increases to eight carbon atoms, this action is lost; since, however, the drug occupies the specific receptors, it is able to antagonise acetyl choline.

According to this hypothesis acetyl choline also is anchored by its $Me_3N$-group and owes its peculiar potency of action to some special configuration of its side chain.

The chief difficulty about this hypothesis is the fact that a drug such as $Me_3NBu$, which produces 50 per cent. inhibition of the frog's heart in a concentration of about $10^{-4}$ molar, produces an addition or even potentiation with acetyl choline which produces the same effect at about $10^{-6}$ molar. It might be anticipated that the combination of a drug of low potency with a drug of high potency would reduce the action of the latter if both drugs competed for the same receptors.

This difficulty can however be explained by assuming that the difference in the intensity of action of acetyl choline and of the quaternary ammonium salts depends on differences in the ease with which they combine with the tissue receptors. According to this hypothesis equal effects are produced by the fixation of equal quantities of the different drugs but the concentrations needed to produce equal fixation vary over a wide range.

The facts mentioned above show that many of the phenomena observed with acetyl choline and the quaternary ammonium compounds can be explained on the assumption that the $Me_3N$ group acts as a haptophore group in both cases. This seems to the author to be a promising working hypothesis, although it is obvious that it leaves a number of facts unexplained. In particular it will be noted that the hypothesis provides no explanation why atropine is a more potent antagonist to acetyl choline than any other alkaloid, and still less does it explain the difference in the intensity of action of 1- and d-hyoscyamine.

**(4) Acetyl Choline Antagonism in Different Tissues.** The variations observed in different tissues for the adrenaline-ergotoxine antagonism have already been described. Such variations are found with many other examples of drug antagonism. For example LANGLEY (1905, 1914)[4] estimated the concentrations at which curare antagonised the action of nicotine on frog's muscles and found

---

[1] HUNT, REID: J. Pharmacol. Baltimore **1**, 303 (1910).
[2] BLANKART, A.: Festschrift E. C. Barell, p. 284. Basel 1936.
[3] ING, H. R., and W. M. WRIGHT: Proc. roy. Soc. B. **109**, 337 (1932).
[4] LANGLEY, J. N.: J. of Physiol. **33**, 374, 380 (1905); **48**, 73 (1914).

that the curare/nicotine ratio was 1/50 with the sartorius and 2.5/1 with the rectus abdominis. Similar erratic effects are observed when any form of drug antagonism is studied carefully.

The acetyl choline-atropine antagonism is a suitable example because it is so well known. Most of the actions produced by acetyl choline on vertebrate tissues are antagonised by atropine, and the same is true for some actions of acetyl choline on primitive forms of invertebrates. For example RIESSER (1931)[1] found that acetyl choline contracted holothurian muscle and that the action was antagonised by atropine. On the other hand, the following actions of acetyl choline are not antagonised by atropine. Contracture of leech muscle (GADDUM, 1936[2]) and inhibition of heart of *Helix pomatia* (JULLIEN and MORIN, 1931[3]).

Similarly muscarine produces a typical inhibition of the hearts of *Helix pomatia* (EVANS, 1912[4]) and of *Aplysia limacina* (STRAUB, 1907[5]), but neither of these actions is inhibited by atropine. Muscarine also depresses the rhythmic contraction of the blood vessels of *Hirudo*, and this effect is antagonised by atropine (PANTIN, 1935[6]).

The acetyl choline contractures produced in vertebrate muscles show a remarkable variation as regards the influence of atropine. HESS (1923)[7] showed that in the perfused frog's gastrocnemius, acetyl choline caused a contraction which was not inhibited by atropine in a concentration of 1 in $10^6$, although inhibition was produced by high concentrations. The contracture produced by acetyl choline in the isolated sartorius or rectus abdominis of the frog immersed in Ringers fluid is, however, antagonised by atropine in low concentrations (RIESSER and NEUSCHLOSS, 1921[8]; CLARK, 1926[9]). In the case of denervated mammalian muscle in situ, FRANK, NOTHMANN and GUTTMANN (1922, 1923[10]) showed that the acetyl choline contracture was not antagonised by atropine, a result confirmed by GASSER and DALE (1926)[11], but DALE and GADDUM (1930)[12] found that atropine inhibited the acetyl choline contracture of the cat's denervated diaphragm when this was isolated. The contraction produced by acetyl choline, when given intra-arterially, in normal mammalian muscle is not antagonised by atropine (BROWN, DALE and FELDBERG, 1936)[13], and the same is true of the quick contraction produced by acetyl choline on frog's muscles (RAVENTOS, 1937[14]).

These exceptions do not of course disprove the general rule that atropine antagonises acetyl choline, but they show that curious exceptions occur to this general rule.

Atropine also acts as antagonist to other drugs. For example, OKAMOTO (1918)[15] found that atropine could partly antagonise the motor action of adrenaline on the isolated rabbit's uterus, a result confirmed by OGATA (1921)[16] and by BACKMAN

[1] RIESSER, O.: Arch. f. exper. Path. **161**, 34 (1931).
[2] GADDUM, J. H.: Gefäßerweiternde Stoffe der Gewebe. Leipzig: Thieme 1936.
[3] JULLIEN, A., and G. MORIN: C. r. Soc. Biol. Paris **106**, 187 (1931).
[4] EVANS, G. L.: Z. Biol. **59**, 397 (1912).
[5] STRAUB, W.: Pflügers Arch. **119**, 127 (1907).
[6] PANTIN, C. F. A.: Nature (Lond.) **135**, 875 (1935).
[7] HESS, W. R.: Quart. J. exp. Physiol. Suppl. **144** (1923).
[8] RIESSER, O., and S. M. NEUSCHLOSS: Arch. f. exper. Path. **91**, 342 (1921).
[9] CLARK, A. J.: J. of Physiol. **61**, 547 (1926).
[10] FRANK, E. M., NOTHMANN and E. GUTTMANN: Pflügers Arch. **197**, 270; **198**, 391 (1922); **199**, 567; **201**, 569 (1923).
[11] GASSER, H. S., and H. H. DALE: J. Pharmacol. Baltimore **28**, 288 (1926).
[12] DALE, H. H., and J. H. GADDUM: J. of Physiol. **70**, 109 (1930).
[13] BROWN, G. L., H. H. DALE and W. FELDBERG: J. of Physiol. **87**, 394 (1936).
[14] RAVENTOS, J.: J. of Physiol. **88**, 5P (1936/37).
[15] OKAMOTO, S.: Acta Scholae med. Kyoto **2**, 315 (1918).
[16] OGATA, S.: J. Pharmacol. Baltimore **18**, 185 (1921).

and LUNDBERG (1922)[1]. BEZOLD and BLOEBAUM (1867)[2] noted that large doses of atropine in a cat paralysed the sympathetic as well as the vagus. HILDEBRANDT (1920)[3] and WEHLAND (1924)[4] found that atropine antagonised the action of adrenaline on frog's vessels and UHLMANN (1930)[5] obtained the same result with the perfused rabbit's ear. RIESSER and NEUSCHLOSS (1922)[6] found that atropine antagonised the nicotine and veratrine contractures of the frog's rectus abdominis, but in this case very high concentrations of atropine (1 in 1000) were used. ROTH (1923)[7] found that atropine antagonised the action of barium on the isolated mammalian intestine, whilst CAMERON and TAINTER (1936)[8] found that atropine antagonised the contracture of the dog's bronchioles produced by histamine.

The selective antagonistic action produced by atropine is particularly famous and it is therefore of interest to note that atropine does not antagonise all the actions of acetyl choline, and that it antagonises some actions of some other drugs.

GASSER (1930)[9] reviewed the action of drugs in producing contractures of muscles and tabulated certain outstanding antagonisms. Tables 26 and 27 show some of the results collected by GASSER, together with certain additional antagonisms. In respect of the actions ascribed to nicotine, it must be noted that this drug in high concentrations produces a general paralysis of tissues. In low concentrations it produces a contracture of the rectus abdominis and also antagonises the action of acetyl choline. In high concentrations it produces a contracture followed by relaxation, and then the tissue is insensitive to acetyl choline and also to further additions of nicotine.

Table 26. Antagonism of Acetyl Choline.

| | Atropine | Novocaine | Nicotine | Curarine |
|---|---|---|---|---|
| Leech muscle[10] . . . . . . . . . . . . . . . | 0 | + | + | + |
| Rectus abdominis (frog)[11] . . . . . . . . . | + | + | + | + |
| Denervated mammalian muscle[12] . . . . . . | 0 | + | . | . |
| Heart (frog)[13] . . . . . . . . . . . . . . | + | + | 0 | + |
| Heart Helix pomatia[14] . . . . . . . . . . . | 0 | . | . | . |
| Hen's gut[15] . . . . . . . . . . . . . . . . | + | . | 0 | 0 |

The nicotine effects are therefore more complex than the effects of most of the other antagonistic drugs.

Certain actions of acetyl choline are stated to be nicotine-like, but Table 27 shows that the action of nicotine is certainly as complex as is that of acetyl choline.

[1] BACKMAN, E. L., and H. LUNDBERG: C. r. Soc. Biol. Paris 87, 475 (1922).
[2] BEZOLD, A. VON, and F. BLOEBAUM: Würzburg. physiol. Untersuch. 1867.
[3] HILDEBRANDT, F.: Arch. f. exper. Path. 86, 225 (1920).
[4] WEHLAND, N.: Skand. Arch. Physiol. (Berl. u. Lpz.) 45, 211 (1924).
[5] UHLMANN, F.: Arch. int. Pharmacodyn. 36, 253 (1930).
[6] RIESSER, O., and S. M. NEUSCHLOSS: Arch. f. exper. Path. 92, 254 (1922).
[7] ROTH, G. B.: Arch. int. Pharmacodyn. 27, 337 (1923).
[8] CAMERON, W. M., and M. L. TAINTER: J. Pharmacol. Baltimore 57, 152 (1936).
[9] GASSER, H. S.: Physiologic. Rev. 10, 35 (1930).
[10] GADDUM, J. H.: Gefäßerweiternde Stoffe der Gewebe. Leipzig: Thieme 1936.
[11] RIESSER, O., and S. M. NEUSCHLOSS: Arch. f. exper. Path. 91, 342 (1921) — CLARK, A. J.: J. of Physiol. 61, 530 (1926) — RAVENTOS, J.: Quart. J. exper. Physiol. 26 (1937).
[12] FRANK, E., M. NOTHMANN and E. GUTTMANN: Pflügers Arch. 197, 270; 198, 391 (1922); 199, 567; 201, 569 (1923).
[13] RAVENTOS, J.: Quart. J. exper. Physiol. 26, 361, 375 (1937).
[14] EVANS, G. L.: Z. Biol. 59, 397 (1912). — JULLIEN, A., and G. MORIN: C. r. Soc. Biol. Paris 106, 187 (1931). — GAUTRELET, J., and N. HALPERN: C. r. Soc. Biol. Paris 118, 412 (1935).
[15] KURODA, S.: Z. ges. exper. Med. 39, 341 (1923).

Table 27. Antagonism of Nicotine.

| | Atropine | Curarine | Novocaine |
|---|---|---|---|
| Leech muscle . . . . . . . . . . . . . . . . . . . . . | 0 | + [1] | + |
| Rectus abdominis of frog . . . . . . . . . . . . . | + [2, 3] or 0 [4] | + [5] | + [2] |
| Denervated mammalian muscle . . . . . . . . . . . . | 0 [6, 7] | + [8] | + [6] |
| Hen's Muscle | | | |
|     Normal . . . . . . . . . . . . . . . . . . . . . . | . | + [9] | . |
|     Denervated . . . . . . . . . . . . . . . . . . . . . | . | 0 [9] | . |

A quaternary ammonium salt such as Me$_4$N appears simpler than acetyl choline, but in fact its action is more complex when its relations to other drugs are considered. For example, Me$_4$N produces a curariform action on motor nerve endings and yet curare antagonises its action both on the frog's heart and on the rectus abdominis. On the other hand, Et$_4$N antagonises the action of Me$_4$N and acetyl choline on the frog's heart (Külz, 1923[10]), but not on the leech (Raventos, 1937[11]), whilst its action in the mammal is still more complex. Burn and Dale (1914/15)[12] found that the nicotine-like action of Me$_4$N on the cat's blood pressure was antagonised by Et$_4$N, whilst Hunt and Renshaw (1925)[13] and Hunt (1926)[14] tested the action of Et$_4$N and several other quaternary ammonium compounds, and in no case found any atropine-like action in the cat.

The writer is unable to formulate any simple statement regarding the acetyl choline antagonisms found in different tissues, since every tissue seems to be a law unto itself.

The only certain impression obtained is that drug antagonism is an even more complex problem than the selective action of drugs and the results certainly indicate that the form of the receptors in different tissues must vary widely.

It may indeed be said that the chief point demonstrated by the comparative study of antagonism in different tissues is the extreme complexity of the phenomena observed.

(5) **Analysis of Drug Actions by Drug Antagonisms.** In some cases the antagonism of one drug by another gives interesting information regarding the nature of drug action.

The antagonism of acetyl choline by methylene blue (Cook, 1926[15]) is an example of this kind, because the colour of the methylene blue facilitates the determination of its site of action. A frog's heart exposed to methylene blue becomes deeply dyed. The process occurs slowly and is practically irreversible since the dye is not removed by prolonged washing. The action of methylene

[1] Führer, H.: Pflügers Arch. **129**, 107 (1909).
[2] Riesser, O., and S. M. Neuschloss: Arch. f. exper. Path. **92**, 254 (1922). — Rückert, W.: Pflügers Arch. **276**, 323 (1930/31).
[3] Matsuoka, K.: Pflügers Arch. **204**, 51 (1924).
[4] Raventos, J.: Quart. J. exper. Physiol. **26**, 361, 375 (1937).
[5] Langley, J. N.: J. of Physiol. **33**, 374, 380 (1905). — Hill, A. V.: J. of Physiol. **39**, 361 (1909). — Boehm, R.: Arch. f. exper. Path. **58**, 267 (1908). — Veley, V. H., and A. D. Waller: Proc. roy. Soc. B. **82**, 333 (1909).
[6] Frank, E., M. Nothmann and E. Guttmann: Pflügers Arch. **197**, 270 (1922).
[7] Gasser, H. S., and H. H. Dale: J. Pharmacol. Baltimore **28**, 288 (1926).
[8] Heidenhain, R.: Arch. f. Physiol. Suppl. **133** (1883).
[9] Langley, J. N.: J. of Physiol. **33**, 374, 380 (1905).
[10] Külz, F.: Arch. f. exper. Path. **98**, 339 (1923).
[11] Raventos, J.: Quart. J. exper. Physiol. **26** (1937).
[12] Burn, J. H., and H. H. Dale: J. Pharmacol. Baltimore **6**, 417 (1914/15).
[13] Hunt, Reid, and R. R. Renshaw: J. Pharmacol. Baltimore **25**, 315 (1925).
[14] Hunt, Reid: J. Pharmacol. Baltimore **28**, 367 (1926).
[15] Cook, R. P.: J. of Physiol. **62**, 160 (1926).

blue in inhibiting acetylcholine is, however, half completed within 1 or 2 minutes and can be reversed in 5 or 10 minutes by washing the heart with clean Ringer's fluid. This proves conclusively that two processes are occurring, firstly the inhibition of acetyl choline, which is a rapid and easily reversible process, and secondly the entrance of the dye into the cells, which is a slow and irreversible process. Furthermore the deeply dyed heart can be made sensitive to acetyl choline by being washed out, and can be again desensitised by a small concentration of methylene blue. These facts are difficult if not impossible to reconcile with the potential theory of drug action, but they agree very well with the hypothesis that the dye forms a reversible compound with some component of the cell surface and thus prevents the fixation of acetyl choline.

The examples of drug antagonism described above have been selected because they appear to throw a certain amount of light on the possible nature of drug action. There are of course innumerable examples of drug antagonism; indeed it may be taken for granted that when two drugs are administered simultaneously they are more likely than not to interfere with each other's actions. In most cases, however, the presence of two drugs instead of one merely represents an increase in the number of uncontrolled variables. Hence there is little profit in attempting any general review of drug antagonisms. One general point may, however, be mentioned, namely, the fact that a drug acts as an antagonist to another drug does not exclude it from producing other pharmacological actions. For example ergotamine antagonises the action of adrenaline but also it produces a variety of other effects on isolated muscles and it is not justifiable to regard an ergotaminised muscle as a tissue which has been deprived of certain receptors but is otherwise unchanged.

In general drug antagonism is a more complex problem than the action of a single drug. The well known examples of specific antagonisms of drugs (e.g. acetyl choline and atropine, adrenaline and ergotamine) have led to the assumption that it is easy to classify the actions of a drug by a study of its mode of antagonism. The actions of acetyl choline are, for example, classified as muscarine-like actions which are antagonised by atropine (but not by nicotine) and nicotine-like actions which are not thus antagonised.

An examination of evidence of the type shown in Tables 26 and 27 indicates that such classifications are of doubtful validity. For example, acetyl choline and nicotine both produce contracture of the leech and of the frog's rectus abdominis, but of these four actions, the only one antagonised by atropine is the rectus abdominis contracture produced by acetyl choline, an effect which also is antagonised by nicotine.

The selective actions of acetyl choline and of adrenaline and their antagonism could be accounted for very readily by the old theory of specific nerve endings which were either stimulated or paralysed by the various drugs. The modern theories of humoral transmission necessitate the assumption that both the humoral transmittor (e.g. acetyl choline) and the antagonist (e.g. atropine) act on the tissue directly. Hence it is improbable that the antagonistic drug produces no effect on the tissue other than that of impeding the combination of the drug which it antagonises.

The hypothesis adopted by the author is that these drugs unite with specific receptors; furthermore in order to account for specific antagonism, it is necessary to assume two processes, (a) fixation of drug, (b) selective action after fixation. It is suggested that the antagonist drugs either prevent fixation or else alter the pattern of the receptor so that the active drug no longer fits in a manner that will produce its specific effect. If this view be adopted, it is easy to conceive that small differences in the pattern of the receptors in different tissues may easily alter not only the intensity of action of the active drug but equally the intensity with which the antagonist drug inhibits this effect.

Relations between chemical constitution of drugs and pharmacological action have been examined so extensively that we have a fairly clear idea of the extent of our ignorance. No one with experience of this subject would care to prophesy the change in pharmacological activity likely to be produced by even a trivial alteration in the structure of a drug. It appears to the writer that the structure of the receptors on which drugs act is probably a subject of similar complexity, but that the complexity has been masked by the fact that special attention has been paid to the action of acetyl choline and adrenaline, which are hormones widespread throughout the animal kingdom. In these peculiar cases a wide variety of tissues happen to possess receptors of similar pattern with which these drugs can react, and since the pattern is standardised, a fair regularity is observed as regards the action of antagonists: a systematic investigation of other drugs would probably reveal in most cases more erratic actions and antagonisms.

Pharmacology is a complex subject and there is a natural human desire to find simple general rules. Consequently once a general rule of drug antagonism has been formulated, there is a tendency to ignore awkward exceptions. Examination of the literature shows, however, that these are fairly numerous in all cases. For these reasons the author believes that the classification of drug actions according to the manner in which they are antagonised is a very uncertain method of analysis.

**(6) General Theory of Drug Antagonisms.** A consideration of the more striking examples of specific drug antagonisms shows that these in many cases follow recognisable laws, both in the case of enzymes and cells. If drug $A$ is antagonised by drug $B$, then if the concentration-action curve of drug $A$ alone follows the dissociation formula $Kx = \dfrac{y}{100 - y}$, the addition of drug $B$ does not alter the shape of the curve, but alters the value of $K$. The simplest interpretation of this fact is to suppose that drug $B$ alters either the rate of association or dissociation between drug $A$ and certain cell receptors. This antagonism by occupation of the active group can be proved to occur in the case of the antagonism by carbon monoxide of the uptake of oxygen by haemoglobin.

STEDMAN and STEDMAN (1931)[1] have advanced the hypothesis of the occupation of a common receptor by an inert compound to account for the inhibition of the activity of acetyl choline esterase by physostigmine and synthetic muscarine.

Amongst a group of allied chemical compounds, some may act as synergists and others as antagonists of a single drug, e.g. acetyl choline and $Me_3NR$ series (RAVENTOS, 1937[2]).

LOEWE's (1927)[3] results which showed that a large proportion of cycloethane amines antagonised the action of adrenaline can be interpreted by the same general hypothesis. Experiments with acetyl choline-atropine and with adrenaline-ergotoxine show, however, that in these cases it is necessary to postulate a complex receptor with which one drug can unite without displacing the other drug. The antagonist drug must be assumed to alter the receptor configuration in some manner so that either the rate of association of the antagonist drug is decreased or its rate of dissociation is increased. Even in the relatively simple

[1] STEDMAN, E., and E. STEDMAN: Biochemic. J. **25**, 1147 (1931).
[2] RAVENTOS, J.: Quart. J. exper. Physiol. **26** (1937).
[3] LOEWE, S.: Klin. Wschr. **6**, 1077 (1927).

case of enzyme poisons, the study of drug antagonisms has necessitated the similar assumption of the existence of accessory groups in the active group of the enzyme.

It appears to the writer that the most important fact shown by a study of drug antagonisms is that it is impossible to explain the remarkable effects observed except by assuming that the drugs unite with receptors of a highly specific pattern. This assumption makes a large proportion of the results intelligible and it even is possible to express the results quantitatively by simple physico-chemical formulae. No other explanation will, however, explain a tithe of the facts observed.

## Chapter 19
## Alternative Theories of Drug Action.

The hypothesis adopted by the author is that drugs which have powerful and selective actions combine with receptors in the cell, that these receptors are frequently situated on the cell surface and that the combination is frequently of a reversible character.

The chief support for this hypothesis is the similarity between the action of drugs on living cells, the action of enzyme poisons on enzymes and the combination of haemoglobin with gases. Another important fact is that this theory provides an explanation for many of the outstanding features of drug antagonism. The theory outlined above is derived from EHRLICH's theory of the action of chemotherapeutic agents.

There are, however, various alternative theories of drug action which require discussion. The following are the more important of these theories:—

(1) Monomolecular theory. (2) Potential theory of drug action. (3) Phasic theory of cell response. (4) ARNDT-SCHULZ law. (5) Explanation of all curves as expression of individual variation.

These theories have all been mentioned and discussed in various chapters of this monograph, but it is convenient to review them briefly in turn.

(1) **Monomolecular Theory.** This theory supposes that the lethal action of a drug on an organism such as a bacterium is an all-or-none process. The action produced is assumed to be due to the combination of one or a few molecules with some vital centre in the cell. The action of the drug is non-cumulative, the lethal event is equally likely to occur at any period during the exposure, and the cells show no important individual variation in the manner in which they are affected by drugs.

This theory was advanced to account for the fact that populations of cells exposed to drugs sometimes show a constant death rate, and hence the time-action curve follows the same course as a monomolecular reaction.

The objections to this theory have been stated in Chapter 12. The essential objection is that the theory involves a series of assumptions, all of which are highly improbable and many of which verge on the impossible. In general the theory is opposed to all the evidence provided by quantitative pharmacology.

The only advantage gained by accepting this theory is that it explains a certain proportion of curves of a single type, and it has been shown that this type of curve can be equally well explained by other methods which do not involve assumptions that violate probability.

The object of the present monograph is to try and explain drug actions as far as possible without postulating properties for the living cell, which are unknown in physical chemistry. The monomolecular theory, however, involves the assumption that the life of a cell depends on a single molecule.

These reasons appear to the writer to be adequate for the rejection of this theory.

**(2) The Potential Theory of Drug Action.** This theory was advanced by STRAUB to account for certain mysterious features in the action of muscarine.

STRAUB (1907)[1] found that when the *Aplysia* heart was exposed to muscarine it was arrested, but the heart recovered after a few hours although it was still in contact with the drug. The heart had acquired a tolerance to further additions of the drug. Moreover when the heart was washed out with drug-free fluid, the inhibition reappeared. These effects could also be shown with the heart of torpedo, but very little tolerance could be demonstrated with the heart of the frog.

STRAUB explained these results by the hypothesis that when a tissue is exposed to a drug it will only continue to act as long as a potential difference is maintained between the concentrations of the drug inside and outside the cells. Hence if the drug penetrates the cell, its action will gradually cease.

It is generally agreed that the theory only applies to a certain number of drugs. For example, the narcotics certainly do not produce this type of action because they can maintain an action for an indefinite period and yet penetrate cells fairly rapidly.

The theory implies that drugs, after they have penetrated the cell wall have an action different from their action outside the cell, and this has been shown to be correct in a wide variety of cases. The potential theory, however, depends chiefly upon whether it can be shown that the effect produced by a drug on a tissue ceases if during prolonged exposure the drug accumulates within the tissue.

The action of acetyl choline on such tissues as the leech muscle and the frog's heart has been studied very carefully. The drug produces a sustained action both in normal and in eserinised tissues. Relatively large quantities of acetyl choline can be extracted from the untreated frog's heart, but the evidence shows that this is fixed in some manner and is released by the process of chemical extraction (BEZNAK, 1934[2]; VARTIAINEN, 1934[3]). The response of the frog's heart to acetyl choline can therefore be explained on the assumption that any of the drug which enters the cells is fixed there in an inactive form and hence a constant potential difference is maintained. Any effects produced by adrenaline can be explained along similar lines, whether the effects be transient, constant or polyphasic.

The action of histamine on the intestine appears to be one of the best established examples of tolerance produced by constant exposure to a drug. FELDBERG and SCHILF (1930)[4] described the manner in which large doses of histamine rendered plain muscle insensitive to additional doses, and concluded that if the concentration of histamine were increased sufficiently slowly, it produced no response.

DEUTICKE (1932)[5] found, however, that a given concentration of histamine produced the same effect on a guinea pig's uterus whether it was added in a single or in four divided doses. BARSOUM and GADDUM (1935)[6] found that histamine caused a contraction of the fowl's caecum, which was followed by

[1] STRAUB, W.: Pflügers Arch. **119**, 127 (1907).
[2] BEZNAK, A. B. L.: J. of Physiol. **82**, 129 (1934).
[3] VARTIAINEN, A.: J. of Physiol. **82**, 282 (1934).
[4] FELDBERG, W., and E. SCHILF: Histamin. Berlin: Julius Springer 1930.
[5] DEUTICKE, H. J.: Pflügers Arch. **230**, 537 (1932).
[6] BARSOUM, G. S., and J. H. GADDUM: J. of Physiol. **85**, 1 (1935).

relaxation, and in this condition the muscle was insensitive to further additions of histamine, although sensitive to other drugs. A similar effect could be obtained, but much more slowly, with the guinea pig's intestine. This appears to be one of the clearest cases of a phenomenon that can most simply be interpreted as a potential action. ING and WRIGHT (1932)[1] studied the paralysis of nerve endings of the frog's sciatic by quaternary ammonium salts. They found that ammonium chloride produced paralysis which was followed by complete recovery in an hour, whilst tetramethylammonium chloride also showed recovery, but this was incomplete after four hours. These effects were seen when the drug solution was changed during the course of the experiment, and hence were not due to changes in the external concentration of the drug.

These examples suffice to show that in some cases prolonged exposure of a tissue to a constant concentration of drug results in a tolerance developing. Such effects have been very frequently described, but in the majority of cases the possibility of experimental error cannot be excluded. For example, a tissue exposed to adrenaline may recover because the drug is oxidised. There is furthermore a large literature on the effects produced by drug wash-out, a large proportion of which are probably due to the process of washing out altering either the temperature of or the tension on the tissue.

The examples selected do not appear to be subject to such errors and they can most simply be explained on the potential theory of drug action. On the other hand the study of ferment poisons shows that equally mysterious examples of development of tolerance of enzymes to poisons may occur, and these effects cannot be explained on the potential theory of drug action. For this reason the author hesitates to accept a theory, which, although it explains satisfactorily certain aspects of drug tolerance, yet on the other hand assumes that the mechanism by which drugs produce their action is of a type which cannot be related to any known physico-chemical process.

The tolerance produced by exposure to a drug can in fact be explained on the hypothesis that the drug unites with complex receptors, if EHRLICH's toxoid theory be adopted with slight modifications. Fig. 78 illustrates the nature of the explanation. It is assumed that a drug produces its specific action when it combines with two receptors (A in combination with a circle and cross). The drug can

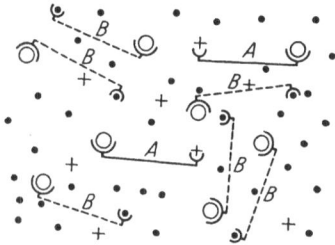

Fig. 78. Scheme of drug fixation and action. (A) Drug fixed and acting. (B) Drug fixed and occupying receptors, but not producing effect.

however combine with other receptors, in which case it does not produce its specific action (B in combination with a circle and a dot). If both these forms of combination are reversible, if the dots are more plentiful than the circles or crosses, but if both the rate of combination and of dissociation are much slower in the case of combination B than in the case of combination A, then prolonged exposure to a drug will tend gradually to produce saturation of the circles with the drug in an inert combination and hence tolerance will be produced. This hypothesis is of course wholly unproven but none of the assumptions appear to be obviously improbable.

**(3) Phasic Response of Cells.** Drugs frequently produce phasic responses in isolated tissues. The initial effect, which may be either stimulation or inhibition, disappears and the drug then produces either no action or a reversal of its initial

---

[1] ING, H. R., and W. M. WRIGHT: Proc. roy. Soc. B. **109**, 337 (1932).

effect. Such results can easily be produced by experimental error but they may occur even when adequate precautions have been taken to maintain the drug concentration constant.

These irregularities of response are not confined to living cells, for they have frequently been observed in the case of enzyme poisons. EULER and SVANBERG (1920/21)[1] found that if mercury perchloride and invertase were mixed and equal portions of the mixture were taken after various times for investigation, the activity was found to increase with the time. They compared this with the DANYSZ effect observed in immunity experiments. They explained it as due to deviation of poison by inert materials. EULER and MYRBÄCK (1923)[2] found that no self-regeneration occurred when pure saccharase was poisoned with metallic salts. Since, however, the amount of silver fixed by pure urease is ten times as much as is needed to inactivate the enzyme (SUMNER and MYRBÄCK, 1930[3]), this distinction between partly purified and pure ferments is unlikely to be a general law. MYRBÄCK (1926)[4] showed that self-regeneration of invertase and mercuric chloride could be intensified by addition of gelatin to the mixture. EULER and WALLES (1924)[5] found very marked self-regeneration when they studied the inactivation of saccharase in the living yeast cell by means of silver nitrate. The time relations of self-regeneration by deviation are noteworthy. MYRBÄCK (1926)[4] found that mercuric chloride was inactivated by sodium cyanide too rapidly for measurement. If, however, invertase was poisoned with mercuric chloride and cyanide was added subsequently, then the full regeneration of activity took 30 minutes.

These examples show that a simple enzyme poison such as mercury or silver will only maintain a constant action on an enzyme if the conditions are the simplest possible. If any substance is present that can cause deviation, this will occur. The deviation will, however, occur slowly even when a substance such as cyanide is added, which is capable of combining with free mercury at a rate that is practically instantaneous.

Since it is difficult to maintain the action of an enzyme poison on an enzyme at a constant intensity, it is not surprising that phasic responses are frequently found with living cells. The ideal response of an isolated tissue to a drug would be an immediate change in the activity of the tissue and thereafter no alteration in activity for as long as the concentration of the drug was maintained unaltered. Needless to say, such responses are rare exceptions and prolonged exposure to a drug usually results either in intensification of the action or else a partial or even a complete recovery; these variations are often termed phasic actions.

The ideal tissue would show a constant response during exposure to the drug and when the drug was removed would simply return to a normal level of activity. This again is a relatively rare event and all kinds of effects are recorded in the literature as a consequence of washing out. The literature on phasic actions and effects of wash-out is very extensive, but much of it is unsatisfactory. It is a difficult matter to maintain a perfectly constant concentration of drug and still more difficult to remove the drug from the tissue without producing any other change. A few of the more obvious and commoner errors are as follows.

Acetylcholine is destroyed by esterase and unless this esterase is inhibited by physostigmine, the concentration of a solution of acetylcholine in contact with

[1] EULER, H. VON, and SVANBERG: Fermentforsch. **3**, 330 (1920/21).
[2] EULER, H. VON, and K. MYRBÄCK: Z. exper. Med. **33**, 483 (1923).
[3] SUMNER, J. B., and K. MYRBÄCK: Hoppe-Seylers Z. **189**, 218 (1930).
[4] MYRBÄCK, K.: Hoppe-Seylers Z. **158**, 160 (1926).
[5] EULER, H. VON, and E. WALLES: Hoppe-Seylers Z. **132**, 167 (1924).

a tissue will decrease steadily. Apart from this acetylcholine decomposes in weakly alkaline watery solution and this may be an important source of error when high dilutions are employed. Similarly adrenaline is rapidly oxidised in high dilutions and it is difficult to maintain around a piece of isolated gut a uniform concentration of adrenaline. BACQ (1936)[1] has shown in the intact animal that while adrenaline in small doses produces a transient effect on the normal animal, yet if reducing agents such as hydroxyhydroquinone be previously administered, adrenaline produces a long continued response. In the case of isolated organs, FRITZ (1928)[2] showed that many of the phasic and wash-out effects described with adrenaline were due to experimental errors. PRASAD (1936)[3] arranged conditions such that the isolated gut would continue to contract regularly for long periods when deprived of oxygen. He found that adrenaline produced an action of indefinite duration under these anaerobic conditions. These results show that oxidation of adrenaline is the chief factor in terminating its action upon isolated tissues.

The examples of adrenaline and of acetylcholine have been considered specially because these drugs have been the subject of intensive experiment. The general impression of the author is that many if not the majority of so-called phasic actions disappear when the experimental conditions are satisfactory.

Wash-out experiments are peculiarly subject to error because the usual method of emptying a bath results in a gross change both in temperature and in the tension on the preparation. All kinds of wash-out effects have been described, but the majority of these can be eliminated by adequate care in experimental technique.

Apart from gross errors of the type indicated above, there are special errors associated with the peculiarities of muscle. WINTON (1930)[4] showed that the course of contraction of the retractor penis indicated the existence of at least two mechanisms, one which resembled an undamped elastic spring, and one which showed high viscosity. Adrenaline caused increase of tonus but at the same time produced a speeding up of relaxation due to a load. With a system as complex as this, it would be fairly easy to arrange conditions such that the addition of adrenaline would cause a diphasic effect.

NANDA (1931)[5] showed that by varying the mechanical conditions the response of the isolated gut to drugs such as adrenaline and acetylcholine could be made to appear either as a more or less uniform response terminated by wash-out or alternatively as a transient response which returned to normal and finally showed a second response on washing out. The mechanical response of skeletal muscle also may show curious irregularities. For example the addition of 0.04 mol KCl to the rectus abdominis muscle when measured under isotonic conditions produces a slow contraction which is maintained for a considerable period, but isometric measurements show a quick rise of tension followed by a fairly rapid fall (fig. 32). In this case the one method of measurement indicates that potassium chloride produces a continued effect and the other method that it produces a much more rapid and temporary action.

Another type of error is dependent on the fact that a change in the condition of an isolated tissue may cause a series of changes, some of which are rapid and others slow. For example, asphyxiation of an isolated frog's heart in contact

[1] BACQ, Z. M.: Arch. int. Physiol. **42**, 340 (1936).
[2] FRITZ, G.: Pflügers Arch. **220**, 495 (1928).
[3] PRASAD, B. N.: J. of Physiol. **86**, 425 (1936).
[4] WINTON, F. R.: J. Physiol. **69**, 393 (1930).
[5] NANDA, T. C.: J. Pharmacol. Baltimore **42**, 9 (1931).

with a small amount of perfusion fluid causes an immediate slight diminution in response associated with the change from aerobic to anaerobic activity, and this is followed by much slower changes due to the accumulation of lactic acid causing a change in the reaction of the perfusion fluid.

Some of the errors associated with experiments on isolated tissues have been indicated above, but with intact animals, the number of uncontrolled variables is much greater, and in the latter case it is unlikely that the administration of a drug will produce a change in activity that will remain constant for any length of time.

RENTZ (1929, 1930)[1] made an exhaustive study of the phasic actions of drugs and particularly of the action of local anaesthetics upon frogs' blood vessels. He concluded that plain muscles very frequently gave complex polyphasic responses to drugs. His general conclusion (1930) was that there was a natural tendency of living tissues to respond to any sudden change in conditions by wave-like opposed processes succeeding each other.

The phasic theory of drug action is indeed little more than the statement of the fact that when a drug acts on a living cell, the complexity of the organisation makes it unlikely that a constant response will be obtained. This statement is undoubtedly in accordance with observed facts, but it is rather a statement of experimental difficulties than a possible basis for any theory of drug action.

(4) ARNDT-SCHULZ Law. This law states that any drug which causes stimulation at low concentrations will cause inhibition at high concentrations. This law is in accordance with homoeopathic doctrines and hence has maintained a certain popularity. The law is true in so far that nearly all drugs if given in sufficiently high dosage or concentration will produce injury or death in living cells.

The chief objection to the law is that it is obviously untrue in the case of most drugs that have been studied carefully. For example, acetyl choline produces graded responses over a more than 1000 fold range of concentration on the frog's heart and rectus abdominis. Over the whole of this range it inhibits the heart and causes contracture of the rectus abdominis.

Many of the effects which appear to support this law have found simple explanations. For example a small concentration of cyanide may benefit an organism or isolated organ in a solution made up with metal-distilled water because the cyanide inactivates the traces of metal present. In the case of lethal agents acting on small organisms, a partial destruction of the population may accelerate the growth of the survivors, because the dead bodies provide food for the latter.

The complex phasic responses that are often produced by drugs have already been discussed, and it is of course easy to find amongst these examples which support the ARNDT-SCHULZ law. There seems, however, no more reason to pay more attention to those cases in which stimulation is followed by inhibition than to the cases where inhibition is followed by stimulation.

(5) Drug Responses as Expression of Individual Variation. This hypothesis which was discussed in Chapter 14 is almost impossible to disprove. All populations of living cells vary extensively and the variation in response to drugs frequently has a markedly skew distribution. Since a wide variety of distributions of variation can be demonstrated, it is easy to proceed a step further and to say that all measured responses of cells to drugs are expressions of cell variation.

---

[1] RENTZ, E.: Arch. f. exper. Path. **141**, 173 (1929) — On Phasic Introductory and Release Effects of the Cocaine group etc. Inaug. Dissert. Riga 1930.

The objection to this hypothesis is that it is so unfruitful, since, if the response to drugs is attributed to a peculiarity of living tissue, there is no means of linking up such responses with the known laws of physical chemistry.

The writer has shown that it is possible, although sometimes difficult, to explain the skew distributions of variation which are so frequently observed as being due to a variation symmetrically distributed over an ordinary range which has been distorted and spread out by a logarithmic relation. The frequency of non-linear relations, which often approximate to logarithmic relations, in hetero-geneous systems is assumed to be the reason for the frequency with which skew variations of a similar type are observed in a wide variety of the responses of cells to drugs.

(6) WEBER-FECHNER Law. WEBER discovered that the response of a sense organ increased by arithmetic progression when the stimulus was increased by geometric progression, and that consequently there was a linear relation between the response and the logarithm of the stimulus. It has been shown that this same relation very commonly occurs over a considerable proportion of the total curve relating the concentration or dose of a drug with the response of a tissue or animal. A number of workers have noticed this fact and have concluded that drug responses followed the WEBER-FECHNER law.

During recent years it has been shown that the WEBER-FECHNER law does not express fully the stimulus-sensation relation in the eye. HECHT (1931)[1] showed that the complete curve resembled a dissociation curve and explained it on the theory that light acting on the retina caused the formation of an unstable chemical substance, which stimulated the nerve. This explanation accords with modern theories of humoral transmission.

The general resemblance between the relations of stimulus and sensation and of drug concentration and cell response can be explained on the hypothesis that in both cases the effect is due to the formation of some reversible chemical reaction.

It must be mentioned, however, that in the case of light acting on the retina, there is a doubt as to how far the curves relating stimulus and effect express a physico-chemical process and to what extent they are modified by individual variation of the receptors.

The statement that drug action follows the WEBER-FECHNER law cannot, however, be considered a reasoned explanation of drug action since it merely states a resemblance between two sets of phenomena, without advancing an explanation for either.

(7) Discussion. A consideration of the various theories which have been advanced to account for the mode of action of drugs on cells, shows that in most cases these theories are unsatisfactory, because they postulate peculiarities in the organisation of cells of a character unknown in physical-chemistry. Hence they close rather than open avenues for further research.

The evidence collected in this monograph shows that a surprisingly large proportion of the phenomena of drug action can be accounted for by the ordinary laws of physical chemistry. It is necessary to recognise clearly that there are many phenomena that cannot at present be explained by these laws, but it seems preferable to admit the present limits of knowledge rather than to cloak our ignorance by postulating inexplicable properties for living cells.

The alternative theory of drug action which attributes all relations to individual variation is to some extent exempt from the criticism that it is completely

[1] HECHT, S.: Erg. Physiol. **32**, 243 (1931).

unfruitful, because it emphasises the fact that all relations obtained with living cells must be modified by individual variation.

The study of the response of cells to drugs is the study of the action of a chemical on a coarsely heterogeneous system, the units of which show extensive variation. It appears to the author that the chief present need of quantitative pharmacology is more detailed knowledge regarding the physico-chemical laws operative in such a system.

## Chapter 20

## Quantitative Aspects of Chemotherapy.

(1) Introduction. Chemotherapy is a subject of such great therapeutic importance that it deserves special consideration. Its position in relation to general pharmacology is peculiar and indeed somewhat exasperating. In the first place it may be said that EHRLICH, working on the general theory of drug action which has been followed in this article, obtained practical successes, so brilliant and important that they initiated a new science, namely that of the treatment of parasitic infections by the use of synthetic organic compounds. This line of research has during the last quarter century made numerous advances of the greatest importance to humanity. This history would suggest that chemotherapeutic results should provide basic evidence for any theory of the action of drugs based on quantitative studies. Unfortunately, however, the history of chemotherapy has repeatedly shown the curious paradox that theories which have provided brilliant practical successes have subsequently been shown to be incorrect. Chemotherapy has in fact developed as an empirical science and until recent years little has been known for certain regarding the mode of action of chemotherapeutic agents on organisms. The study of the mode of action of an organic arsenical on trypanosomes involves a whole range of difficult problems, such for instance as to whether the host activates the drug, the factors on which drug tolerance of the organism depends, etc. For these reasons it has seemed preferable to the author to treat this important but difficult problem separately and to defer its consideration until the end of this article.

The chief reason why empirical knowledge in chemotherapy developed so much more rapidly than did theoretical knowledge is that the earlier chemotherapeutic research was concerned with the action produced by drugs when injected into infected animals. This method gave satisfactory practical results, but the number of unknown factors in such a system was too great to permit much advance in knowledge regarding the mode of action of the drugs used.

The rate of growth of a trypanosome population in a rat represents the algebraic sum of the rate of growth of the organisms and the rate of their destruction by the defence mechanisms of the body. The introduction of a drug alters this rate of growth in a manner that can be measured accurately, but the alteration may be due to a number of causes, e.g. direct lethal action on the organism by the drug, lethal action on the organism by the drug after this has been altered by the host, action of drug in stimulating defence mechanisms of the host, etc. These factors led to the curiously irregular development of chemotherapy that has already been noted.

Techniques for the measurement of the intensity of drug action have been developed to a high level of accuracy, and these methods have been used to test thousands of compounds. Brilliant practical successes have been obtained but relatively little advance has been made in the solution of the fundamental problem as to the manner in which chemotherapeutic agents kill organisms.

Similarly the tolerance that organisms can acquire for drugs can be measured fairly accurately, but there is still an unsettled controversy regarding the elementary problem as to whether or not an organism fixes a drug for which it has acquired tolerance.

Chemotherapy therefore is an imposing edifice, the foundations of which are hidden and unknown. It may indeed be said that most of the exact knowledge regarding the fundamental problems of chemotherapy has been provided by researches on the action of drugs on trypanosomes in vitro, a subject for which a satisfactory technique has only been developed in recent years.

The great practical importance of chemotherapy has caused the subject to develop into a special branch of medical science with an extensive literature. Considerations of space forbid any attempt to give a general review of such a science, but certain special points will be considered which are of interest in relation to the general problem of the mode in which drugs act on cells.

Chemotherapeutic agents can be divided into the metallic compounds and the non-metallic compounds and it is convenient to consider these two classes separately.

(2) **Action of Metallic Compounds.** (a) *Action on Enzymes.* The action of heavy metals on enzymes was considered in Chapter 6. They may be regarded as general enzyme poisons since they act on a large number of enzymes. Their action can be interpreted as being due to the formation of a reversible compound between the metal and the active group of the enzyme. Although reversible these compounds have a very low dissociation coefficient and hence the heavy metals may produce measurable effects on enzyme activity at dilutions of the order of $10^{-9}$ molar. The chief factor limiting the activity of heavy metals is the ease with which they are deviated by combination with impurities present in enzyme solutions.

The toxic action of arsenic compounds on enzymes is more restricted than is that of the heavy metals. HEFFTER and KEESER (1927)[1] mention for instance that $As_2O_3$ in concentrations as high as 0.4 per cent. does not inhibit erepsin, pancreatic diastase and various other ferments. On the other hand, inorganic arsenites have a powerful action in inhibiting autolysis and can produce this effect at a concentration of 1 in 100,000.

RONA and his co-workers examined the action of various arsenic compounds on a number of enzymes and found that the relations were extremely complex. For example 10 mg. p. 100 c.c. sodium arsenite did not affect maltase, nor did 2 mg. of atoxyl, whilst 3 mg. methyl arsinoxide produced 50 per cent. inhibition. Methyl arsinoxide in a concentration as high as 0.3 g. p. 100 c.c. did not, however, inhibit invertase, whilst atoxyl also had no action on invertase but inhibited liver lipase in a concentration of 0.0002 mg. per 100 c.c. Serum lipase was however much less sensitive (RONA, AIRILA and LASNITZKI, 1922[2]). RONA and HAAS (1923)[3] found that the concentration-action relation of atoxyl acting on kidney lipase followed the dissociation curve shown in fig. 79. RONA and GYORGYI (1920)[4] found that arsenious acid and atoxyl had no action on Soya bean urease, whilst methyl, phenyl and diphenyl arsenoxide produced powerful inhibitory effects.

[1] HEFFTER, A., and E. KEESER: Heffters Handb. exper. Pharmakol. **3**, 463 (1927).
[2] RONA, P., V. AIRILA and A. LASNITZKI: Biochem. Z. **130**, 582 (1922).
[3] RONA, P., and H. E. HAAS: Biochem. Z. **141**, 222 (1923).
[4] RONA, P., and P. GYÖRGYI: Biochem. Z. **111**, 115 (1920).

These examples suffice to show that arsenical compounds have a highly selective toxic action on enzymes. The concentration-action relations (fig. 79) suggest the formation of a reversible compound with the active group.

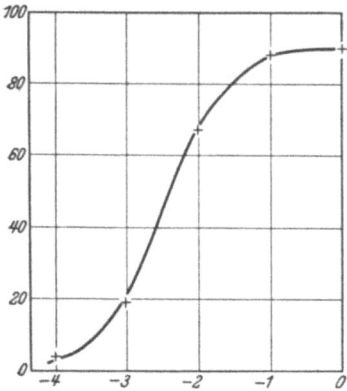

In general pentavalent arsenicals both inorganic and organic have a much weaker action on enzymes than have trivalent arsenicals.

(b) *General Action on Living Cells.* The powerful lethal action produced by heavy metals on all forms of living cells was discussed in Chapter 6. The results suggested that at least two separate processes could be recognised, namely:— (a) adsorption of metal on cell surface; (b) penetration of cell by metal.

It was shown that the so-called oligodynamic action depended on the fact that many forms of cells in presence of watery solutions of metallic salts adsorbed metals so that the concentration of metal on the cell surface was thousands of times greater than the concentration in solution. The variation in the rate of poisoning of free living bacteria and of spores illustrates the manner in which the toxic actions

Fig. 79. Action of atoxyl on kidney lipase. Abscissa:— log. conc. atoxyl (mg. per 28 c.c.). Ordinate:— per cent. inhibition. Curve drawn to formula
$$kx = y/90 - y.$$
(RONA and HAAS, 1923[1].)

of metals are modified by differences in the case of penetration.

The exact manner in which heavy metals kill cells is unknown, but in many cases the amounts adsorbed are sufficient to produce general injury to the cell protoplasm and it is not necessary to assume any form of selective poisoning of enzymes.

The action of arsenicals on cells is more complex than that of heavy metals. Arsenious acid has a strong toxic action on most forms of plant life. There are certain striking exceptions to this general rule, since *Mucor mucedo* and *Penicillium glaucum* will grow on moist arsenious acid. CHATIN in 1845 showed that cryptogams were more sensitive than phanerogams and that monocotyledonous plants were more sensitive than dicotyledenous. BRENCHLEY (1927)[2] measured the action of sodium arsenite on the growth of barley seedlings and showed that in some cases a measurable effect was produced by a dilution of 1 part in $2.5 \times 10^8$. Her figures show a graded action over at least a 100 fold range of concentrations. She also found that 1 part of sodium arsenate in $10^5$ produced no effect on the growth of barley plants.

The sharp distinction between arsenates and arsenites is seen therefore with plants as well as with animal cells.

FRIEDBERGER and JOACHIMOGLU (1917)[3] found that sodium arsenite in relatively high concentrations (0.1 per cent.) inhibited the fermentation of yeast, and MEIER (1926)[4] obtained similar results. ARXMACHER (1936)[5] found that atoxyl did not affect the fermentation of yeast cells or of cell free extracts of yeast.

MEIER (1927)[6] measured the action of arsenious oxide and of methyl arsenoxide on the respiration of goose erythrocytes. In both cases 50 per cent. inhibition was produced by concentrations between 1 in 10,000 and 1 in 100,000 and the concentration-action relations approximated to a dissociation curve.

[1] RONA, P., and H. E. HAAS: Biochem. Z. **141**, 222 (1923).
[2] BRENCHLEY, W. M.: Inorganic Plant Poisons, 2nd Ed. Cambridge: Univ. Press 1927.
[3] FRIEDBERGER, E., and G. JOACHIMOGLU: Biochem. Z. **79**, 135 (1917).
[4] MEIER, R.: Biochem. Z. **174**, 384 (1926).
[5] ARXMACHER, FR.: Arch. f. exper. Path. **180**, 142 (1936).
[6] MEIER, R.: Arch. f. exper. Path. **122**, 129 (1927).

VOEGTLIN (1925)[1] put forward the general theory that the toxic action of arsenic was due to it causing the inactivation of gluthathione, the reaction proceeding according to the following equation

$$2(\text{RSH}) + \text{RAs} + \text{O} = \text{RAs}\Big\langle{}^{\text{SR}}_{\text{SR}} + \text{H}_2\text{O}.$$

Arsenical compounds react with gluthathione in vitro, but the function of gluthathione in cell metabolism is still uncertain and hence this attractive hypothesis cannot be regarded as fully established. Moreover it must be remembered that arsenic compounds exert a toxic action at high dilutions on other enzymes, e.g. liver lipase.

Iodo-acetic acid is another toxic substance which is believed to inactivate gluthathione; and SMYTHE and REINER (1933)[2] compared the actions of arsenic and of iodo-acetic acid on trypanosomes. They concluded that it was difficult to account for the effects observed on the simple hypothesis that the toxic agents produced their effect by inactivating glutathione.

The actions of arsenic derivatives that have been described show that these have a very wide action, since they poison plants as well as animals in low concentrations. On the other hand the actions are extremely selective since some compounds poison some cells in high dilutions whilst other combinations produce no effect. In all cases, however, pentavalent arsenicals have a weaker action than have trivalent arsenicals.

(c) *Action on Trypanosomes and Spirochaetes.* The course of development of chemotherapeutic knowledge is exemplified by the history of the use of mercury in syphilis, since the curative action of this metal was discovered 400 years before the cause of the disease was recognised. Early experiments on the action of mercury salts on spirochaetes in vitro increased the mystery regarding their mode of action since it was found that concentrations of the order of 1 part of mercury perchloride in 1000 were needed to produce rapid destruction of the parasites, and similar paradoxical results were obtained with most other chemotherapeutic agents.

Improvements in chemical technique and in methods of cultivation of organisms have in recent years yielded results which provide a basis for a working hypothesis regarding the chemotherapeutic action of metallic compounds.

PAPAMARKU (1927)[3] showed that, provided a period of exposure of 24 to 48 hours was allowed, trypanosomes and spirochaetes could be killed in vitro by organic arsenicals at a dilution of 1 part in 1 million, and that the same was true in the case of acridine derivatives. He noted that trypanosomes were more readily killed than spirochaetes and found an extraordinary difference in the case of tartar emetic which killed trypanosomes in a dilution of 1 in 30 million but did not kill spirochaetes in a concentration of 1 in 300.

The action of metallic agents on trypanosomes in vitro has been reviewed by YORKE (1932, 1934)[4], and he mentions the following outstanding facts.

Experiments with trypanosomes in vitro show that although agents such as neosalvarsan produce no rapid effect, yet if the exposure be continued for 24 to 48 hours the drug will produce a lethal action at a dilution of 1 part in $10^8$. Furthermore it can be shown in such experiments that measurable quantities of arsenic are fixed by the organisms (REINER, LEONARD and CHAO, 1932[5])

[1] VOEGTLIN, C.: Physiologic. Rev. **5**, 63 (1925).
[2] SMYTHE, C. V., and L. REINER: Proc. Soc. exper. Biol. a. Med. **31**, 289 (1933).
[3] PAPAMARKU, P.: Z. Hyg. **107**, 407 (1927).
[4] YORKE, W.: Brit. med. J. **1932 II**, 668 — Arch. Schiffs- u. Tropenhyg. **38**, 55 (1934).
[5] REINER, L., C. S. LEONARD and S. S. CHAO: Arch. int. Pharmacodyn. **43**, 186 (1932).

Experiments on trypanosomes in vivo have shown that in this case also the parasites fix arsenicals (SINGER and FISCHL, 1935[1]).

In the case of experimental rabbit syphilis, LEVADITI and MANIN (1927)[2] showed that infection did not occur when the tissues contained 1 part per $10^6$ of bismuth. In the case of human syphilis, a mercurial cure produces a similar concentration in the blood.

The action of chemotherapeutic agents can therefore be interpreted as being a slow action that is produced by high dilutions of the drug. Moreover there is evidence that the drug is directly fixed by the parasite.

The results obtained in vitro and in vivo still show certain discrepancies, but it has frequently been noted that chemotherapeutic agents in dilutions which are insufficient to kill trypanosomes may nevertheless render them incapable of producing infection. This suggests that the first effect produced by the drug is either to render the parasite incapable of multiplication or to reduce its resistance to the defence mechanisms of the host.

It may be said therefore that the mode of action of metallic chemotherapeutic agents is no longer a mystery but has been brought into line with other actions of metals such as the poisoning of enzymes and their "oligodynamic" action on cells. The primary action in all cases is a selective adsorption of the metal by the enzyme or organism.

Experiments with trypanosomes in vitro have incidentally explained a puzzling result which was obtained at the commencement of chemotherapeutic research. The first effective trypanocidal arsenical agent to be discovered was the pentavalent compound soamin and this result suggested that trypanosomes differed from all other living cells in that they were more susceptible to pentavalent than to trivalent arsenicals.

Experiments with trypanosomes in vitro have however shown that pentavalent arsenicals have little or no toxic action upon these organisms, and the effects produced by these compounds in vivo must be due to their reduction to the trivalent form.

YORKE and MURGATROYD (1930)[3] working with *Tr. rhodesiense* showed that pentavalent organic arsenicals were inactive in vitro since the minimal lethal concentration was about 1 part in 1600, whereas when these drugs were reduced to the trivalent state they acted in a dilution of 1 part in 200 million. LEVADITI and CONSTANTINESCO (1932)[4] also showed that pentavalent arsenicals were much less toxic than trivalent arsenicals not only to trypanosomes in vitro but also to spermatozoa and to cells in tissue culture. They found also that neoarsphenamine had a much feebler action on spirochaetes than on trypanosomes. Trivalent organic arsenicals such as neoarsphenamine acted in a dilution of about 1 in 100 million, whilst sodium arsenite acted at a dilution of 1 in 5 million. In the case of organic arsenicals, the concentration required to kill spirochaetes (S. recurrens) was about 10 times that needed to kill trypanosomes.

Their results show also that the action of the drugs is a fairly sharp all-or-none effect. After any particular period of exposure (e.g. 8 hours) the concentration of arsenical which produces a high mortality (95 to 100 per cent.) is only about 4 times as great as the concentration which produces a just measurable mortality (less than 1.0 per cent.).

[1] SINGER, E., and V. FISCHL: Z. Hyg. **116**, 36 (1935).
[2] LEVADITI, C., and Y. MANIN: C. r. Soc. Biol. Paris **97**, 655, 1687 (1927).
[3] YORKE, W., and F. MURGATROYD: Ann. trop. Med. **24**, 449 (1930).
[4] LEVADITI, C., and N. CONSTANTINESCO: C. r. Soc. Biol. Paris **109**, 283 (1932).

These results agree in showing that only trivalent arsenicals are active trypanocides in vitro. The figures do not show any obvious difference in rate of action between inorganic arsenites and trivalent organic arsenicals.

Various workers have made quantitative studies of the uptake of arsenic by trypanosomes. REINER, LEONARD and CHAO (1932[1]) found that there was a sharp distinction between pentavalent and trivalent organic arsenicals. They exposed *Tr. equiperdum* to arsenical solutions for 30 mins. and obtained the results shown in Table 28. These results show that pentavalent organic arsenicals are not fixed by trypanosomes, whereas fixation occurs with trivalent organic arsenicals.

Table 28. Fixation of arsenic by Trypanosomum equiperdum.
(REINER, LEONARD and CHAO, 1932[1].)

| Drug | Concentration in solution g. atoms of arsenic per 10⁴ litres | Micrograms of arsenic fixed by 10¹⁰ trypanosomes |
|---|---|---|
| Sodium aminarsonate (soamin) . . . . . . | 50 | trace |
| Arsenoxide . . . . . . . . . . . . . . | 0.33 | 20 |
| Neoarsphenamine | | |
| (a) Normal strain of trypanosomes | | |
| (I) alive. . . . . . . . . . . . . . | 0.85—4.1 | 13.5 |
| (II) dead . . . . . . . . . . . . | 2.5 —4.1 | 66 |
| (b) Resistant strain of trypanosomes. . . | 2.4 —10.2 | 13.4 |

LEVADITI (1909)[2] concluded that atoxyl was activated by the liver, and the activation of this drug by red blood corpuscles has been demonstrated by TERRY (1912, 1915)[3] and by LOURIE, MURGATROYD and YORKE (1935)[4].

The results shown in Table 28 demonstrate certain interesting points concerning the mode of action of trivalent arsenicals. They show that dead trypanosomes fix much more arsenic than do live trypanosomes. This explains the rapid increase in fixation of arsenicals which occurs when lethal concentrations are approached. The results indicate a rapid adsorption of the arsenic followed by some slower toxic process which finally causes a breakdown of the cell resistance and also results in the fixation of relatively large amounts of arsenic by the dead cell. The process therefore bears a striking resemblance to the disinfectant action of heavy metals upon yeast or upon bacteria.

The authors calculate that the volume of a trypanosome is about $10^{-10}$ cu.cm. and that its surface is $10^{-6}$ sq.cm. The average amount of arsenic bound they take as 0.1 micro equivalents per $10^{10}$ trypanosomes. On the assumption that each molecule of the phenyl arsenious oxide type occupies 300 sq $A$ ($3 \times 10^{-14}$ sq. cm.) they calculate that the surface of a trypanosome would be occupied by $3 \times 10^7$ molecules arranged in a monomolecular layer. This is five to ten times the amount found and hence the figures show that the amount of arsenic bound is only sufficient to cover one tenth of the surface of a trypanosome. The amount of arsenic adsorbed by dead trypanosomes is of the order of that required to cover the surface with a monomolecular layer.

As regards the intensity of adsorption, their figures show that not more than 5 p.c. of the arsenic present in solutions of neoarsphenamine was fixed by the trypanosomes and that the concentration in the solution and in the trypanosomes

---

[1] REINER, L., C. S. LEONARD and S. S. CHAO: Arch. int. Pharmacodyn. **43**, 186 (1932).
[2] LEVADITI, C.: Ann. Inst. Pasteur **33**, 604 (1909).
[3] TERRY, B. T.: Proc. Soc. exper. Biol. a. Med. **9**, 41 (1912) — J. of exper. Med. **21**, 258 (1915).
[4] LOURIE, E. M., F. MURGATROYD and W. YORKE: Ann. trop. Med. **29**, 265 (1935).

was similar (10—20 $\gamma$ per c.c.). In the case of arsenoxide, however, the adsorption was much more intense. The amount fixed was 40 to 50 per cent. of the total present and the final concentrations were 1 $\gamma$ per c.c. in solution and 20 $\gamma$ per c.c. in the trypanosomes.

The activation of pentavalent arsenicals by the host has been proved with some certainty, and similar theories have been advanced in relation to other metallic compounds. VOEGTLIN (1925)[1] observed that arsenious acid when injected intravenously produced an immediate reduction in the trypanosomes in the blood stream, whereas neoarsphenamine acted after a latent period of some hours. He concluded that the drug was changed to a more active form. The *in vitro* results prove that the activation by the host is not necessary in the case of trivalent organic arsenicals, but the long period of exposure before any action occurs suggests the possibility that the drug is activated after it has been fixed by the parasites.

LEVADITI believes that drugs such as bismuth are activated by the host by conversion into some lipoid soluble compound.

The results quoted show with some certainty that the primary stage in the action of arsenicals upon trypanosomes is the fixation of the drug on the surface of the organism, and that only trivalent arsenicals are thus fixed. The fixation is not a simple adsorption since dead organisms fix much more of the drug than do living organisms. The chief point of uncertainty is the form in which the drugs are fixed, and whether they act in the form in which they are introduced or whether they are metabolised to some active form. The results obtained with arsenicals acting on trypanosomes *in vitro* make doubtful some of the forms of activation that have been postulated, but show that activation does occur in certain cases.

**(3) Action of Non-metallic Compounds.** Many of the non-metallic chemo-therapeutic agents are dyes and this fact has facilitated the study of their mode of action. GONDER (1912)[2] showed that the dye oxazin first stained trypanosomes and that death followed the staining. YORKE (1934)[3] showed that trypaflavine killed trypanosomes *in vitro* in a dilution of 4 parts per $10^8$.

In the case of dyes as in the case of metal compounds the *in vitro* and *in vivo* experiments in some cases show paradoxical results. For instance germanin is four times as effective against *Tr. rhodesiense in vivo* as is trypaflavine, but *in vitro* germanin is inert (YORKE, 1934[3]). This effect may reasonably be attribut-ed to the activation of germanin by the host.

HAWKING (1934)[4] showed that, both *in vitro* and *in vivo*, acriflavine was adsorbed by Tr. rhodesiense. The experiments *in vivo* showed that, when the dye concentration in the blood was 0.05 per cent., the concentration in the parasites was 20 times as great (1 per cent.).

SINGER, FISCHL et al. (1935)[5] studied the action of various fluorescent parasit-ocidal dyes and showed that these were fixed by such parasites as trypanosomes and plasmodia. For example they demonstrated the fixation of atebrin by parasites of bird malaria.

OSTERLIN (1936)[6] put forward the interesting suggestion that the activity of malaricidal dyes was associated with fluorescence. He suggested that the presence

[1] VOEGTLIN, C.: Physiologic. Rev. **5**, 63 (1925).
[2] GONDER: Z. Immun.forsch. **15**, 257 (1912).
[3] YORKE, W.: Arch. Schiffs- u. Tropenhyg. **38**, 55 (1934).
[4] HAWKING, F.: Ann. trop. Med. **28**, 67 (1934).
[5] SINGER, E., V. FISCHL et al.: Z. Hyg. **116**, 133, 138 and 683 (1935).
[6] OSTERLIN, M.: Klin. Wschr. **15**, 1719 (1936).

of a strongly basic group was necessary for the fixation of the dye and that the subsequent lethal action was associated with the properties causing fluorescence. This interesting hypothesis is mentioned as an example of the lines of advance that at present are being explored in chemotherapy. The fixation of the agent by the trypanosome is now generally assumed and the problems that are now being attacked are the manner in which the drugs produce their toxic effects on the parasites and the factors influencing the resistance of the parasites.

(4) **Drug-resistance.** Tolerance to chemotherapeutic agents may be either natural or acquired. The natural specific variation of organisms as regards susceptibility to chemotherapeutic agents is an outstanding feature of chemotherapy. Although this problem has been studied exhaustively, yet very few general rules have been discovered, and in most cases the reason why a drug kills one species of organism and not another is completely unknown.

The power of trypanosomes to acquire resistance to drugs was discovered soon after the commencement of chemotherapeutic research (EHRLICH, 1907[1]) and it has been found that drug resistance can be produced both to metallic and to non-metallic agents. YORKE (1934)[2] has given a systematic review of this subject and the following points amongst his conclusions are of particular interest.

The tolerance that can be produced is remarkable as regards its extent. For example the concentrations of reduced tryparsamide needed to kill tolerant and normal *Tr. rhodesiense* are 10 parts and 0.04 parts per million respectively, which is a 250 fold difference. The tolerance is not sharply specific for YORKE found that if tolerance was induced for either organic arsenicals or trypaflavine, the organism became resistant to both agents. Such organisms were not resistant to germanin and organisms made germanin-tolerant acquired no tolerance for the other drugs. The nature of this striking tolerance is however still a matter of doubt.

EHRLICH (1909)[3] concluded that dye-resistant organisms were not stained, and on this fact he based his theory of chemotherapeutic action. This has been confirmed by many workers subsequently.

In the case of arsenicals, YORKE found that drug-resistant parasites did not fix arsenic and this has been confirmed by other workers. PEDLOW and REINER (1935)[4] found, however, that arsenic resistant trypanosomes *in vitro* fixed the same amount of arsenic as did normal parasites, although *in vivo* they fixed a somewhat smaller amount. The arsenic resistant parasites *in vitro* fixed slightly less acriflavine than did normal parasites, but *in vivo* the arsenic resistant parasites fixed much less acriflavine than did normal parasites. FELDT (1934)[5] found that the binding of arsenic *in vivo* was the same with normal and with resistant parasites.

There is therefore an unsettled controversy as regards experimental fact concerning this question, which is of fundamental importance in any theory of drug-resistance. FISCHL and SINGER (1935)[6] showed that dyes were fixed equally well by species of parasites which they killed and by species on which they produced no effect. This shows that the action of chemotherapeutic agents must depend on at least two separable factors, firstly, fixation, and secondly, the toxic action produced after fixation.

[1] EHRLICH, P.: Berl. klin. Wschr. **44**, 233 (1907).
[2] YORKE, W.: Arch. Schiffs- u. Tropenhyg. **38**, 55 (1934).
[3] EHRLICH, P.: Münch. med. Wschr. **56**, 217 (1909).
[4] PEDLOW, J. T., and L. REINER: J. Pharmacol. Baltimore **55**, 179 (1935).
[5] FELDT, A.: Zbl. Bakter. I Orig. **131**, 137 (1934).
[6] FISCHL, V., and E. SINGER: Z. Hyg. **116**, 348 (1935).

As regards the nature of acquired drug resistance, one striking feature is the firmness with which it is retained through thousands of generations after it has once been established. EHRLICH (1907)[1] and BROWNING (1907)[2] noted this fact which has been confirmed repeatedly.

The ease with which tolerance can be established varies greatly with different drugs. Tolerance to organic arsenicals is easy to induce, tolerance to germanin is difficult to induce, and no certain tolerance can be induced to inorganic arsenic or antimony.

The production of tolerance involves selective destruction of a variable population over an enormous number of generations, and the process appears to be the establishment of a new type by the selective destruction of all susceptible individuals. There is therefore no close connection between the drug resistance acquired by trypanosomes and the resistance acquired by an animal to a drug such as morphine.

**(5) Discussion.** The introduction of accurate methods of study of drug action has greatly enlarged our knowledge of chemotherapeutic action in recent years. The general trend of recent advances has been to bring the subject more into line with the remainder of pharmacology and there are striking resemblances between the action of drugs on trypanosomes and their action on bacteria, on enzymes and on measurable functions of higher organisms.

Trypanosomes and bacteria share however the common disadvantage that normally they are multiplying populations, and quantitative studies are more difficult in multiplying than in static populations. Trypanosomes are peculiar as regards their power to acquire drug resistance; this phenomenon is for example much less marked amongst bacteria. Unfortunately, however, the mechanism by which drug resistance is acquired is a matter of dispute and consequently no general deductions can be drawn from our present knowledge of this subject.

The fact that naturally resistant organisms fix malaricidal dyes in the same manner as do susceptible organisms proves however that the destruction of organisms must depend on two factors:— (a) fixation, and (b) action produced after fixation, and that tolerance may be associated with the latter of these factors.

In general it may be said that from the quantitative aspect the results of chemotherapy do not present any exceptional difficulty. Chemotherapeutic agents act in high dilutions (e.g. 1 part in $10^8$), but these dilutions are similar to those at which heavy metals kill bacteria in watery solutions, and many hormones produce effects at much lower concentrations. The quantity of chemotherapeutic agents fixed by the organisms is moreover considerable, for it is equivalent to a concentration of about 1 part of drug in 100,000 parts of organism.

As in the case of the "oligodynamic" action of heavy metals, delicate methods of quantitative analysis have made the action of chemotherapeutic agents much less mysterious.

The mode of action of chemotherapeutic agents is unknown, but the virulence of trypanosomal infections depends on the rate of multiplication of the organism and rapid growth implies a high rate of metabolism. Arsenicals are known to inhibit many forms of enzyme activity at high dilutions and hence it is not surprising that the concentrations of arsenicals in organisms that are known to occur should produce lethal effects, and there are many forms of interference with enzyme activity to which the lethal effect might be due.

[1] EHRLICH, P.: Berl. klin. Wschr. **44**, 233 (1907).
[2] BROWNING, C. H.: Brit. med. J. **1907 II**, 1405.

Considerable advance has therefore been made in the solution of certain quantitative problems of chemotherapy, but much less is known regarding the more intricate and much more important qualitative problems. As is the case in other fields of pharmacology, the relation between chemical constitution and pharmacological action remains a mystery.

There are certain general indications associating activity with certain types of structure, but few if any general laws have been established.

Chapter 21

## Conclusion.

The general aim followed by the author in this monograph has been to determine the extent to which the effects produced by drugs on cells can be interpreted as processes following known laws of physical chemistry.

The ground covered has been very wide and this has necessitated summary and even superficial treatment of important subjects which are still highly controversial. Inspection of the literature shows, however, that a general survey of pharmacological problems is essential at the present stage of knowledge. The general tendency in the past has been to devise an ad hoc explanation for any striking phenomenon observed, without stopping to consider whether the explanation was remotely possible, when the pharmacological evidence was considered as a whole.

The theory that a cell reacts and is killed by one or a few molecules of drugs is an example of this type. This "monomolecular" theory was advanced to explain certain-time-action curves which followed a singular course. The hypothesis explains these curves but is at variance with the whole of our knowledge regarding the quantities of drug which actually combine with cells.

In other cases striking phenomena have been regarded as manifestations peculiar to living cells, although they can be explained by the ordinary laws of physical chemistry. The "oligodynamic" action of heavy metals is an example of this type.

Quantitative analysis has shown that cells adsorb relatively high concentrations of heavy metals from dilute solutions. Moreover the study of the action of such metals on enzymes has shown that these actions can be interpreted as an exceptionally simple form of chemical reaction.

In other cases laws have been enunciated which merely state that certain phenomena frequently occur, without providing any explanation for their occurrence. The ARNDT-SCHULZ law and the law of phasic variation are examples of this type and so also is the statement that drug actions follow the WEBER-FECHNER law. In the last mentioned case it is certainly true that a linear relation between the logarithm of the cause and the effect is frequently observed both with sensations and with drug actions. This fact does not however advance knowledge unless some reason be found for the relation in one or other of the cases.

The chief dangers attending any attempt to make a general survey of pharmacological evidence is that of unfair selection of material. Pharmacological data in general are of a low standard of accuracy as compared with physical chemistry or even with biochemistry, and the results obtained by different workers often differ completely. The author has selected results which he believes to be reliable but in cases where the results are in disagreement it is very difficult to maintain exact impartiality and to avoid favouring those which agree with an interesting hypothesis.

Quantitative pharmacological data suffers not only from a low standard of accuracy but also the evidence it provides is usually ambiguous; this is an inevitable consequence of the large number of uncontrolled variables that are present in even the simplest of cell-drug systems.

In most cases there are several possible alternative explanations for any particular relation, and the author has simply selected the explanations which appear to involve the fewest improbable assumptions.

Such considerations raise the obvious question as to whether it is worth while attempting physico-chemical interpretations of cell-drug reactions. The author believes that such attempts are worth while, even in our present incomplete state of knowledge, because the formulation of provisional hypotheses provides an object for further research. The only danger is when such provisional hypotheses are mistaken for definitely established laws, and as a result inhibit rather than stimulate further investigation. For this reason the author wishes to emphasise the provisional nature of all the hypotheses outlined in this article.

Regarding the evidence as a whole, the author has found that a somewhat surprisingly large proportion of the more accurate quantitative data can be interpreted as the expression of a chemical reaction between the drug and specific receptors, which latter in a large number of cases appear to be situated on the cell surface. Quantitative resemblances can be traced between the action of drugs on inorganic catalysts, on purified enzymes, on the enzymatic activity of cells and on cellular activities the nature of which is unknown. It is an interesting and significant fact that the author in 1926 found that the quantitative relations between the concentration of acetyl choline and its action on muscle cells, an action the nature of which is wholly unknown, could be most accurately expressed by the formulae devised by LANGMUIR to express the adsorption of gases on metal filaments. The surprising fact is that formulae devised for a system of such extreme simplicity should be of any value for describing the behaviour of a system of such infinitely greater complexity. This example suggests that the mathematical formula which expresses as a first approximation the action of the drug on the cells probably represents an extreme simplification of the processes that actually occur. The simple end result is probably due partly to a wholesale mutual cancellation of independent variables and partly to the fact that the data are too inaccurate to demonstrate small deviations from the formulae.

In general the writer regards the mathematical formulae used as convenient methods for describing briefly the general form of the relations observed. In no case where living tissues are involved are the uncontrolled variables sufficiently limited to permit of a proof that would be accepted in physical chemistry of the occurrence of any particular form of reaction.

Even when these limitations are recognised fully, the evidence provided by quantitative pharmacology is still of great interest, because the quantitative relations found in the action of drugs on cells are of several kinds and in many cases are of unusual forms. It has been shown that many of these forms can be explained as the expression of reactions between drugs and receptors.

The chief alternative theories of the mode of action of drugs, alternative to the one outlined above, are the potential theory and the theory of individual variation. The potential theory has the disadvantage of assuming processes unknown in physical chemistry and the writer believes that the facts on which it is based are capable of alternative explanations.

The theory that all quantitative phenomena in pharmacology are expressions of individual variation cannot be disproved, but has the disadvantage of being unfruitful since it does not link phenomena observed in living cells with phenomena observed in simpler systems. It is of course true that the whole theory of mass-action is based on individual variation of the kinetic energy of atoms, but in order to explain quantitative pharmacological data as the expression merely of individual variation it is necessary to assume peculiar skew forms of distribution of variation.

There is no doubt that individual variation modifies a large proportion of the quantitative data in pharmacology, but the writer has endeavoured to show that the peculiar skew forms of variation observed can be interpreted as the result of moderate variation being distorted and spread out by logarithmic relations between cause and effect. The manner in which the increased accuracy in the study of drug actions has revealed a previously unsuspected range of individual variations is one of the most striking modern developments in pharmacology and one which should have an important effect on medical practice in the future.

The most interesting feature of drug action is the extraordinary specificity of the actions of drugs and the manner in which slight changes in chemical constitution alter their action. Unfortunately the relation between chemical constitution and pharmacological action was found to be a subject much too large to be dealt with in the present article. The writer believes, however, that quantitative methods should in the future throw more light on this interesting and important problem. One of the features of this subject, that hitherto has been regarded as mysterious, is that in a homologous series of drugs some members may not only fail to produce the action typical of the series but may even antagonise the action of other members. The conception of specific receptors explains this fact, since a drug which occupies the receptors without producing an action will antagonise the action of other members. Another general principle of drug action appears to be that the receptors in different tissues vary slightly in their pattern and hence the relative extensity of the actions of related drugs and also drug antagonisms differ with every tissue studied.

The most hopeful line of advance for the future in this most important study would appear to be the careful analysis of the mode of action of series of related drugs in the case of the simplest cell-drug systems that will give an easily measurable response.

# Index of Authors.

# Index of Subjects.

Dehydrogenase, 179.
Diamond, 32.
Diastase, 207.
Di-chloro-benzene, 163.
Di-chloro-phenol, 55, 56, 89.
Diffusion of drugs
  in fluids, 98, 130.
  in cells, 100, 129, 130.
Digitalis glucosides
  action of — on heart,
    125ff., 161.
  characteristic curves of —
    with cats, 142, 143.
    with frogs, 167ff., 174.
  massive dosage of —, 168.
Dimensions
  of cells, 17.
  of molecules, 17.
Di-nitro-α-naphthol, 38.
Di-nitro-phenol, 37, 38, 54ff.,
  89, 161.
Diphasic actions
  of alcohols, 57.
  of cyanides, 49, 55.
  of enzyme poisons, 35ff.,
    202.
  of heavy metals, 48.
Disinfection,
  time-action curves of —,
    108ff.
  time-concentration rela-
    tions of —, 136ff.
  see also under names of
    drugs.
Distribution coefficient see
  under narcotics.
Donnan equilibrium, 13.
Drosophila, 121.
Dyes,
  action of —
    on enzymes, 50.
    on trypanosomes, 212ff.
  rate of penetration of cells
    by —, 101, 123, 124, 130.
Dysentery toxin, 147, 148,
  158, 163, 173.

Ear, rabbit's perfused, 195.
Echinoderm eggs,
  action on — of drugs, 49,
    60, 84, 89, 174, 179.
  dimensions of —, 17.
Egg albumen, dimensions of
  molecule of —, 18.
Electrolytic solution pressure, 46.
Enzyme poisons
  amounts of — reacting
    with enzymes, 34, 40.
  antagonism of —, 181ff.
  concentration-action curves
    of —, 37ff., 42ff., 50ff.
  deviation of —, 41, 202.
  diphasic actions of —, see
    diphasic actions.

Enzyme poisons
  minimum effective con-
    centrations of —, 35, 36.
  rate of action of —, 37, 100,
    104.
  selective action of —, 35,
    207.
Enzymes,
  activity of —, 34.
  cell content of —, 19, 20.
  structure of —, 27, 33.
Erepsin, 207.
Ergotamine, 107, 171, 184,
  186, 187, 189, 197.
Ergotoxine, 95, 191, 198.
Erythrocytes,
  amounts of drugs fixed
    by —, 20.
  dimensions of —, 17.
  haemolysis of —, see hae-
    molysis.
  inhibition of oxygen uptake
    by —, 52, 53, 55, 208.
Eserine see physostigmine.
Esterase, acetyl choline see
  acetyl choline liver, 36.
Ether, ethyl, 82, 91, 140, 141,
  159, 160, 161, 174.
Ethylene, 32.

Ferments see enzymes.
Fluorescence and chemotherapeutic activity, 212, 213.
Fluorides, 35.
Formaldehyde, 11, 25, 39,
  110, 176.
Freundlich's adsorption formula, 6, 67.
Fundulus, 91.
  eggs, 47.
  embryo, 21, 69.

Ganglion, superior cervical,
  71, 94.
Gases, irritant, 141.
Gauss' formula, 144, 172.
Gelatine, 130, 132.
Germanin, 212.
Globulin, dimensions of mole-
  cule of —, 18.
Glomerella cingulata, 162.
Glucose metabolism, 76, 77.
Glutathione, 209.
Glycolysis, 16, 48, 102.
Gold, 47, 49.
Graphite, 32.
Gut, isolated, action of drugs
  on —, 70, 76, 79, 88, 95,
    107, 136, 186, 187, 191,
    192, 195, 200, 201.

Haemocyanin, 18.
Haemoglobin
  combination of —
    with carbon monoxide,
      27ff., 180, 181, 189.

Haemoglobin
  combination of —
    with oxygen, 27ff., 34,
      83, 100.
  dimensions of molecule of
    —, 18.
  structure of molecule of —,
    26, 27.
Haemolysis, 8, 20, 85, 98, 108,
  119.
Heart of frog
  action on —
    of acetyl choline see ace-
      tyl cholin.
    of cyanides see cyanides.
    of iodo-acetic acid, 102.
    of narcotics see narco-
      tics.
    of potassium salts, 88.
  amount of drugs fixed by
    —, 21, 69, 70, 80, 91.
  dimensions of cells of —,
    17, 69.
  structure of —, 99.
  of mammal, 74, 126, 127.
  of tortoise, 60.
Heat, action
  on enzymes of —, 33.
  on proteins of —, 110.
Heat production of muscles,
  88.
Helix pomatia, 95, 194, 195.
Henry's law, 58.
Hirudo see leech.
Histamine, 22, 86ff., 107, 136,
  200.
Holothurian muscle, 95.
Homoeopathy, 26.
Human populations, varia-
  tion of — in response to
    drugs, 166, 169ff.
Humoral transmission of
  nerve impulses, 90ff., 177,
    197.
Hydrochloric acid, 131.
Hydrocyanic acid see cy-
  anides.
Hydrogen ion concentration,
  action on organisms of, 128.
  influence of — upon drug
    action, 73, 128, 181ff.,
      188, 189, 192.
Hydroxy hydroquinone, 187,
  188, 203.
Hypersensitivity, 171ff.

Idiosyncrasy, 171ff.
Imbibition, 132.
Individual variation see va-
  riation.
Insulin, 22, 76, 77, 149, 159,
  169, 174, 175.
Intestine see gut.
Invertase, 19, 33ff., 50ff., 84,
  178, 181ff., 191, 202, 207.

Herstellung: fotokop wilhelm weihert, Darmstadt
Einband: Konrad Triltsch, Grafischer Betrieb, 87 Würzburg